Natural Healing

*Alternative/Complementary Resources
for Total Health*

S. Jeanne Gunn

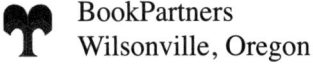
BookPartners
Wilsonville, Oregon

Natural Healing: Alternative/Complementary Resources for Total Health was written to awaken and enlighten mankind in his daily quest for a quality life and purpose. This book contains the facets of the Body/Mind/Spirit connection working together to create a life of fulfillment and good health, available to each and every one of us.

The book section "Reiki—A Natural Method of Healing" is about healing and explains how this simple technique of healing can work for everyone. The Reiki portion can be used by anyone. Initiation into Reiki comes through a Reiki III Master teacher administering attunement symbols activating the chakra centers with the universal life energy force.

Note: The information contained in this book is offered as a guide and not intended to prescribe or diagnose in any way, nor to replace the licensed health care professional of your choice. Resources are for reference and help only; not all information listed has been used by this author.

A small portion of this book was printed in 1994 under the title
Reiki and Beyond—Healing Manual. ISBN 0-9643 41204
Library of Congress Cataloging-in-Publication Data
Gunn, S. Jeanne
Bibliography, Glossary, Index
Alternative/Complementary Therapies, Aromatherapy
Ayurveda, Environmental Health, Herbs, Vitamins and Nutrition
Chakras and Energy Fields, and Reiki Natural Method of Healing

© 1999, revised and amended
All rights reserved
Printed in the United States of America
Library of Congress Catalog 98-72445
ISBN 1-58151-013-6

Cover design by Richard Ferguson
Text design by Sheryl Mehary

This book may not be reproduced in whole or in part, by electronic or any other means which exist or may yet be developed, without permission of:

BookPartners, Inc.
P.O. Box 922
Wilsonville, Oregon 97070

This book is dedicated to all Earth people,
Our gateway and inheritance to One Planet ♥ One People, and the Universe!

Table of Contents

List of Diagrams and Charts vii
Acknowledgments ix
Introduction 1
    Great Spirit 1
    Earth People—Hear This Call! 2
    The Council Meets 3

1 Alternative or Complementary Therapies 5
    Alternative/Complementary Medicine Becomes Mainstream 5
    Therapies—New Choices for a New Reality 6
    Book Resources 14

2 Energy and Medicine—Personal Experiences of Professionals 15
    Transition into the Twenty-First Century 15
    Bodywork, Massage, and Spiritual Healing—Practitioners' Experiences 16
    Best Ways to Find a Healer 23
    Bodywork and Massage 23
    Healers at Work 29
    Book Resources 34

3 Nature's Medicine—Herbs, Vitamins, Minerals, and Food 35
    Herb Resources 42
    Antioxidants/Minerals/Amino Acids 42
    Vegetarianism 44
    Pantry Checklist 48
    Quick and Healthy Vegetarian Meals 52
    Nutrition 56
    Oils and Fats 58
    Food Additives 59
    Food Combining 61
    Book Resources 66
    Recipe Books 66
    Magazines for Better Health 66
    Resources 67
    Product Resources 67
    Sources: Organic Seed Catalogs 67

4 Natural Earth Healing—Physical Body 69
    Aromatherapy and Natural Body Products 69
    Natural Product Resources 80
    Book Resources 80
    Organizations 80

5 Ayurveda—Wisdom of the Ancients 81
    Book Resources 92

6 Natural Earth Healing—Environmental 93
    Environment on the Web 104
    Book Resources 104
    Environmental Product Resources 105

7 Toxic-Free Health 107
    Parasites, Candida, and Dental Amalgams 107
    What Do We Do? 109
    Book Resources on Amalgam Toxicity 115

8	Body Awareness and Detoxification	119
	Understanding Detoxification	124
	Book Resources	127
9	Chakras and the Human Energy Fields	129
	The Fields of Energy	130
	Chakra System	132
	Root Chakra	133
	Sacral Chakra	135
	Solar Plexus Chakra	137
	Heart Chakra	139
	Throat Chakra	141
	Third Eye or Brow Chakra	143
	Crown Chakra	145
	Link between Heart and Thymus Gland	147
	Chakra Imbalances	148
	Cords That Bind Us	149
	Our Character Structures	150
	Hara Vital Center	152
	Inner Light or Core Star	154
	Crystal Information and the Body	158
	Purification Techniques for Personal Healing	160
	Elements Used in Purification	161
	Energized Baths	162
	Blessings	162
	Smudging	163
	Book Resources	163
10	Fears, Stress, and Worry as Emotional Diseases	165
	Fears—How They Affect Us	165
	Positive Motivations	174
	Book Resources	174
11	Reiki—A Natural Method of Healing	175
	What Is Reiki?	175
	Origins of Reiki	177
	Working with Reiki	183
	Preparation for Giving a Reiki Treatment	193
	Procedures for Treatments	199
	Reiki—Hand Positions	203
	Initiation into the Power of Reiki	210
12	Nature and the Sacred Space of Man	227
	The Rainbow Legend	227
	The Lakota Ten Levels of Consciousness	238
	Golden Light Alignment	240
	Creating Our Own Sacred Space	241
	Book Resources	243
	Appendixes	245
	Glossary	253
	Index	260
	Resources	263
	Poem: An Earthling Mission—To All Earth People	267
	Angelic Guidance through a Time and Space Warp!	269
	About the Author	271

Diagrams and Charts

Therapeutic Approach to Alternative Traditions—Chart	Chapter Two	21
Vitamin Reference Chart	Chapter Three	35
Herb Reference and Body Symptom Chart	Chapter Three	36
Natural Herb Chart	Chapter Three	38
Natural Vitamin Chart	Chapter Three	39
Pantry Checklist	Chapter Three	48
Fat, Fiber, and Carbohydrates—Chart	Chapter Three	52
Food Combining for Easiest Digestion—Diagram	Chapter Three	62
Mediterranean Diet Pyramid	Chapter Three	63
Acid and Alkaline-Forming Foods—Chart	Chapter Three	63
Mineral-Rich Foods—Chart	Chapter Three	64
Ayurveda Dosha Chart	Chapter Five	85
Ayurveda Vitamins and Minerals—Chart	Chapter Five	86
Uses of Chemicals for Water Treatment—Chart	Chapter Six	95
The Auric Field—Fields of Energy Diagram	Chapter Nine	130
Location of Seven Chakras—Diagram	Chapter Nine	133
Hara Line Diagram	Chapter Nine	153
Core Star Diagram	Chapter Nine	155
Polarity Diagram	Chapter Nine	156
Emotional Sources of Disease—Chart	Chapter Ten	172
Reiki Hand Positions—Front of Body—Diagram	Chapter Eleven	204
Reiki Hand Positions—Back of Body—Diagram	Chapter Eleven	207
Reiki Closure Technique—Diagram	Chapter Eleven	209
Reiki Master Symbols—Diagrams	Chapter Eleven	217
The Ten Levels in Lakota Language—Chart	Chapter Twelve	238
Golden Light Alignment Symbols—Diagram	Chapter Twelve	240
Feng Shui Diagrams	Chapter Twelve	244
Dental Chart	Appendix A	245
Chart of Effects of Spinal Misalignments	Appendix B	246
Location of Major Body Organs—Front View	Appendix C	247
Location of Major Body Organs—Back View	Appendix D	248
The Lymph System	Appendix F	249
The Endocrine System	Appendix E	250
Reflexology—Hands	Appendix G	251
Reflexology—Feet	Appendix H	252

Acknowledgments

I thank my family for their love and support, my children Daryl, Dennis, and Jennifer; my mother, Shirley; my sister, Susan; other family members CJ, Barbara, James, John, Marlene, Kim, Del; and grandchildren David, Jared, and Ashlyn.

Kudos to the friends listed below for their experiences, insights, and participation.

I am forever grateful for the spiritual guidance given to me throughout this project and in my daily life.

I thank and bless you all. I am forever grateful.

S. Jeanne Gunn, Author.

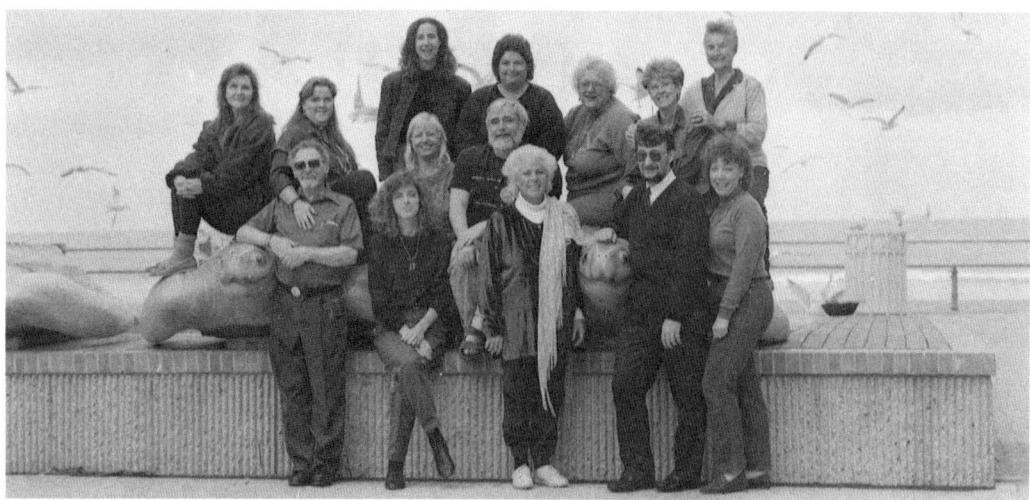

Contributions (Illustrations, research, personal experiences, case histories, computer guidance, and charts):

Marius J. Broekhuizen	Jennifer A. Link
Daniel Cunningham	DuLois Lee
Deborah Edholm	Dr. Light Miller
Joan Essig	Suban Potijinda
Barbara Fraser-Duthie	Bobbee Rickard
Lucinda Fury	Linda Schiller-Hanna
Dr. Mark A. Gellasch	Brenda Stone
C. E. Hamblin	Usha and Dr. Vasant
Ruth Hutton	Dr. John T. White
Kathyrn Thiele Jones	Dr. Albert Zehr
Dr. Dean H. Kent	Claire Zieman
Joseph Kuehling	Lumis Two Hawks
Rich Lanigan	Wind Dancer

Introduction

This book introduces you to many ways of healing the physical body, intellectual mind, and soul or spirit. It also shows you how we can come into the purity of all we can be, and how to become awakened to what is happening around us in our environment. We are the only ones who can heal ourselves, help our families and save the only place we have to live. This book is my service to mankind, an opportunity to share information with you that will help encourage us all, and to create thinking beyond pain and our material world.

Great Spirit

Great Spirit, Beloved Creator, you who dwell in the All
Beloved, mighty, and majestic you fill the sacred space
You who are of sky, the sun, stars, moon and the light
You who are earth, lush and radiant gardens abloom
You who are rock, earth, wind, water, insect, tree and animal
Holy are your infinite names, chanted, sung and whispered
By every language, tongue, and native upon the land
You are the heaven and earth, the above and below
You are the glory, wisdom, power, grace and the light
Forgive my inconsistencies and help me forgive
Others who have transgressed against me, and all of mankind
Help me not to stray into darkness, ego and greed
But keep me on my pathway and intended purpose of this life stream
Guide our hands to the soil, see out thoughts with your loving light
Let us remember your abundance and share with all who hunger
Guide my heart into balance, harmony, courage and strength
For the days that are coming — restore the Great Law of Peace
Making conscious choices rather than frustration, desperation and need
Striving to be in the stillness of inner mind, the place where you dwell
That I may manifest within my soul all that you are. Forever, Amen.

S. Jeanne Gunn

Earth People—Hear This Call!

It has taken us until this twenty-first century
To wake up to the fact that our life is based upon
Knowing we have a body, a mind, and a spirit
Which we are totally responsible for, you see!

We have been blessed spiritually and physically by a Divine Creator,
Been given this planet called Earth, which was to be like living in a Garden of Eden.
Mother Earth has sustained us with her abundant resources, and unceasingly
Loved us through eons of evolutionary changes to be sure.

Now we face the most important task in our lives,
Awakening to realize a truth so simple,
One to help our bodies become whole and free from pain,
Finding a balance between healing the body and the mind.

Why does this reality seem to escape into the back of our minds?
Because we think we are already whole, and that from this Earth we have gained,
But we have taken and taken, and what have we given in return?
With the healing of our soul—the lesson was so simple
Learning the Balance of Living on Earth and the Universal Laws of our own Universe.

No matter what your race or culture, gender or creed
We face enormous planetary devastation, caused by our pollution and greed,
Our misuse of nature and technical inventions galore.
We will soon face the essential task of our own shortsightedness and abuse.

Unless we sign on the dotted line,
To become what are known as Earth people in this vast universe,
To face our responsibility with dignity and determination,
To rediscover our relationship, with who we are, and with our Living and Loving
Mother Earth…

So this balance we speak of—in terms oh so simple
Is to free your body and mind from pain,
Knowing we treat ourselves, and others, as we treat our beloved Mother Earth.
Do not waste your time here—beleaguered with greed and profit and gain—
Or you will not become one of the Earth people in this vast universe
Known by the Rainbow Legend as …
One Planet ♥ One People.

The Council Meets

Source: Dancing with the Wheel *by Sun Bear and* Earth Medicine *by Kenneth Meadows*

The Thunder Stick Story

The Thunder came. The Elder spoke.
The Council is called
The concerned Earth people gather.

In a respectful and direct manner they form the circle that will be the meeting. The elder enters, coming to the far side of the circle. He is holding an array of colorful decorated sticks. They are tied with many ribbons: red, yellow, black, and white.

The elder will tell a story this day, a story of great importance about Mother Earth, and all of Mankind. It is a story of peace and healing, a story that will be handed down from generation to generation.

As the story starts, one of the decorated sticks is handed to the first person in the circle. He must remember the first part of the story as the Elder tells it. It is his to know and remember and repeat.

As the story continues, other sticks are passed clockwise and each person knows that they are to pass on that part of the story that their stick represents. In this way, the story is complete, many people carrying out a part of the whole.

I see the spiritual awakening today being like this council meeting. Each person who awakens the healing energy within is being given a stick. We are part of the whole story. Together, all over the world, we can work in harmony, balance, and unity. We can pass this Divine Love along to Mother Earth and all of the Earth people. Perhaps we shall one day work and act together in unity, as a united Earth people. We can then achieve the prophecy of peace, for which all of our ancestors have worked, and accomplish the legend of One Planet ♥ One People. HO!

Medicine Wheel

The four races of man:	white	red	yellow	black
The four directions:	North	South	East	West
The four archangels:	North-Uriel	South-Michael	East-Raphael	West-Gabriel
The four elements:	North-earth	South-fire	East-air	West-water
The four animals	North-buffalo	South-coyote	East-eagle	West-bear

Chapter One

Alternative or Complementary Therapies

Alternative and complementary therapies:
- Reawaken—creates, opens—us to Earth medicine
- Create healing through our human energy fields
- Open the One-Heart to more trusting and loving relationships
- Reawaken our being and awareness to the Creative Force
- Assist the physical body in overcoming crisis
- Help relieve painful conditions
- Aid in recovery from surgery or traumatic experiences
- Help uncover our discontentment
- Balance feelings in the healing of our mental/emotional body fields
- Guide us in letting go of the anger, fears, worries, and stresses of life
- Open the doors to viewing our masks
- Create the doorways for healing past, present, and future events
- Unwind and transmute the crystallized thought patterns that have limited us
- Connect us to the Divine Source; help raise the vibrational rate of the lower ego-body chakras

Alternative/Complementary Medicine Becomes Mainstream

Dr. C. Everett Koop, former Surgeon General of the U.S.A., speaks of being flexible when treating patients. He points out that eighty percent of the world's population depends on what Westerners consider "alternative" care. He also says, "We need to do more to conserve the plants from which modern medicines are derived. We will not be able to afford a high-tech, drug-based medical system for much longer."

In 1994 one out of three people (425 million) were using some type of alternative therapy, for stress, for pain, or to help cure an ailment. Newly aware physicians are concerned with finding the most effective synthesis of conventional and alternative medicines for their patients. The public's interest has been so strong that the National Institute of Health created an Office of Alternative Medicine. As a result there are approximately thirty medical schools—including Harvard, Columbia, Stanford and Georgetown—that offer courses in alternative medicine, and several schools that offer naturopathic certification.

Information is readily available for those who are searching for the means to good health; books, magazines, workshops, nutritional guides, vegetarian cookbooks, vitamins, and minerals have flooded the marketplace.

Homeopathy stimulates the body at an energetic rather than a physical level. Homeopathy is achieving worldwide support and acceptance in countries such as Australia, Belgium, Denmark, France, India, the Netherlands, South Africa, the United Kingdom, and the United States, according to the *New England Journal of Medicine*. The word homeopathy comes from Greek origins and means "like treatment of diseases."

Good health, disease or dissatisfaction, life and its cycles, and repetitions, all go the full circle, and the circle's meanings are to be treated as One. This is what is known as the mind-body-spirit connection. One in thought, one in action, one in deed—physically, emotionally, mentally, and spirituality—our being revolves around all of this, as the One reaction within us.

There are many varied types of therapy. What type is best for you? Check the reference books, magazines and sources listed in this book for more information. Otherwise, some of the more popular therapies being used today are listed alphabetically below.

Naturopathic Doctors—Naturopathic medicine is based essentially on natural substances and natural processes. Physicians are trained in natural medicine, involving four years of postgraduate study, and two years of medical sciences and a collection of natural therapies, including vitamin and herbal medicine, hydrotherapy, nutrition, and homeopathy.

Holistic Physicians—These medical doctors are trained in some type of natural therapy, i.e., nutrition or homeopathy. They analyze all levels of the patient's state of heath: nutritional, emotional, spiritual, environmental, and life style. The goal is to achieve some unified sense of well-being.

Medical notice: We, not the doctors, are responsible for our own health. It is up to each individual person to follow through and check any pharmaceutical prescriptions by reading the labels for any side effects or warnings about taking two different prescriptions at the same time. It is time to become aware of what chemicals we are digesting and breathing, and what we put into our bodies.

Therapies—New Choices for a New Reality

Aromatherapy and Essential Oils Therapy

The pure essences of aromatic plants have been recognized for more than six thousand years for healing, cleansing, preservative, and mood-enhancing properties. These essences utilize the therapeutic powers of essential oils and help relax muscles and work with restorative bodywork massage. These properties are being rediscovered to restore balance in everyday life. Stress, pollution, unhealthy diets, etc. — these factors have adverse effects on our bodies and spirits. Aromatherapy harnesses the potent, pure essences of plants, flowers, and resins to work on the most powerful senses—smell and touch—to restore the harmony to body and mind. There are many excellent books available on aromatherapy. One is *Ayurveda and Aromatherapy* by Drs. Light and Bryan Miller, which lists many essential oils and their purposes and has the Marma body charts, indicating which oils to use for problem areas. There are great differences between essential oils and mixtures of aromatherapy oils. Essential oils last without becoming rancid. Read labels.

Aromatherapy Examples
- Walnut acts as a coordinator and balances the nervous system.
- Sesame is ideal for stretch marks.
- Sweet almond oil is neutral and non-allergenic, so it is ideal for baby massages.
- Lavender is very popular to use when meditating; it enhances the mind and allows better sleeping.
- Geranium eases anxiety, stress, and mood swings.

Acupressure

From China, acupressure is a method of contact healing that creates a smooth flow of vibratory energy throughout the body. A deeper pressure on meridians in the body releases the flow of nerve fluid and stimulates the body's cells to normalize and heal where there is disease. Meridian lines of concentrated energy run from the brain to the toes.

See charts in chapter 9, Chakras and the Human Energy Fields

Acupuncture

There are 741 tiny, invisible, concentrated center points of energy and intelligence in the body that act as transmitters. They are located in the nervous system (your "electrical" system), which distributes your emotional load. In working with these congested and diseased points, once the flow is restored where these blockages are, the body can heal itself more easily. These points accept the vibrational frequency that comes into them and then change the frequency that goes to the various organs and tissues of the body. Meridian lines are in a universal pattern and run throughout the human body. Because of the connection with the electrical system (emotion), our emotions clog up and cause imbalances in the natural body flow, thus manifesting disease (or dis-ease). Acupuncture is very useful to facilitate muscle relaxation, decrease pain, or promote soft tissue healing. Methods used are: needles, finger pressure, massage, ointments, and sound.

Ayurveda

More than five thousand years ago a group of holy men known as the Rishis compiled the ancient Hindu philosophical and spiritual texts called the Vedas. This knowledge comprises the science of life, as revealed to the Rishis through what today we call divine inspiration. The Vedic science includes self-knowledge, yoga, Vedic astrology, and Ayurveda. Built on the concept of life force energy called Prana, Ayurveda is the science dealing with physical healing, diet, herbs, and bodywork or massage. At the heart of Ayurveda is the concept that all of existence comprises five basic principles or elements: earth, air, fire, water, and ether. See chapter 5, Ayurveda—Wisdom of the Ancients.

Biofeedback

Biofeedback is the detection of information about your biological functions. Biofeedback means what is "fed back" from an imperceptible physiological process, and is picked up by electrodes and electronically amplified on a monitor. This shows what is happening within the body with regard to thoughts and emotional states. The signals can be amplified in colors, sounds, lights, digital displays, and graphical recordings. Subjects learn about self, their emotional states, attitudes, and traumatic experiences in this life at present or in the past. Biofeedback serves as a tool for learning to control one's attitudes, thoughts and emotions. It is most useful in behavioral disorders, accident trauma, pain disorders, nervousness or stress disorders, anger, gastrointestinal disorders, and various phobias.

Breath Work

Breath work is designed to assist in breaking free from old behavior patterns, which prevent us from demonstrating or reflecting purity in heart, mind, and body. The breath exercises work with the kundalini, which in turn moves upward through all the chakras and helps bring a harmony and balance to the body-mind connection. Focus is on the emotional body, where suppressed crystallization (material) and denial is stored. Denial of any emotion, positive or negative, can make that emotion take the form of addictive habits; this disguising of our emotions gives us the illusion that we are in control of them. Breath work is a type of energy work.

Chiropractic

The science of chiropractic deals with the study of the body's structure. Chiropractic manipulation and adjustments (alignment) deal primarily with the spinal cord and the nervous system. The nervous system controls and coordinates all organs and structures of the human body. Concentration in these areas affects the mental body's kundalini (energy) and in turn affects the physical organs in the body. Misalignments of spinal vertebrae and discs may cause irritation to the nervous system, which could affect the body's structures and the organs and their functions. An alignment allows the body to normalize; malfunctions in turn heal themselves.

For a diagram of the spine and its effects in the body, see Appendix B.

Colon Therapy

Colon therapy or colonics is the process of flushing the large intestine, or colon, with water. The colon is the only internal organ that can be easily cleaned. The most universal aspect of colonics is the release of toxins. Even when bowel movements are regular, toxins build up in the colon, and be reabsorbed into the blood stream or create problems in the colon itself. The flushing of toxins frees up the movement of energy in the body. For some, colonics is a regular health maintenance program, and it was highly recommended by Edgar Cayce in his health readings through the Association of Research and Enlightenment (ARE) in Virginia Beach. Supportive of other organs, colon therapy is reported to be helpful with headaches, skin eruptions, PMS, mood swings, parasites, and toxins.

For further information see chapter 4—Body Awareness and Detoxification; and Iridology in this section.

Color Healing

Color healing had its foundations in Egypt and Greece. In using color to promote a natural body healing, you are affecting wavelengths known by their colors, tones, and hues. This has an effect on the body tissue, and can be used in cooperation with or regulation of the chakras or etheric double. Each chakra has a pattern which vibrates to a different color and sound, which in turn stimulate the physical body by normalizing its cells, Then the body can more easily heal itself. Color healing is very helpful in visualization techniques, meditation, and healing with Reiki.

For more information see chapter 9—Chakras and the Human Energy Fields.

Contact Healing

Magnetic healing, known as contact or touch healing, is where the practitioner works with the client's auric field to promote a change in body chemistry so that the body can more easily heal itself. The magnetic energy passes through the practitioner into the client's emotional and nervous systems affecting the disease. Clients can sometimes feel hot or cold, tingling, and physical sensations within the body. The application is not harmful and the client usually leaves with a feeling of well-being. For more information about healing, check paragraphs on Reiki, No-Touch Healing, and Healing Science Therapy.

Also see chapter 11—Reiki, The Natural Method of Healing.

Core Energetics

Three main theses are woven together in what Pierrakos calls core energetics. The first is that the human person is a psychosomatic unity. The second is that the source of healing lies within the self, not with outside sources, whether physician, God, or powers of the cosmos. The third is that all of existence forms a unity that moves toward creative evolution. Geared to help people move beyond tragedy and destructive conflicts and focus their lives on creativity, core energetic work with patients demonstrates that every part of the human person, from the structure of the body to the clarity of perception, is molded by what we call internal energy.

Pierrakos Pathwork Center is located in New York.

Dreams for Health

A dream is an uninitiated process occurring during a person's sleep in which their mind shows them moving or still pictures relating to life style, personality, or health. These pictures bring intent of activity, but without actual conversation. They are a human function vital to maintaining balance, a way of bringing the hidden truth in the subconscious mind to the surface to reveal itself (between the lower beta and upper alpha levels). Dreams are in symbolic language and provide help for new decisions, activities, health, etc. Dreams are a form of psychic energy originating from the guiding divine source. The symbols are unconsciously chosen by the dreamer, and can have multiple meanings pertaining to all phases of the dreamer's life. Keeping a log of one's dreams is helpful and gives continuity of thought. A symbol or image about a health issue could give a diagnostic clue to one's prevailing ailment or show how one could heal oneself. For example, the faulty electrical system (troubled nerves) in one's car (you) could be due to the stress of emotions in the body.

Hair Analysis

The condition of the hair is a duplication of the entire body's health. A small section of healthy hair is used to determine how a person's body is assimilating its food and drink. The practitioner is then aware of any necessary minerals or vitamins the body is lacking. The assessment shows concentrations of metals and minerals in the body, those that are toxic in any amount, and those that are essential and necessary. The correlation between mineral concentrations in the internal organs of the body and mineral levels in the hair is more reliable than the same comparison using urine specimens.

Please note: results may not be totally accurate if you have been using bleaches, hair dye, or perms, or are a heavy coffee drinker, on medications, and so forth. In these cases you would be better off using a pubic hair specimen.

Healing Science Therapy

Author Barbara Brennan, founder of the Barbara Brennan School of Healing, teaches theories and instruction in what she calls healing science, aimed at manipulating and rebalancing the human energy field, or aura. Healing science is based on belief in the process of diagnosing and treating illness through what she calls High Sense Perception (HSP), a form of extrasensory perception that resembles clairvoyance but can be studied and clinically practiced. This work helps dissolve the imaginary veil between the spiritual and material worlds that human beings create in their bodies through their thoughts. Personal inner study and work with many clients guided Brennan into understanding our defensive energy systems, our angry energy systems, and much more.

Her two books *Hands of Light* and *Light Emerging,* teach the advanced methods of the generally known hands-on healing with many photographs of our energy system, how we use it, and how we misuse it. Brennan's *Light Emerging* also describes the basic body types in a different language than *The Celestine Prophecy.* It explains how we manipulate our own physical body's attitude and how this affects other peoples' energy fields, 'dramas.'

Herbal Medicine or Earth Medicine

Herbal medicine (herbology) has been around as long as civilization, and it is still the most common healing modality on our planet. In India and Asia, it is a true science. In the United States, herbology has been rejected by much of the mainstream medical and scientific establishment. That is beginning to change. An herbal practitioner understands plants for their medicinal use, and which herbs are helpful in healing various kinds of diseases. All cultures around the world have known and used the healing powers of leaves, barks, roots, flowers, seeds, and oils of plants to improve digestion, relax muscles, balance hormones, control control, stimulate immunity, and achieve other healing effects. The theory is that there is no illness, mental or physical, that nature's herbs cannot aid in healing. Natural medicine, nutrition, and life style counselors are usually listed in phone books under Naturopathic Physicians, who are licensed professionals. Herbal or Earth medicine is using the natural vital life force energy of the plant kingdom to heal another vital life force, called humans.

Native Americans, Chinese, South Americans, East Indians, and Asians are very versed in information about healing herbs. There are classes on edible leaves and survival courses training with information about the fruits of the forest. There is book upon book in which we can glean information on how to help heal our physical bodies with herbs and essential oils, which are made from nature's plants. More and more people are turning to growing their own herbs for cooking and looking for natural ways to a healthier life.

Hypnotherapy

Hypnotherapy uses hypnosis to help develop constructive changes in a person's life style. The theory is that the mind works on two levels, the conscious and the subconscious. The conscious level is responsible for our everyday thinking and represents about twelve percent of the mind. The subconscious level occupies the other eighty-eight percent, and without conscious thought, runs our functions such as breathing, walking, and digestion.

Hypnosis is a natural state of increased suggestibility, and it is through our mental process of suggestibility that we learn our habits and behaviors. Through hypnosis techniques, the conscious mind relinquishes its role of decision making. A hypnotherapist must have a thorough knowledge and understanding of the five minds and karma, in case a client regresses into a past life without suggestion. Hypnotherapy works well with weight problems, smoking, destructive habits, emotional disorders, sleep disorders, pain, and so forth.

Readily available throughout the country; hypnotherapists are required to be certified.

Iridology

Iridology is the study of the eyes and their corresponding body parts. The iris area of the eyes corresponds to and reveals structural defects, toxic weakness, assimilation problems, parasites, and the past and present activity of body organs. It helps to determine the locations of blockages or congestion and the depth or stage of the congestion. Some common recommendations would be proper vitamins, minerals, and colonic therapy.

There are charts and books from which to study this therapy. Iridology eye readers, are people who take picture slides of your eyes and do a health study, recommending vitamins and herbs for any problems they foresee. This can also be done with a magnifying glass and small flashlight.

Iridology is considered to be a road map for discovering unhealthy situations in the human body.

Kinesiology

The science of kinesiology deals with the interrelationship of physiological processes and the anatomy of the human body. The theory is that humans are equilateral triangles and good health is achieved when the structural, chemical, and emotional sides of that triangle are harmoniously balanced. This is accomplished by aligning the meridian lines.

The method is to locate a malfunctioning nerve by testing the client's own hand and then using it to add or subtract energy from nerve centers, correlating the total nervous system. This method can be used to evaluate nutrition and the functioning of the vascular, lymphatic, and nervous systems.

The kinesthetic feedback method is a normal function in which body consciousness information is given to the senses via the nervous system and the brain. This is useful to test for minerals, foods, vitamins, or herbs that the body may want or not want.

Massage Therapy

Massage therapy originates from Rome, China, Egypt, and Hippocrates in Ancient Greece. Massage is an art that manipulates the soft tissue for therapeutic purposes, including restoring and improving balanced circulation and general body tone. Massage relieves mental and physical fatigue, tones the soft tissue, and creates a relaxation of muscles. Massage aids in the elimination of toxins and stimulates nerve activity relating to all internal organs, especially when doing reflexology on the hands and feet. Massage hand movements work with the energy circuitry of the body and act as a mechanical cleanser in reducing wastes and accumulated toxins, replenish the body with fresh blood, and increase oxygenation of the tissues. Massage is very useful for any human being, including infants; it is the touch of loving kinship.

Body awareness is enhanced during massage to restore balance between body and mind frequently lost in stressful situations. The circulation to tight muscles is increased and pain associated with chronic tension is relieved because increased circulation brings more oxygen and nutrients needed for relaxation to muscles. Additional blood and oxygen flow aids the function of the digestive and immune systems.

Many therapists use either hot or cold packs, salt glows, aromatherapy, or essential oils to relate back to certain organs in the body for healing.

Massage therapists are required to be certified and in some areas are licensed by the local government. This is an inexpensive way of helping the body-mind, and is available throughout the country.

For more information see chapter 2, Energy and Medicine—Personal Experiences of Professionals.

Meditation

Meditation is maintaining a disciplined mind technique for an allotted time, the purpose is to achieve a high state of consciousness, concentration on an unbroken flow of thought, and visual awareness of the object of concentration. This has been very effective in working with cancer clients and those with other deeply rooted disease. The objective is to quiet the emotions, control the mind, and relax the physical body to where the conscious mind awareness is narrowed down to a focal point, the subconscious mind is bypassed, and the superconscious mind becomes activated.

It is most beneficial to take a few minutes to meditate before rising in the morning or before retiring at night when the mind is in a peaceful mood. Meditation creates a unifying healthful and loving experience of the inner self, improved general health, mental alertness, positive attitude toward life, and a feeling of well-being. Medical testing has found mediation to cause definite changes in body chemistry. Many relationship therapists use it. There are clinics throughout the country that help people overcome disease using many of the techniques listed here.

Nutritionists

Nutritionists use diet as therapy. They analyze the patient's individual requirements and check for food allergies. They then prescribe food supplements such as vitamins or minerals, and a health maintenance program. Most common conditions can be treated very effectively by dietary measures.

Past-Lives Therapy

If an individual dies and is suppressing feelings of resentment, anger, or fear for a person or a situation, this will be carried over into other lifetimes. These suppressed feelings bring about unwanted painful behavioral patterns or physical illnesses in each lifetime until the charge is taken out of the original experience. A trained practitioner traces self-destructive patterns through several lives with the objective of finding incidents in other lives that are influencing the present life. Repeated phrases by the subject are keys for questions asked by the practitioner.

Many techniques are used to help the client regress to the life in which the experience occurred and to dissipate the charge either over a period of time or all at once by revivification in a hypnotic state. It may be necessary to work out verbally and emotionally until the client resolves the attitude of the trauma and can then manage, or change, the behavioral pattern in his present life. Many therapists have this training and use it along with other modalities of healing.

Polarity Therapy

The positive and negative aspects of the body, which are necessary for balance work simultaneously with vibrations and human thought—thought directs them. Vertical polarity is the belief that the human body's right side is positive and the human body's left side is negative. To horizontal polarity the upper body is positive and the lower body is negative. This applies to all organisms.

The female gender reflects the energy essence of Mother Earth and is receptive and respected. The male gender reflects the essence of the Sun and is full of energy and giving. The practitioner moves his fingers over the top of the body to create an energy circuit, developing a polarity of electromagnetic charge. This works with the meridian lines bringing a balanced flow (between positive and negative) through these currents, and breaks up the blockage of energy flow. Practitioners are knowledgeable in how to place the fingers or hands to create the circle of energy flow between them and the client. This represents the circle of energy or continuity of flow.

See chapter 9, Chakras and the Human Energy Fields, for polarity chart.

Practitioner or Therapist

Practitioner or therapist is a title for one who knows and understands his profession and practices it proficiently. It is a name frequently used today for spiritual healers, alternative/complementary therapists, nurse practitioners, etc. A professional is one who is willing to take time to prepare his thoughts and attitude before a session. When versatile in several methods of therapy, he must have a clear understanding of which method the client would prefer. The therapist and practitioner are dedicated to performing a service without allowing their ego to interfere.

Rebirthing

The rebirthing technique is used to simulate the birth process to make the subject relive their birth trauma. This helps to work out negative feelings regarding one's birth process and can help transform a traumatic subconscious impression of a birth to one of pleasure. The practitioner guides the client in a rocking motion and counsels them through the process. This may need several sessions, as our soul mind contains memory records of many births on planet Earth in the physical body.

Reflexology

An ancient foot and hand therapy, reflexology is used for healing physical ills. Compression and massage on various parts of the hands or feet release a flow of electrical energy to the blocked nerve endings. The massage or compression, normalizes the cells of the diseased area and hastens the ability of the body to heal itself. Areas sometimes have the sound or feeling of crystallization; acupuncture may be necessary. Hands and feet correspond back to the area of the body that is affected or congested. Aromatherapy or essential oils are also helpful.

Reflexology charts are found in appendixes G and H.

Reiki

From Ancient Tibet, Reiki is a method of healing using the universal life force energy. It is a philosophy that was handed down from the ancient tradition of the Sanskrit text through the teachings of the Vedas. A Japanese teacher, Dr. Mikao Usui, rediscovered Reiki in the late 1800s. Accepted internationally, this is a simple method of being attuned and initiated (connected) into your own life force (fields of energy and chakras). The Reiki method responds to any person's pathway, whether it is health-related, spiritual, or physical.

The principal, or concept, of Reiki is observed in all cultures, although known by different names. The universal life force energy is transmitted from Divine Source through the practitioner (channeled) into the client. The Reiki practitioner works with the conscious intention of being centered or grounded when giving a treatment. The practitioner's own energy is not used.

Reiki works in harmony with nature, the geographical environment, one's pets and animals, plants, vegetable and herb gardens, Mother Earth, the weather patterns, and, of course, people. Reiki is the essence of all elements that man is made of—fire, air, earth, water, and spirit/ether. Reiki helps unlock wisdom and psychic ability and can be learned by anyone. Reiki instructions, meditations, personal insights, and case histories by spiritual healers and Reiki masters are widely available.

See chapter 11, Reiki—A Natural Method of Healing

Rolfing or Structural Integration

Rolfing is a method of manipulating the fascia (connective tissue) to align the body's structure with the earth's gravitational field. It is designed to help the body heal itself by working with the layers and layers of fascia to restore structural balance. The body's tissues store within themselves unresolved negative thoughts. Rehydration of the connective tissue loosens the trapped negation, helping the client to be free of the cause of the ailment. Ten-session series work with a specific theme that emphasizes exact anatomical goals; an identifiable layer of connective tissue is addressed in each session. Clients will have a transformational experience that occurs on the physical, the psychological, and the environmental levels to the basic core line. Practitioners are required to be certified and are available throughout the country.

See chapter 2—Energy and Medicine—Personal Experiences of Professionals.

Sleep Learning

Sleep learning is the playing of cassette tapes repeatedly during the night or at the onset of sleep when the mental levels of awareness are highly suggestible. One can learn new material, reprogram one's life style, or change one's behavioral patterns. This has been suggested, along with meditation, by many clinics that are teaching alternative therapies to deal with major disease cases.

Sounds of Music—Toning

Scientific research shows coherence and harmony in brain wave patterns from certain sounds, suggesting that the two brain hemispheres are synchronizing. The older brain structure surfaces to mingle with the new tones and this synchrony changes nerve cells, permitting physical hearings, psychic experiences, and inflow of higher intelligence. Different tones and colors are identified with the chakra centers. These tones influence, or change, the vibrational frequency of a person or object while awakening one's spinal centers, and bring forth a dim memory of divine origin fed by the superconscious mind.

Native Americans developed effective sound rituals to control such things as wind and rain. Hindu music is a subjective, spiritual, and individualistic art aimed at personal harmony. Native Americans and Africans use drums to carry messages.

Sound is a primary energy that moves us from third dimension to fourth dimension. Sounds—music, vowels, drums, chanting, singing, and nature are used in everything we do. Each of the four elements—earth, air, water, and fire—have a sound. When we are attuned to the higher dimension, we can literally hear the music of the universe.

Recently, sound has been used with material objects to create a new art form. The sound of laughter has been introduced to help heal major illnesses. Massage therapists and healers frequently use sound.

Therapeutic Touch Healing

"Therapeutic Touch," a term coined by D. Krieger, refers to a transfer of healing energy from the practitioner to the patient to promote normal healing more quickly. A special technique is used to unruffle the energy field of the congested area in the patient, which comforts and relaxes the client and their energy field. Not considered to be offensive, it is now being used by many in the nursing and medical field. The patient's body can show a change in body chemistry. Krieger's thinking centers on the human being as an energy system, and bringing the disarray of energy fields present during illness or disease back into balance. The balancing of these energy fields is produced by the positive intention of the "healer" or the person administering the treatment.

Book Resources

Alternative Methods (380 choices of complementary/alternative healing) by Dr. Deepak Chopra
Merck Manual physician's desk reference book of medicine 1-800-659-6598
801 Prescription Drugs: Good Effects, Side Effects and *Natural Healing Alternatives*

Chapter Two

Energy and Medicine—
Personal Experiences of Professionals

*When health is absent, wisdom cannot reveal itself,
creativity cannot become manifest, strength cannot be exerted,
wealth is useless, and reason is powerless.*

Herophilies, 300 B.C.E.

Transition into the Twenty-First Century

Each year more emphasis is being placed on the importance of learning about lifestyles, diet, and exercise for our own personal health. We are moving from the crisis thinking of "fix me" to becoming responsible for our actions. The day-to-day routines of how we eat, what we eat, exercise, the stress and tension we believe are necessary in our relationships and our careers, have an affect on our quality of health. This pattern of thinking has been slow to change in our current environment.

Changes have come about from media, computers, the Internet and Web communications, magazines and books promoting knowledge of the physical body's health, professionals and scientists looking at the mind-body-spirit connection, and professionals participating in learning energy modalities.

Each year more and more people are thinking that the alternative way is more therapeutic than the operation along with prescription drugs. Doctors are becoming more aware of patients' needs on an emotional level, besides the physical level. People are looking toward the medical profession to help them with alternative therapies that would compliment conventional treatment methods.

More and more professional clinics, hospitals, nursing homes, corporations, chiropractors, dentists, and medical doctors are aligning themselves with specific techniques of "energy workers." One of the main techniques has been to recommend therapeutic massages in these settings. Many massage therapists are nurses changing roles; their knowledge of anatomy, massage, and energy work has become invaluable. The knowledge of Rolfing, or Structural Integration—working with the fascia of the body—has become invaluable and works well in the chiropractic practice.

The visionary role of hospitals in integrating massage therapy into a wellness program for employees has been a very innovative way to bring health into the lives of these caregivers. Massage therapy is also available to patients at some hospitals and is covered by some health care insurers.

Many hospitals contain chapels, and prayer groups have become a more common element, existing along with the traditional medical care. Doctors are accepting miracles as commonplace in this atmosphere. Rescue squads see the miracles on a daily basis. The spiritual aspect of man is becoming more accepted, and with this knowledge and the common sense of our physical body's needs, we are on track to a positive pattern of healing.

This transition of the medical world has occurred rapidly. In seminars given throughout our country, a new knowledge is addressing the needs of our ever-changing environment. Attention is being directed towards abusive and explosive family situations, and relationship counseling is reestablishing healthy family environments. Vitamin and herbal remedies have resurfaced from our grandmothers' day. Nutrition is being addressed with cookbooks relating to herbs and safe foods to eat, and books of preventive measures and helpful guides are available on almost any topic questioned. Help is here; we only have to reach out. Do not accept runarounds from any modality or professional field that does not address your health in a way that you are comfortable with.

Bodywork, Massage, and Spiritual Healing—Practitioners' Experiences

Physician Assistant

by Mark A. Gellasch, PA-C, Portsmouth ,VA

As a physician assistant practicing for more than twenty years, I am pleased and refreshed to see many medical, nursing, and other health-care colleagues become more open to reading about the various non-traditional approaches to the "healing arts." Dr. Deepak Chopra and Barbara Ann Brennan have been leaders in bringing this information to the forefront. The newly formed committee appointed by President Clinton, Alternatives to Traditional Medicine, hopefully will bring about a balance of health techniques.

Reiki and Therapeutic Touch (TT) are two such approaches that have slowly been adopted by nurses, massage therapists, nursing homes, and some dental and chiropractic centers. However, Reiki has not been given the clinical research validation that traditional medicine has. But under close observation, Reiki provides a positive margin of hope and, therefore, relief of various kinds of pain and suffering. I have attended many sessions of non-traditional healing art forms over the years. Some are without any value, while others appear to have a tremendous calming effect on persons distraught with great emotional anxiety and depression, presenting many observable organic signs and symptoms.

The support group of individuals practicing Reiki gives a strong, positive, visible web of security to those in desperate need of emotional comfort. The release of tension, stress, anxiety, and fear by the patient, once they recognize such an enormous force of caring people focusing all their energy upon them, soon allows rapid disappearance of somatic complaints, and over time eliminates physical signs. It is this "focused visible caring," only one of the many positive facets of Reiki, that has become the catalyst for many traditionalists in medicine to reach out and provide for their patients' greater emotional needs.

Overview of the PA Profession

The AAPA, American Academy of Physician Assistants, provides an overview of the PA profession that gives a thumbnail of the background of what I do in the traditional medical arena. The mixture of Reiki and traditional medicine has been beneficial to many. Each year, modern medicine is spending more research dollars on non-traditional modalities like Reiki.

Physician assistants practice medicine with the supervision of licensed physicians, providing patient services that range from primary medicine to very specialized surgical care. Educated in a medical program, PAs are qualified to perform eighty percent of the duties most commonly done by primary care physicians.

Physician assistants perform physical examinations, diagnose and treat illnesses, order and interpret lab tests, counsel on preventive health, suture wounds, set fractures, and assist in surgical operations.

There are more than 30,000 physician assistants in the United States. In some rural areas, where physicians are in short supply, PAs serve as the only providers of health care, under supervising physicians. Eighteen percent of all PAs practice in rural communities with 50,000 to 100,000 people, and a third practice in towns with fewer than 50,000 people. Many hospitals, faced with a shortage of physician residents, employ physician assistants as house staff in medical and surgical departments.

Insurance
The following are insurers that promote alternative and complementary therapies:
- American Western Life Insurance Wellness Plan 1-800-925-5323
- Alternative Health Plan 1-800-966-8467
- Mutual of Omaha 1-402-342-7600
- Common Well Health Plan 1-617-566-9355.

Nursing in the Emergency Room
by Jennifer A. Link RN, BA, CEN, SANE, RP, Rochester, NY

The body-mind-spirit connection is permeating the medical community in the same manner that new ideas always do, slowly. The difference here is that this is a return to the basics, or full circle. I have seen the practice of, specifically, Reiki evolve over the past eight years from totally rejected, seen as some form of mysticism, to its current status of a specialty, requiring training and knowledge.

As an emergency room certified nurse working in a busy emergency/trauma center, I find many uses available for the Reiki training I received. The ability to center oneself prior to approaching a patient, child or adult, has noticeable effects. It is reflected in one's tone, demeanor, excitability in crisis and overall ability to instill a sense of confidence in the patient. I often find that a poor attitude is transferred to my colleagues or patients before I say or do anything.

When I take a few moments to align my thoughts to the activity at hand, I am much more effective in my interactions. Nothing is more satisfying than to work with the chakras of a toddler to allay fear. I never fail to be amazed by the difference in the level of anxiety displayed by children who are, compared with those who are not, exposed to the soothing effects of Reiki.

In the adult population, I have used the same techniques in violent aggressive patients. The result is usually a person who forgets why he is angry or who decides he is now ready to discuss the underlying problem. Reiki can be performed with hands on the person or at a distance with the same benefit. The advantage to using Reiki over a method requiring close contact is evident in the scenario of an emergency room. Personal safety is a priority in a frequently explosive environment.

I recall one particular case of an older gentleman who was physically and verbally abusive to the staff. He eventually had to be restrained for the safety of all, including himself. Despite numerous attempts, nobody could get near him to render care without receiving a barrage of insults and verbal filth. I stood outside his door for a moment and concentrated on care, compassion, and calming thoughts. I picked up a sense of loss from him. I was then able to approach the bedside without incident only to discover that the tears were just below the surface of anger. He had recently lost his spouse.

I also function as a sexual assault nurse examiner. Due to the fast pace expected in the emergency room, there is a limited amount of time allotted even to cases where a strong bond is essential to the emotional welfare of the patient. My role as patient advocate, primary caregiver, and the person in charge of evidence collection for prosecution is greatly enhanced by the ability to form a rapid empathetic bond with my patient.

A less-promoted use of Reiki is the ability to use the available or universal energy on one's self. Nurses are forever searching for more effective ways to care for their patients, often at their own health expense. A well-aligned spirit-mind creates excellent stress reduction. It offers a means of self-debriefing.

Although specific techniques often vary from person to person, depending on their need, the knowledge criteria is the same, the intention to do no harm.

Spirit of Caring

Source: Article in Advances in Nursing Science *17, no. 1 (September 1994), by Anita Beckerman, ARNP, CS, EdD*

Today's struggle for a greater awareness of the meaning of spirituality is very significant in these times. Many materialistic foundations of our culture have proven to be disappointing. In this search for an acceptable basis for spirituality, the field of nursing has demonstrated great leadership in its investigation of caring. Nursing scholars and researchers present evidence that within this simple and universal human act, there is much that has spiritual significance. These investigations have also shown that our depth of understanding affects the very methodology used in researching human concerns.

To care means to be aware of another person, to reach out and make contact with that person. To be in contact with another can mean actual touching, but primarily it is a willingness to experience an interconnectedness with that individual, a willingness to be touched or moved emotionally by that person. In caring there is also humility, because feelings of responsibility, hope, and sadness mingle with those of doubt about one's personal adequacy and competence to respond appropriately. There is also a fluctuation between being bound in oneness with the other person and experiencing a separation or distance. In the struggle to do what is necessary to be of help there can be a certain stiffness in our sense of connectedness, when what is required may be unpleasant and not what the patient wants.

Caregivers use their daily presence to closely involve themselves with their patients' well-being. The nurses thus feel that they aid by listening and helping the patients and their families to find meaning in these circumstances.

At the heart of spirituality in the nursing field, the image of oneness, that we are interconnected beings, comes through. The caring for one another, defined in the Golden Rule, is a basis reached through compassion born of intuitive empathy, experiencing the other's needs within oneself. A helpful way for caregivers to release or understand emotions from work is "journaling." This writing down of inner feelings to gain a deeper understanding of the inner spirit, the daily presence working and caring for these patients, and the rewards given back from a nursing career.

Rescue Squad and Natural Healing—Reiki

by Lucinda Fury, RP, Virginia Beach, VA

"Eve" works in the paramedical field as a volunteer with a local rescue squad. Their job is to care for those people in need of emergency medical treatment prior to and during transport to a hospital. In most cases, people are frightened and suffering from shock after a sudden onset of illness or injury. Eve has found her natural healing touch invaluable in assisting people in emergency situations. While I listened to her describe what she does how she tunes into the injured person, how she centers herself and feels the energy flow with a prayerful attitude, I realized that she was describing a form of Reiki. Eve has been doing this healing from instinct. Some people are in fact "connected," with a type of healing touch even before they understand what it is. Her paramedic job calls for immediate assessment of the trauma and delivery of the proper pre-treatment for transport. Her ability to calm a person in emergency situations has given her a reputation, one which her co-workers call upon in more critical situations. Obviously, Eve's practice of Reiki or a related form of healing, has provided a benefit to those who have needed reassurance, calmness, and healing.

Chiropractic
by Dr. John T. White, DC, Virginia Beach, VA

Holistic health care is more than addressing all the systems of the body. To be whole is to be balanced in mind, body, and spirit. I use a gentle, specific chiropractic technique to align the spinal structure of the body and take pressure off of the spinal nerves. This increases the neurological potential, thus enabling the body to use its own innate healing properties. I have had thousands of people lay on my table in front of me. It has been my experience that there is an electromagnetic field around the body and that can be affected by other electromagnetic fields. This force has been called prana, chi, or life force. The method of working with this energy is called Reiki, Quigong, Polarity, Therapeutic Touch, and many other names. In chiropractic, it is called the body's own innate intelligence.

What is healing? Why do some people heal while others do not? There are times when the structure is stabilized and the neurological system is properly functioning and yet the person's innate healing force is still blocked. I often find that a person's innate healing will not awaken because of an emotional block. An entanglement of thinking, which causes an emotional aberration like fear or guilt, can block the natural healing of the body.

I find polarity and Reiki to be extremely valuable when treating patients with migraines and emotional stress. With migraines I put my left hand on the forehead and my right hand on the base of the neck. With emotional stress I put my left hand on the forehead and my right hand under the navel and rock their hips while talking to them about relaxing and visualizing. My advice is to learn the techniques, and your intuition will tell you when to use them. They work!

My responsibility to my patients is to do everything I can to enable them to heal themselves. They will receive chiropractic adjustments, massage therapy, neuromuscular therapy, and many times polarity or Reiki.

A couple of years ago, my mother died from her treatment for cancer. She would come into my office, but there wasn't a lot I could do because the chemotherapy had devastated her immune system and the radiation had turned her skin into something like wood. She was tired of being sick and weak and saw no future where she would be whole again. I would have her lie face up on my adjusting table. With my left hand on her forehead and my right hand on her navel, I would gently rock her hips. She would noticeably relax as I continued the treatment. She would breathe deeper, become calmer and feel more centered and at peace. When she walked out of my office, her attitude was better and she felt stronger. Since that time I have seen many people on my table who were not at peace and centered in their bodies. I've used my electromagnetic field to calm and center theirs. Using polarity has added depth to my practice of holistic chiropractic.

California Chiropractic
by Bobbee Rickard, RM, Livermore, CA

I recently began working with a chiropractor who is very open-minded to alternative forms of healing. After we discussed Reiki and the benefits of having this powerfully loving vibration in one's life, as well as in the work environment, he decided that he would like to be attuned to this energy. Within the first two months of doing so, he commented to me on how others had noticed something different about him, and that his energy vibrations were more vibrant. He is feeling great about his experience and has recommended it to his staff, friends, and clients. His patients are benefiting, as is his chiropractic work, by being embraced through the Reiki "universal life force energy."

Dental Practice with Reiki Energy Application
by Dr. Dean H. Kent, DDS, Virginia Beach, VA

I have been a practicing dentist for the past eighteen years. Like all dentists, I was trained in a traditional school and learned traditional forms of treatment. The healing art of dentistry was taught almost exclusively on a physical level. My dental school was very good at teaching its graduates the biological processes and the physiological functions of the human body. We learned how to recognize all forms of dental-related diseases and how to treat most of them. It was, however, weak at teaching dentists how to cope with a patient's mental and emotional state and was completely remiss in teaching anything about a person's spiritual dimension, and how it may be related to the emotional and physical state of that person.

Throughout my life, I have been interested in that aspect called the spiritual. I have done extensive reading in metaphysics and spiritually related topics and have attended many lectures on the like. I have been trained in Reiki (universal life force energy), and have also learned other forms of spiritual healing. I have been fortunate to have attended Delphi (an institute for spiritual development in Georgia) and have taken classes from many local spiritual teachers.

I found it difficult, at first, to apply my knowledge and experience of healing in the dental profession. Since my patients came to me specifically for dental problems, I was obligated to treat such problems on a physical level. I found, however, that if I consciously applied the Reiki principles, and allowed this energy to channel through me, the results of the treatment were better. My procedure consisted of attuning myself first, by stating my intention of being a channel for healing. As I felt the energy flow through me, I would send this universal life force energy from my heart chakra and engulf the patient with it, producing a calming effect.

When performing more difficult dental procedures, I again would allow this universal life force energy to flow through my hands to the patient. I found that the more extensive dental procedures, which would normally be uncomfortable, were completely painless. An example of this is the injection. The injection of lidocaine in the mouth to achieve anesthesia, which is often painful, was nearly painless when Reiki energy was present.

A healing treatment with Reiki can reduce postoperative pain, inflammation and swelling. The most significant result of receiving Reiki is the calming effect on the patient's mental and emotional state. The method of using this healing energy seems to relieve a lot of anxiety and reduce the stress levels during a dental treatment.

The results I have described to you are not documented, but are personal observations noted over the years of dental practice. Reiki has been a wonderful tool as an adjunct in the treatment of my patients. I am able to treat on all levels, using a holistic approach to dentistry. A person's physical needs are met, as well as satisfying their emotional and spiritual needs.

Dental Chart
Source: From a dental professional friend in South America. See appendix A.

Usually if you have teeth missing (e.g., wisdom), it is important that the cavitation be thoroughly cleaned. The periodontal membrane must be properly removed in the area, or this area does not heal and infection could be ongoing. Example: At a young age, I had bronchial problems, sore throats, and coughing, almost like whooping cough. In looking at the teeth associated with the throat and bronchus on the chart, this theory is supported in my case.

Therapeutic Approach to Alternative Traditions

Tradition	**Somatic**	**Herbal/Nutrition**	**Energetic**
Chinese Medicine	Acupressure Massage Tai chi	Chinese herbs Diet	Acupuncture Acupressure Tai chi
Ayurveda	Massage Pranayama Yoga	Ayurveda herbs Diet for Vata, Pitta, Kapha	Massage Pranayama Meditation
Homeopathy	None	None	Homeopathic
Naturopathic Medicine	Massage Bodywork Manipulation Hydrotherapy	Eastern herbal Western herbal Diet	Methods from all traditions
Mind/Body Medicine	Exercise, yoga, tai chi, chi kung Breathing	Diet guidelines used by other traditions	Imagery Biofeedback Relaxation
Osteopathic Medicine	Manipulation of all bones, tissues, and organs of body	Individual training and interest	Individual training and interest
Chiropractic	Manipulation of skeletal system and soft tissue	Individual training	Recommended: Polarity, Reiki, or Rolfing
Bodywork/Massage Therapy	Traditional European Contemporary Western Structural, Functional Movement Oriental Energetic Reflexology Other approaches	Individual training	Individual training, Recommended: Reiki, TT, Polarity Aromatherapy Breathing Visualization

Structural Integration (Rolfing) Practitioner
by DuLois Lee, CMT, SIP, North Carolina

As a structural integration practitioner or Rolfer, I am daily entering, experiencing, and working in other people's energy fields. Focus is the physical manipulation of their fascia (connective tissue); the restoration of balance, space, and length through this tissue to their spines, heads, limbs, organs, and joints is the body's ultimate goal.

My intent is to create space to allow the body to effect its own healing. The results are astonishing. The body's intelligence communicates infinite amounts of information to every layer of tissue, cells, bones, thoughts, memories, emotions, and all related energy fields from a single release of stress, or a restored space. This immediate shifting of energy is not only felt in a client's system and energy field, it is also felt in the person who is helping to effect the changes (practitioner). The hands don't have to be touching the body to assist with energy fields. It is almost as if our minds and hearts can direct a flow of healing energy into another's field. However, the actual "laying on of hands" seems the most powerful and fastest mode for me.

As I work from day to day, I feel more and more connected to all fields of healing. This is not to say we all recognize each other's efforts that are still to come. However, there are many areas of healing work, such as Reiki, that are similar to mine, and many friends in these fields strive for and communicate the same ideals that inform my work. We all feel, sense, see, or work toward the total uplifted, wholly functioning, human man, woman, and child.

When I am Rolfing a person, I can see lifting and straightening and I can see, as well as feel with my hands, the integration of the body's segments, now working together in movement and grounded in stance, being lifted by gravity like a plant stretching toward the sun. In such a balanced state, a person's energy field must surely expand and flow through them with every breath, promoting growth and attainment of their fullest potential.

In structural integration, this ideal is called "being on your line of gravity." In Reiki, it is Hara, vital center around which your whole body is centered. Most Eastern beliefs strive for balance in the flow of energy through these centers, or lines for homeostasis. Even massage promotes a more balanced flow of energy. A structurally integrated body, as proven in photographs before and after, shows a marked change in the posture and balanced segments of the torso and body. The walk and stance are more balanced, and the use of the body is affected. The skin tone is noticeably lighter afterward. The personality changes. The subject has a sense of empowerment, is usually calmer and less easily disturbed or upset, and has less need for abusive behavior. The changes are innumerable and varied, but always remarked upon as better.

These changes begin in the first session as the whole outer envelope of the body fascia is "fluffed up." This allows space for the deeper layers to move out. The subject usually feels lighter afterward, and very relaxed. The second session is from the knee to the plantar surfaces of the foot. This is the foundation that all of the structures will rest upon. The lower leg is of vital import in the stability of the foot. Most report a very different stance and walk. No wonder, they are now coming from a very different place in their universe! The miracles begin as sessions three through ten, each one on a different part of the body, build on each other to stack themselves into an integrated, balanced body, comprised of four sides.

Each session creates space for the next layer of fascia to unwind itself. Tissues and joints are freed from frozen states and interstitial fluid flows more freely. Old wounds, injuries, and traumas, both emotional and physical, can now be released. The body begins to heal itself.

Many chronic back, neck, and shoulder complaints have been relieved during a single session, such as five, six, or seven when the spine (anterior and superior) becomes integrated, "the head is put on," and the spine is realigned. For the first time, the proper support systems for the upper body are coaxed into use. The strain is removed from the unbalanced structure.

These tissues will continue to move and lengthen for several months to a year after the initial series of ten sessions. Post-ten work and advanced sessions are available for even more growth as needed.

There is no rule that you receive only ten sessions of structural integration. Dr. Ida Rolf, who perfected the Rolf technique, felt that ten sessions were what most people needed. Some ongoing structural integration clients may be, for example, new mothers post birth to restore the pelvic floor, recent physical or emotional trauma victims, people with chronic illness, athletes, or very physical people who use their bodies strenuously in work. There are numerous occasions where the Rolfer is needed, just like the family doctor. It has been brought to my attention many times, however, that the chronic need for chiropractic treatment, massage, pain pills, and drastic medical procedures has been eliminated by Rolfing. The body is better able to hold chiropractic adjustments and less apt to be injured, or to become ill after structural integration.

I am always amazed at the "miracles" I see in my studio, and hear about from Reiki practitioners, massage therapists, color and essence therapists, and other energy workers I know and work with. I feel very happy to be in this field of beautiful energy work.

Best Ways to Find a Healer

Are you ready to explore alternative methods of healing? Keep in mind that a good healer, just like a good doctor, can be hard to find. Try the following sources:

Primary care physicians—More and more doctors are incorporating alternative therapies into their practices. Check your local directory for the listings Health and Medicine, Homeopathic or Naturopathic, or under Dental and Chiropractic doctors, for caregivers who are now using these methods.

Medical schools—Currently, there are more than two dozen medical schools in the United States offering courses devoted to the topic of alternative medicine.

Friends and family—Each year Americans spend more than ten billion dollars on alternative treatments. Chances are, someone you know has experimented with one or more alternative forms of healing and they could refer you.

Government—The Office of Alternative Medicine at the National Institute of Health, (301) 402-2466, (888) 644-6226, has a listing of professional associations grouped by type of alternative treatment.

American Association of Naturopathic Physicians
2366 Eastlake Avenue, Suite #322, Seattle, WA 98102
(206) 298-0126
(provides a directory listing of naturopathic physicians)

Bodywork and Massage

Facts about Bodywork Massage

Massage therapy is the manipulation of soft tissue for therapeutic purposes. Two strong hands smooth sweet-smelling oil onto your body, and with long gentle strokes, move along the sore muscles on either side of your spine, around your shoulder, and along the neck, releasing tensions built up in the body. These strokes may include effleurage, petrissage, tapotement, compression, vibration, friction, and other Swedish movements. Massage therapy does not include diagnosis or any service requiring a license to practice medicine; however, many massage therapists have been trained in other modalities, such as: polarity, breathwork, Rolfing, nutrition, aromatherapy, reflexology, counseling, past life regression, etc. Massage enhances the function of the joints and muscles, improves circulation and general body tone and relieves mental and physical fatigue. Time passes by as you float in the experience and let go of stress.

Applications of Therapeutic Massage

Circulatory system—Massage increases the blood supply and nutrition to muscles without adding to their load of toxic lactic acid, produced through voluntary muscle contraction. Massage helps to overcome harmful fatigue resulting from strenuous exercise. Massage can compensate, in part, for lack of exercise and muscular contraction resulting from injury or being bed-ridden.

Nervous system—Massage has a tranquilizing effect on the central nervous system. Effects from massage induce the body's own painkillers, called endorphins, and directly aid in dealing with over-stressed lifestyles in today's society.

Muscular system—Massage works to relieve chronic tightness around the neck and shoulder areas, whether from poor posture or job-related functions. Massage (1) frees the lower back from stiff or aching muscles, (2) helps legs from poor circulation, cramps, and soreness from athletic training, (3) increases blood flow to the feet and stimulates the organs through reflexology of the feet, (4) acts as a mechanical cleanser in the abdomen pushing along waste and accumulated toxins and replacing them with fresh blood and increased oxygenation to the tissues, and (5) helps address tension from headaches often found to come from facial muscles (TMJ), through facial and scalp treatment.

Lymph drainage—The lymphatic system plays a vital role in the human immune system. This branching network of vessels transports lymph, a thin, milky fluid. The lymphatic system removes toxins, waste products, and excess fluid from our tissues. Lymph is purified of foreign substances through lymph nodes, which contain disease-fighting cells and eventually empty into the bloodstream. Olszewski and Engeset (1979) found that massage of the feet increases the contraction frequency of the lymphatic system and the rate of lymph flow in humans. Feather-light strokes rather than the normal massage strokes, which stimulate circulation, accomplish lymph drainage. Bodywork facilitates the release and movement of the fluids between the cells—the primal soup. It is effective in conditions of decreased immune response or congestion.

Emotional transformation—Bodywork is one of the fastest vehicles for transformation. Our attitudes, beliefs, feelings, fears, and traumas lie trapped in our connective tissues waiting to be released. When bodywork is combined with emotional release, huge changes occur in structure and life style. Emotions are what make us uniquely human, but when they are neglected or suppressed, this can be the largest source of diseases. No one teaches us how to have healthy emotions. It is important to be working in a job that is a source of satisfaction, rather than one that will shorten your life.

Aromatherapy—Along with massage, plant essences can subtly, but powerfully, alter your mental, emotional, and physiological state. Massage is most beneficial with meditative music and a serene massage room, along with an environment of positive energy and a healthy therapist.

Body/Mind/Work Technique
by Joan Essig, CMT, RN, Virginia Beach, VA
Energy is energy is energy, consistently, ever-changing within natural patterns.

As your spiritual self is open and energy fills you, the creative source flows, allowing connectedness and oneness with your client; and, thus, a knowingness of what energy needs facilitation (movement), where, and how.

Inner guidelines may be given, and yet logic is a foundation; but this technique does not allow the logic to interfere with creativeness, the essence of healing, joyfulness and love.

Session

Center Self:
- Connection—State mentally or verbally your intention. This creates a focus of the unconditional love frequency (vibration) that always surrounds us (like water around fish in the ocean).

Opening Stretch, Individual Facilitator:
- With client lying on their back, place fingertips along occipital ridge (base at back of head) and provide slight traction. Place hands on sacral reflex at ankles and, while cupping heels, provide slight traction.

Opening Stretch, Team Facilitation:
- With client lying on their back, one person provides the head hold; one person provides the ankle hold; both provide traction simultaneously.

Scanning System:
The human system is an energy imprint (grid or blueprint) that manifests in physical form (the body). Determine areas requiring balance with an evaluative energy scan. Particularly note knees and ankles.

Interventions:
Intervention techniques are used to balance energy as required through the client's system—within the body and beyond. (See diagrams of Fields of Energy and Chakras in chapter 9.)
- *Knees*—Check that energy flowing through this area is not "leaking out." When leaking, seal with hand "sandwich method" medially and laterally or anteriorly and posteriorly. (See chapter 11—Reiki Hand Positions)
- *Ankles*—Assure that energy flows through the ankles and out the soles of the feet.

Removal of Crystallized Energy:
- *Left hand*—Hold energy of area.
- *Right hand*—Laser with fingertips or focused intention (heats/melts with hand chakra) Can also laser with third eye.
- Lasering is often a spiraling motion, sometimes a "cross-fire." When complete, pluck out and discard misqualified or negative energies to all consuming violet flame (neutralizing) through Saint Germaine of the Ascended Masters.

- Always fill area you removed from, and seal with *left hand* boosted by *right hand*. During this process, instruct client with self-intention, visualization, color, sound, etc.

Placement of Energy Grids:
Balance Area
- Insert via visualization, intention (i.e., time-release capsule or pyramid for pain relief).
- Seal when complete.

Sandwich
- Place hands opposite each other with body between (i.e., one hand on top of body, one hand on bottom of body in direct correlation).
- Focus on energizing area.

Cross-Fire
- Use index and middle fingers of both hands to cross-fire small areas (polarity). (See chapter 9 diagram—Polarity.)
- Connect any chakra point with any area requiring balance.

Torso Energy-Moving Contacts:
- *Right hand*—Connect middle finger with tip of tailbone, exert stronger pressure.
- *Left hand*—Place on any blocked point above right hand position, with intention to draw out contact from blockage (meridian linc).
- *Left hand*—Place index finger on third eye.
- *Right hand*—Place on any blocked point of body below left hand position, with intention to replenish area.
- Keeping *left hand* higher than right *hand,* make strongest balancing contact at any point connected with solar plexus.

Flowing Figure (Infinity) Sacral-Cranial Balance:
Sandwiching technique (posterior/back and anterior/front)
- Start at sacrum/pubic area.
- Balance, alternating bottom hand to top and repeating to next hand width, up the spine.
- Continue process up the body through the third eye area.

Emotional Release from Lifetimes:
- *Left hand*—place over heart.
- *Right hand*—place over navel (solar plexus and sacral chakra area).

Immersion:
- Visualize holding a vessel above the client or surrounding the client (like a cocoon), and allow the energy to pour upon or to envelop the client.

Intention during Session:
- Focus use of energy via hands, fingers, third eye; visualize with the mind.

- Invoke presence of energy imprints of anything needed (e.g., sound, color, crystals, water flowing, plants, herbs, essences).
- Invoke assistance from angels, fairies, Jesus, Buddha, ascended masters, power animals.

Ending Session:
- End after client is in balance.
- Aura brush or ruffle to clear energy field.
- Seal with infinity sweep (see chapter 11 diagram, Closure Technique), ground at feet.

Give Thanks—Detach:

Client self-empowerment is promoted via active participation in their process. This exponential energy thus quickens and intensifies results. Use your voice to facilitate a journey and invoke places of past and future lives. You may have messages come through for the healing.

Encourage participation via: education, music, movement, progressive relaxation, breath work, toning, visualization.

Go with loving tenderness for yourself, for the serving of humanity is a most reverent calling, which first requires self-nurturing.

Learning to receive good also means learning to refuse harm.
It means accepting a life free of physical, mental, emotional, and spiritual abuse.

Massage therapy along with other natural healing,
and aromatherapy (essential oils are plant life energy)
helps release the tensions and core issues we hold in our tissues.
Massage is a gentle way of learning to really "let go."

Experiencing a Combination of Bodywork and Spiritual Healing
by Lucinda Fury, RP, Virginia Beach, VA

Anyone who has been in the presence of "J," even for a few minutes, has felt the serenity that radiates from her very center being. I myself have felt "the presence of angels" around her. It didn't surprise me to find that she indeed works with the angels in many facets of her life, including her professional bodywork massage, her Reiki training, her creative pastel energy paintings, her personal meditations, and her everyday activities.

In her home you may see a tiny angel peeking down on you from a high shelf, or one serenely poised on a table surrounded by various Earth crystals. Throughout her work and living space, many angelic motifs combine harmoniously with Native American influences.

J appears to be as eclectic in her furnishings and decor as she is in her spirituality. Her angels are ever present during her massages. Her gentleness and calmness soothe away the tensions and cares of her clients, as does the Reiki energy that she has incorporated into her bodywork practice and teachings. A Reiki practitioner for the past fifteen years and a Reiki Master for six years, she easily blends the healing energy force with all facets of her spiritual work. But there is evidence of a shamanistic approach to her healing and teaching as well. She successfully combines the essences of Native American, Tibetan, and Western spirituality in all that she does.

J refers to what she does as "a combination of massage, spiritual healing and a connection to a universal energy force." She would tell you the healing comes from Creator and self (client), and that with her angelic guides, she vacillates the healing atmosphere. We are all responsible in part for our own healing; it's people like J who help us get into that space where we can give ourselves to the healing process.

With J's capacity for expanding on knowledge and concepts of spirituality, it isn't surprising that a few years ago her awareness of Earth's needs in healing and people's needs in healing were connected. From the one planet one people concept, an idea germinated and came into full blossomed "knowing" one night, on her journey home from a seminar. A spiritual awakening on that dark night probably saved her life and gave her direction to write a book: a concise, easily understood Reiki manual, with poems to awaken mankind to our environmental needs in relationship to Mother Earth.

Since then, J's focus has turned not only to teaching the Reiki method of healing, but to promoting a purer understanding of a practice and healing life style, that can literally put us back in control of our true spiritual purpose.

When she works in her small garden, you can't help but notice, as she lovingly tends and cares for her flowers, that their colors are a little more vibrant, their greens a little more lush, their fragrances a little more pungent, than they could have otherwise been without her special touch. The same quality lends itself to J's pastel paintings, her healing touch through Reiki, her massage therapy, and the classes she teaches.

Some wonderful energy glows through her being and extends to all those fortunate enough to be around her. I'm not sure exactly what it is, but I know Creator gave it to her and J lovingly, devotedly shares it with us every day.

Bodywork and Counseling Terms

Alexander technique—is a series of lessons helping to identify and correct faulty habit patterns in the body, and reestablishes psycho-spiritual balance.

Bodywork massage—is an art that employs body manipulation by a therapist to restore and maintain balanced circulation, tone of muscles, aid in eliminating toxins, and stimulate nerve activity. There is an energy circuit whereby the electromagnetic energy passes between the client and therapist.

Cranial-sacral therapy and Somato-emotional release—offer gentle unwinding of the spinal column and rebalancing of the autonomic nervous system. Originally a part of osteopathy these approaches have been brought to a wide variety of practitioners through widespread training by the Upledger Institute.

Bioenergetics and Core Energetics—derive directly from the work of Wilhelm Reich as developed by Alexander Lowen and John Pierrakos. The focus is on using special exercises to draw to consciousness and release chronic tensions in a psychotherapeutic setting.

Breathwork—(including holotropic breathwork, rebirthing and others) guides the client through intensive breathing into a state of altered consciousness from which deep emotional and physical release can rise.

Dance therapy—and expressive movement utilize guided movement to access and work with unconscious blockages, bringing to awareness feeling through the direct sensation of the body in motion.

Feldenkrais—can include hands-on painless manipulation of the skeletal structure plus various movements and postures designed to offset restrictive personal and cultural programming.

Hakomi therapy—integrates Gestalt, bioenergetics, and a variety of other modalities to enliven and balance the whole person.

Polarity therapy—builds awareness of whole-person bodywork, energy balancing, vibrational healing, nutrition, and counseling.

Reichian therapy—(including neo-Reichian and post-Reichian) works with breath, patterns of holding in the body, and how emotional or physical trauma or deficits manifest in terms of physical structure. The focus is on the verbal.

Rolfing—(structural integration), postural integration, body synergy, and soma seek to reintegrate physical structure so that it can function more harmoniously and efficiently with gravity. It utilizes deep stretching of connective tissue. The amount of psychological integration depends on the individual practitioner.

Rubenfeld synergy—incorporates Feldenkrais and Alexander work with Gestalt therapy and Ericksonian hypnotherapy. It uses gentle touch and dialogue.

Trager—uses gentle lifting, pulling, and touch to free up different parts of the body in a process of sensory reeducation.

Healers at Work
Source: Association for Research and Enlightenment (ARE) 16, no. 5 (February 1995).

What do spiritual healers experience while performing their various arts? What are the consistent patterns among transpersonal practitioners? A study of published statements by renowned healers and interviews brought about a variety of spiritual healing methods. An analysis of text and personal interviews for a variety of topics—such as elements of the healer's frame of mind, preparation for healing, emotions, and quality of attention and awareness—brought about the following information.

1) Healers notice a self-induced shift in their attentions, their physical functioning, and their thoughts as they prepare to engage in healing.
2) They make their intention to heal a reality, often through invoked imagery or verbalized affirmations or prayer.
3) They shift their attention inward. Referencing to non-ordinary energies, powers, spiritual beings, or paranormal abilities, they transform their consciousness so that it is no longer limited by personal identity and it comes into a state of merger with the healee.
4) Healers make a shift in sensing personal control, making an effect to skillfully letting go to a transcendent organizing principle (Divine Creator). This is accomplished by concentrating and paying attention to becoming absorbed in the flow of the experience.
5) There are often images or intuitions and insights. Time stands still, or the healer may lose all sense of time.
6) There can be physical sensations of warmth, a sensing of the change in vibratory energy flowing like a current, and an alertness of more energy being directed to one area or another.
7) Body images may change, with parts like the hands or feet expanding, the person feeling taller or lighter, or not aware of having a body at all. These changes comprise an altered state of consciousness.

California Reiki Healing Therapist
by Bobbee Rickard, RM, Livermore, CA

Case History: I recently worked with one of my Reiki students who had been diagnosed with breast cancer for a second time. This time she was aware of Reiki Therapy and had recently been attuned to Reiki energy. She had already begun chemotherapy when she came to me to begin Reiki therapy sessions. Shortly after that time she began radiation, too.

The first few weeks we met three times a week, then decreased to two times per week, and then one time per week consistently. The Reiki sessions required more time than usual, due to the depletion her body was experiencing, undergoing both chemotherapy and radiation. Each Monday, she was given a blood test by her medical professional to check her blood count. The purpose of this was to monitor the "fighter cells." Each week her blood count became stronger, to the nurses' amazement, and by the third week, her blood count was stronger than before she had begun chemotherapy.

She began to question the medical doctor about needing to continue the radiation, because of the trauma her body was going through. After each session she felt that her body was fighting and winning. The doctor had her undergo a CAT scan first. The CAT scan confirmed, as she had perceived, that the cancer was gone. This was our visualization in each Reiki session that the day would come when the doctor would give her a clear and clean bill of health. It had been two months since her first Reiki therapy session.

Two months later, she went to a plastic surgeon for reconstructive surgery and he was amazed at her skin. In fact, he thought that she had not had radiation, because the skin looked so well. He had treated more than one thousand cases and he had never seen skin after radiation look so well.

This lady had worked with her medical professionals, as well as taken responsibility for her healing through Reiki therapy. She got to the source of the diseases; healed her inner child; self empowered herself, used nutrition, massage, positive affirmations and prayer; and loved, nurtured and honored herself. She was in my life so that I might experience the power of this gift that we have come to honor—the gift of Reiki!

United Kingdom Healer

by Barbara Fraser-Duthie, RM, MCOH, MAR, ICR, ASK, BABTAC, BHMA, AERP, ITEC
Pegasus Natural Therapy Clinic, United Kingdom

Case History One (Chunky): The beautiful rolling Cotswold hills in Gloucestershire in the Southwest of England have been sheep country for hundreds of years. The limestone escarpment is shallow of soil but springtime presents a glorious scene of gamboling lambs amidst green fields and hills.

In late years, due to the supermarkets insisting on early lamb, many farmers are breeding from their ewes in January. A local farmer's wife came to the back door of my Cotswold home and asked, "Do you heal lambs?" So off we went to view five-day-old "Chunky," a quite enormous single lamb who was very clearly suffering from birth trauma as he lay in his well-strawed pen in the old stables. "He can't get up," she said. The veterinary surgeon had been by on the second day, but, even for excellent stock people who would not allow an animal to suffer, a lamb requiring expensive treatment becomes very uneconomical.

Chunky was extremely stiff all over his back and neck, not least due to the problems of getting him out of the ewe.

Reiki symbols were drawn over the lamb (rather to the bemused interest of the farmer's wife who was acting as surrogate to "muscle test"), and massage offered to his rigid neck and back. I gave him some Bach Flower Rescue Remedy for shock to his chakras. Chunky was still lying fairly lifelessly and offered no resistance as I used the Reiki energy to enable prioritizing of my nutritional "test kits" to assess his obvious deficiencies.

He was exceptionally deficient in magnesium, but also zinc and copper. There were some others, including assorted vitamins, herbs, minerals, homeopathics, etc. He was not expected to survive unless improvement came soon.

The nutritional test kits are intended for assessing the patient's needs and then prioritizing if financially necessary, giving the herb, vitamin, or mineral in tablet, granule, or liquid essence form. The healer's Reiki energy has always enabled direct absorption of the nutrient via the crown chakra whilst the patient or surrogate "therapy locates" or touches the relevant acupuncture/reflex point. (Test kit manufacturers often telephone to inquire why I find their products so entirely satisfactory, but never order any stocks!) The frequency of the vibration of the nutrition appears to correct the problem immediately and patients stay "fixed." The Reiki energy enhances the vibration, or so it seems, for they still correct with one hundred percent efficiency after several years. My pendulum advises when sufficient has been absorbed.

While the farmer's wife and I viewed the triplet lambs next to Chunky and the very unusual quads on the opposite side, he suddenly got up and walked around his pen. "Did you see that? I don't believe it. He just got up and walked around!" said the disbelieving farmer's wife. (One had noticed!) Initially he flopped back down after twenty or thirty steps, but thanks to the Reiki energy and a second healing the next day, he made a full recovery.

Case History Two: "A," born in 1948, first came to see me at the Stratford-Upon-Avon surgery in August 1995, when traveling within forty miles to her son's wedding. The mother of four children, she was a lovely lady, but one of life's "victim scripts."

She had received her Reiki First and Second degrees, but little of the wonderful healing energy seemed present in her life. She was drawn, gray, weary, tense and, totally devoid of energy, and said "that everybody always left her." Her mother had died and left her; the first and second husbands; the children, having grown up, had left her, and daughter "R," the youngest doubtless would as she was fifteen years old now.

A described a catalog of horrors over the telephone and was encouraged to consider a minimum two-hour appointment, which was little enough time.

She came by train with R, who sat in the waiting room looking lost and forlorn and evidently still carrying deep emotional memories of her horrendous birth in 1980. "I wish I could get R to agree to come and see you," said A, "but she won't."

After using the Reiki Master and Tibetan Master symbols over A, also including R outside in the reception room, details of A's problems were listed. To find something that A didn't have wrong with her would have been amazing! All fourteen of the body's main meridians were down, and she had problems or imbalances in her liver, heart, gallbladder, pancreas, small intestine, large intestine, bladder, kidney, hormones, lungs, uterus, throat, and jaw; cranium, spine, neck and shoulders, electrical and lymphatic symptoms, genetic-nutritional makeup, and polarity and chakras to name a few!

Her emotional and loss-of-energy problems were due in fact to A carrying eleven entities. Perhaps four could be described as "shadowing" of the aura, but the remainder were attached more specifically to various parts of the body's energy fields. (Many entities, being "lost souls" rather than the Hollywood version of satanic possessors, tend not to realize that their presence depletes the host's energy levels, often very dramatically, as I had seen with post-natal depression in my experience with patients.)

A smiled as I told her she was a "walking disaster" and I didn't know where to start with her. If in doubt, give Reiki! Because of the time factor and A living more than one hundred miles away without transport, it seemed appropriate to ask Dr. Usui himself and Hayashi, plus Takata and any other available ascended masters, to help. The result was truly amazing. As A lay on the couch listening to the relaxing music, I just held her head in the appropriate manner and all was rebalanced before my eyes. As I held her head giving Reiki, I was aware of the very clear presences of Drs. Usui and Hayashi, actually peering into A's crown chakra.

It is said that the investment one makes in paying for Reiki attunement initiation will come back to the initiate. And so it was with A, unable to work by virtue of her totally depleted energy fields and on benefit from the government.

"No wonder you had a lot of head pain and migraines," I related to A, as this entire strange scene unfolded as I held her head in my hands. "You had an absolute armory of things in your etheric energy field." For those not into past life karma, the foregoing may seem extremely strange (as indeed it would have been very suspect to the writer in previous years of traveling internationally). Subsequent training in later life in this field has awakened old memories, and the training has become second nature in current work practices.

After perhaps three-quarters of an hour of Reiki, all the past life weapons had appeared to leave A. Her energy fields, when tested for the next step in realigning her body electrically, nutritionally, emotionally, physically, structurally, etc., were all absolutely one hundred percent strong. "You are a very lucky lady," I told A.

Following a December 1995 meeting with both A and R, who agreed to work with her birth trauma, both were greatly improved. R, using Reiki energy from me, released the black stuff covering her infant body at birth. A said her three older children were born without problems but R's birth had lasted seventy-two hours. "She was born covered in black yucky gunk," was her mother's description.

The yucky gunk was past life poisons in R's subtle energy fields, which had been dramatically affecting her current life emotionally and at other levels. Her bowels were now improving and her leg pains were much better. R agreed to come again in the spring to continue working with her considerable past life blockages.

A also needed ongoing Reiki healing and much help with her own past life problems. Her entities were gone, but she still felt a deep feeling of being left in a prison cell scratching for food on the floor. She would give herself and R lots of Reiki healing until our next visit.

Case History Three: "L" first came to see me in my surgery at Rother House Medical Center, Stratford-Upon-Avon, Warwickshire, United Kingdom in July 1993.

She then worked as a consultant for a well-known insurance office in Stratford-Upon-Avon, Worcester, and latterly Birmingham in the English West Midlands. Her day started early with travel by train and was extremely taxing and stressful. Our economic recession did little to help willing, responsible people, already extremely overworked, cope with the additional stress of job loss for anyone bold enough to object to current working practices.

Happily married, she was childless due to her husband seeking a vasectomy rather than obliging her to spend years taking the pill.

Present Problems: Back pain, mostly as a result of having size 42G breasts (reduction operation awaited). Stress including tension headaches, stomach and bowel pain, candida, bloating and other allergy-type symptoms. Throat and imbalanced energy in all chakras, non-alignment of central and governing meridians affecting up-and-down energy flow in the body, ileo-caecal and houston valve imbalances, gall-bladder malfunction, leg pain, fluid retention problems, and numbness in the left arm. (The latter was corrected by laser work to metal fillings of amalgam, resulting in release of energy flow to the arm. The top jaw tooth affected aligns with the corabrachialis muscle in the arm.) TMJ energy also had to be corrected, as the internal pterigoid muscle was now tight. L was also weary and lacking in energy generally.

Procedure: Reiki energy assisted with a variety of techniques to rebalance the above. After beginning to walk very early (at six months), L had developed hip problems in childhood as a result of leg problems due to being bow-legged, then knock-kneed, and developing bone spurs. Reiki was also used to assist with a fluctuating weight problem, mostly water retention that was menstrual related. Diet and nutritional back up were discussed, with affirmations and relaxation techniques.

A breast reduction operation of abnormally large breasts, which affected her posture, was done in early 1994, after two years of being on the waiting list. L was asked to telephone the details of the operation, time, and date as soon as possible, so that Reiki healing could be sent to her body in advance.

As this turned out to be short notice, the Reiki symbols were sent the day before, distantly, advising the etheric body or energy field of prospective surgery. As the operation commenced at nine o'clock on Friday morning and (unusually) the writer overslept, this was dealt with by sending Reiki immediately, as Reiki can be sent forwards or backwards in time, as required.

As a past life therapist, I had trained under Dr. Roger Woolger, the leading authority on this subject, and the professional training seminars required addressing many patterns related to the "whole picture." According to my good friend and College of Healing Astrologer, John Pegley, large breasts result from a connection (birth-chart related) with the ancestral patterning to "Juno." L checked as requested, and said her great-grandmother had huge breasts. Her mother was of normal size. The genetic interaction, John said, was as likely to present via the male line as much as the female line.

Past Life Interaction/Karma: While not a requirement of patients presenting themselves for Reiki healing, in any context, the writer has had the privilege of "tuning in" to their energy fields (either current, past, astral, cosmic or even everyday normal). L's previous life revealed the following: In the 1870s, her forebear gave birth to at least five live children in very difficult and frugal circumstances. The babies were starving and the youngest was deprived of breast milk by the lack of money and food for a nursing mother. At her lowest ebb, perhaps at the point of death, she made a vow. Vows and decisions brought through from a previous life of trauma govern many of our thought patterns today. L's great-great-grandmother vowed something like "No baby will ever die from these shriveled breasts ever again! I will, with every fiber of my being, give huge nurturing breasts to those who succeed me and my kin."

Post-Operative Care: Reiki was duly sent to L for her operation. L was scheduled for a normal eleven-day sojourn in the hospital. Due to the body reacting so favorably to the surgery, L was discharged in three days! L had many consultants stopping by her room and asking, "When did you say you had the operation?" Nurses kept showing colleagues L's progress. None could believe her improvement so soon. New consultants viewed the patient in disbelief.

Out of the hospital L could not drive, but came for regular Reiki and laser treatment for her scar tissue at the medical center. Internal stitching was not dissolving easily. The stomach meridian normally being on the nipple area, required re-routing and nutritional supplement, to offset discomfort. All were resolved with the help of Reiki.

Best of all, L gave up her job and was last heard of in Spain, where both she and her devoted husband hope to open a home for the elderly or needy. Postcards come from time to time, from Spain or the United Kingdom, but with love and gratitude for the Reiki received.

Reiki—Natural Healing and Broken Bones

by Lucinda Fury, RP, Virginia Beach, VA

Being at a Reiki eleven level, I knew my son "N"'s broken wrist would benefit from the healing that Reiki provides. I was, however, surprised at some of the results. As I practice Reiki, I am learning constantly about reactions and feelings from clients, as well as from me.

My son was eight years old and this was his first broken bone. I used Reiki to calm his nervousness at the hospital during x-rays and while they put his arm into a cast. The cast would be removed in about six to eight weeks. Later that night N was experiencing quite a bit of pain and requested that I Reiki his wrist. I did, and he had an immediate quieting of pain and went right to sleep. When he awoke in the middle of the night, he complained he had twice as much pain as before. I was alarmed, but continued Reiki, telling him to allow the pain to happen, but to focus on a pleasant place. Finally he drifted off to sleep.

The next morning his wrist was fine and he had no pain at all. At the one-week check-up, the x-ray showed accelerated healing. At three weeks, the healing process was complete and the cast was removed! I know that Reiki played a part in the healing of my son's wrist. I think the increased pain that he felt that first night was due to the accelerated healing process that Reiki triggered.

N experienced no itching under his cast and his arm did not have that flaccid lack-of-muscle-tone appearance that I've seen with long-term casted limbs. The Reiki benefits in this case were three-fold.

Note: I selected this orthopedic doctor due to a prior experience with another of my sons. I watched as he set a finger without local anesthetic. He sat quietly holding the finger for a few minutes. He then closed his eyes, breathed in deeply, exhaled, and pop! The finger was in place. No pain registered on my son's face, only a look of surprise. I didn't question the doctor at the time, but I knew I felt the connection of healing energy he was tapping into that day. It was all I needed to convince me to use his expertise again.

Book Resources

Nurse as Healer Series by Delmar Publishers 1-800-347-7707
   The Nurse's Meditative Journal by Sherry Kahn, MPH
   Healing Nutrition by Lynn Kegan, PhD, RN
   Healing Touch: A Resource for Health Care Professionals by Dorothea Kramer, EdD, RN
   Healing Life's Crises: A Guide for Nurses by Frisch and Kelly, PhD, RN
   Creative Imagery for Nurse Healers by Karlee Shames, PhD, RN
Ayurveda and Aromatherapy by Drs. Light and Bryan Miller
Defense against Mystery Syndromes by DAMS Group
Directory of Alternative Health-Care Resources by Arle Hagberg
Encyclopedia of Aromatherapy Massage and Yoga by McGilvery, Reed, and Mehta
Natural Science of Healing (Rolfing) by Jim Oschman, PhD
Massage by Anne Hooper or *Ultimate Sexual Touch (lover's guide)* by Anne Hooper
Rolfing and Physical Reality by Ida Rolf, PhD
The Book of Massage (Eastern and Western techniques) by Lucinda Lidell
Why I Left Orthodox Medicine: Healing for the Twenty-First Century by Derrick Lonsdale, MD

Chapter Three

Nature's Medicine—
Herbs, Vitamins, Minerals, and Food

The following pages on vitamin and herb reference charts are reprinted with permission from *Healthy Steps* by Dr. Albert Zehr, PhD, developer of the Pure Life Nutritional Programs.

To order contact Abundant Publishers, PO Box 250, 7101C 12th Street, Delta, BC V4E 2A0.

Vitamin Reference Chart

Abbreviations

Acid	Acidophilus	MGlan	Male Multi Glandular
Adren	Adrenal Stimulant Formula	Min	Chelated Multi Mineral
Cal	Calcium	Multi	Multi Vitamin Mineral
Dig	Digestive Supplement	PA	Pantothenic Acid
FGlan	Female Multi Glandular	Pot	Potassium
Lec	Lecithin	Pro	Protein
		Sel	Selenium

Acne E, A, B6, PA, Zinc
Arteries A, B6, C, E, Multi, Sel
Arthritis B, C, E, Calcium, PA, Pro, Multi
Asthma PA, C, A, E, Adren
Backache C, Cal, Pro, Min
Bed Sores B Complex
Blood Clotting C, E, Cal, Min
— Inhibits Clotting Pro, E, C, Lec, Multi
Blood Pressure
— High C, E, Multi, Lec, Sel, Pot
— Low B, C, E, PA, Pro, Sel
Bruising C
Burns B, C, E
Canker Sores B6, Niacin, B

Cholesterol A, B6, C, E, Lec, Multi
Cold Sores PA, C, B6
Colds PA, C, B. Min
Colitis Multi, PA, Min
Constipation Multi, B, E, PA
Diarrhea B6, B. Niacin, Multi, Pot
Digestion Acid, Dig, A, B, C, E, Lec
Eczema Niacin, B, B6, Multi
Eyes A, C, E, PA, B, Pro
Fingernails Pro, A, Cal
Flu C, E, B6, B, Multi
Gout B, C, E, PA, Min
Hair Pro, B, Multi, Zinc
Kidney Stones Cal, B6, Min. C
Liver Pro, A, C, E, B, Min

~ 35 ~

Motion Sickness B6, B
Muscular Cramps B6, Cal, PA,
  Multi, Adren
Nervousness B, Cal, Min, B6
Nosebleeds C
Ovaries C, Min, FGlan
Prostate A, C, Min, Zinc, MGlan
Psoriasis B6, Lec, A

Sinus A, B6, C, E, PA
Stretch Marks E, PA
Throat, Sore C, B
Ulcers A, B, C, E, PA
Varicose Veins B, C, E, Lec, Min
Warts A, E
Wrinkles B6, E, A

Herb Reference and Body Symptom Chart
Reprinted with permission of Dr. Albert Zehr, PhD, from his book Healthy Steps.

Acne	Barley Green, Bee Pollen, Chaparral, Yellow Dock
Adrenal Glands	Licorice Root
Aging	Bee Pollen, Ginseng, Gotu Kola
Allergies	Barley Green, Bee Pollen, Spirulina
Anemia	Alfalfa, Comfrey, Dandelion, Spirulina, Yellow Dock
Appetite Depressant	Chickweed
Arthritis	Alfalfa, Barley Green, Capsicum, Chaparral, Poke Root Sarsaparilla, Yucca
Asthma	Black Cohosh, Lobelia, Mullein, Thyme
Atherosclerosis	Hawthorne Berry
Bladder	Alfalfa, Horsetail, Uva Ursi
Blood	
— Oxygenation	Black Walnut Leaves
— Purifier	Chaparral, Dandelion, Echinacea, Poke Root, Sarsaparilla, Yellow Dock, Yucca
Blood Pressure	
— High	Barley Green, Dandelion, Garlic, Hawthorne Berry Evening Primrose
— Low	Hawthorne Berry, Licorice Root
Bones, Broken	Comfrey, Horsetail
Bronchial	Chamomile, Comfrey, Ginger, Lobelia, Thyme
Chemotherapy	Spirulina
Childbirth	Black Cohosh
Circulation	Capsicum, Ginger
Colds	Capsicum, Garlic, Ginger, Golden Seal, Licorice Root, Safflower
Colic	Chamomile, Wood Betony
Constipation	Cascara Sagrada
Coughs	Ginger, Licorice Root, Lobelia, Thyme
Cramps, Stomach	Barley Green, Black Walnut Leaves, Ginger, Wood Betony
Diabetes	Dandelion, Golden Seal, Spirulina, Uva Ursi

Diarrhea	Mullein, Thyme, White Oak Bark
Digestive Disorders	Alfalfa, Barley Green, Bee Pollen, Garlic, Wood Betony
Drug Withdraw	Chamomile
Drugs, Resistance to	Ginseng
Ears	Chickweed, Garlic, Lobelia, Yellow Dock
Eyes	Eyebright, Spirulina
Fatigue	Bee Pollen, Garlic, Ginseng, Gotu Kola
Female Complaints	Black Cohosh, Damiana, Licorice, Uva Ursi
Female Hormone Imbalance	Damiana, Sarsaparilla
Fever	Chamomile, Safflower
Flu	Capsicum, Ginger
Gallbladder	Safflower, Cascara Sagrada
Gas	Ginger, Sarsaparilla, Thyme
Hair, Nails, Teeth	Horsetail
Headache	Ginger, Thyme, White Willow, Wood Betony
Heart	Capsicum, Hawthorne Berry, Mullein
Hemorrhoids	Mullein, White Oak Bark
Hypoglycemia	(see Blood Sugar - Low)
Impotency	(see Sexual Debility)
Infection	Echinacea, Garlic, Golden Seal
Insomnia	Chamomile, Valerian
Intestinal Tract Inflammation	Licorice Root
Kidney	Alfalfa, Barley Green, Capsicum, Horsetail, Uva Ursi
Lead Removal	Barley Green, Spirulina
Liver	Barley Green, Chaparral, Dandelion, Safflower, Spirulina, Yellow Dock
Lungs	Chickweed, Lobelia, Mullein
Lymphatics	Chaparral
Membrane Inflammation	Chickweed, Comfrey, Golden Seal
Menstrual Flow	
— Excessive	Uva Ursi
— Stimulation	Chamomile, Thyme
Mercury Removal	Barley Green, Spirulina
Motion Sickness	Ginger
Muscles, Cramps	Safflower
Nervous Disorders	Chamomile, Gotu Kola, Thyme, Valerian, Wood Betony
Obesity	Chickweed, Kelp, Poke Root
Pain	Mullein, Valerian, White Willow Bark
Pancreas	Dandelion, Spirulina, Uva Ursi
Parasites	Black Walnut, Cloves, Garlic, Sarsaparilla, Wood Betony, Wormwood
Poison, Resistance to	Barley Green, Ginseng, Sarsaparilla
Prostate Disease	Bee Pollen, Echinacea, Kelp
Psoriasis	Dandelion, Sarsaparilla, Yellow Dock

Radiation	Ginseng, Spirulina
Respiratory	Comfrey, Lobelia, Mullein
Rheumatism	Capsicum, Poke Root, Sarsaparilla, Yucca
Senility	Gotu Kola
Sexual Debility	Bee Pollen, Damiana, Licorice Root, Ginseng
Skin	Horsetail, Sarsaparilla, Yellow Dock, Yucca
Spleen	Dandelion, Poke Root, Uva Ursi
Stomach, Upset	Chamomile, Ginger
Stress	Lobelia
Throat, Sore	Bee Pollen, Garlic, Ginger, Licorice, White Oak Bark
Thyroid	Kelp, Poke Root
Tumors	Chaparral, Chickweed, Echinacea, Yellow Dock
Ulcers	Capsicum, Licorice, Spirulina, Yellow Dock
Urinary Tract	Chaparral, Uva Ursi
Varicose Veins	Black Walnut, Capsicum, White Oak Bark
Viral Infections	Echinacea, Safflower, Uva Ursi

Natural Herb Chart

Herb	Usage	Importance	Essential Oils
Ginseng	adapting	increases mental/physical efficiency, adjusts body's response to stress	rosemary, basil, peppermint
Aswagandha	adapting energy	adapting, adjusts the body's response to stress	clary sage, bergamot, rose geranium
Astragalus Root	cold and flu	enhances immune system, restores peripheral circulation	lemon grass, lavender, rosemary, camphor
Bilberry	eye care	anti-inflammatory, antioxidant, eye disorders, vascular disorders	lavender, bath-eucalyptus
Butcher's Broom	arthritis, sports injuries	anti-inflammatory	frankincense, vetiver, bath-juniper or cypress
Cascara Sagrada	laxative	increases intestinal mobility	fennel, basil, roman chamomile
Chamomile	relaxation	anti-infective, aids digestion	ginger, cumin
Echinacea	cold/flue infections	immune stimulant, antiviral	goldenseal, astragalus root, licorice, ginseng
Feverfew	migraine headaches	anti-inflammatory, reduces severity of migraine headaches	lavender, jasmine, peppermint, chamomile

Herb	Usage	Importance	Essential Oils
Ginger	digestion	nausea, motion sickness, digestive aid, reduces fever	fennel, grapefruit, lime, gold chamomile
Green Tea	cancer	antioxidant, prevents plaque buildup, acts as diuretic	jasmine, lemon grass, juniper + parsley oil
Hawthorne	heart	dilates blood vessels, increases enzyme metabolism	rose, rosemary, lavender, ginger, orange
Milk Thistle	liver detox	antihepatotoxic, protects liver against toxins	roman chamomile, lemon sage, juniper
Saw Palmetto	prostate	anti-inflammatory, helps conditions with benign prostate	ylang ylang, rose, patchouli, nutmeg, clary sage
St. John's Wort	depression	treats nervous unrest, sleeplessness	lime, lavender, orange

Natural Vitamin Chart

Vitamins	Food Sources	Deficiency Symptom
Vitamin A (retinal)	eggs, colored fruit and vegetables, dairy products, fish liver oil	defective teeth and gums, allergies, dry hair and skin, sinus infections
Vitamin B (complex)	whole grains, liver, brewer's yeast	poor appetite, rough skin, fatigue, dull hair, constipation, acne, insomnia
Vitamin B1 (thiamine)	organ meats, nuts, wheat germ, fish, brown rice, egg yolks, legumes	depression, constipation, shortness of breath, fatigue, nervousness
Vitamin B2 (riboflavin)	cheese, milk, egg yolks, brewer's yeast, nuts, whole grains, molasses	inflammation of mouth, eye problems, poor digestion, dermatitis, dizziness
Vitamin B6 (pyridoxine)	cabbage, cantaloupe, legumes, peas, molasses, wheat germ, whole grains	insulin sensitivity, nervousness, acne, depression, muscular weakness, arthritis
Vitamin B12 (cobalamin)	pork, beef, cheese, eggs, fish, organ meats, milk products	tiredness, poor appetite, anemia, nervousness, brain damage
Vitamin C (ascorbic acid)	tomatoes, sprouts, alfalfa, peppers, citrus fruits, broccoli, cantaloupe	muscular weakness, tendency to bruise, slow-healing wounds, bleeding gums
Vitamin D (cholecalciferol)	fat, butter, fish liver oil, sardines, egg yolks, bone meal, organ meats	lack of energy, rickets, diarrhea, soft bones/teeth, low absorption of calcium

Vitamins	Food Sources	Deficiency Symptom
Vitamin E (tocopherol)	whole wheat, sweet potatoes, eggs, dark green veg., oatmeal, wheat germ	fragile red blood cells, dull hair, sterility, enlarged prostate, gastrointestinal ills
Vitamin F (unsaturated fatty acids, linoleic acid)	butter, wheat germ, vegetables, oils, sunflower seeds	acne, dandruff, diarrhea, weak nails, gallstones, low weight, varicose veins
Vitamin H (biotin)	sardines, legumes, egg yolks, mung, bean sprouts, lentils, whole grains	extreme exhaustion, loss of appetite, muscle pain, gray skin, depression
Vitamin K (phylloquinone)	cauliflower, egg yolks, yogurt, kelp, soybeans, leafy veg., alfalfa, molasses	intestinal absorption, nose bleeds, diarrhea, blood clotting, cellular disease
Vitamin P (bioflavonoids, rutin, hesperidin)	buckwheat, black currants, cherries, grapes, fruit	tendency to bruise/bleed easily, vitamin C deficiency
Choline	leafy green vegetables, egg yolks, brewer's yeast, legumes, soybeans	high blood pressure, intolerance of fats, cirrhosis and fatty degeneration of liver
Folic Acid (folacin)	root vegetables, leafy green veg., brewer's yeast, whole grains	B12 deficiency, anemia, graying hair, gastrointestinal disorders
Inositol	citrus fruits, nuts, molasses, lecithin, brewer's yeast, whole grains, vegetables	eye problems, high cholesterol, skin problems, constipation
Niacin (nicotinic acid)	beans, green vegetables, rice bran, whole wheat, brewer's yeast, nuts	nervous disorders, tiredness, loss of appetite, gastrointestinal disorders
Pantothenic Acid	egg yolks, legumes, brewer's yeast, whole grains, wheat germ, OJ	stomach stress, hair loss, diarrhea, kidney trouble, hypoglycemia
PABA (paraaminobenzoic acid)	leafy green vegetables, yogurt, wheat germ, molasses, brewer's yeast	constipation, digestion problems, tiredness, headaches, nervousness

Mixing and Matching Vitamins

Amino acids should be taken on an empty stomach, combining with B6 helpful
Calcium interferes with absorption of iron
Copper should be taken in combination with zinc, selenium, and molybdenum
Iodine available in supplement form as potassium iodide
Iron interferes with absorption of vitamin E
Magnesium interferes with calcium, take at different times during the day
Molybdenum should be taken with copper
Selenium helps vitamin E do its job
Zinc should be taken with copper and selenium

Vitamins
- A (beta carotene) — high intake of vitamin E (greater than 600 IU) can interfere with absorption and utilization of vitamin A and beta carotene
- B take together with A as part of a well balanced vitamin/mineral formula
- C increases absorption of iron
- E best if accompanied by selenium, known to interfere with absorption of iron and vitamin A

Sources of Iron Derived from Plants

Molasses	Tofu	Spinach
Raisin Bran	Bagels	Dried Prunes
Potatoes	Mustard Greens, Broccoli	Peanut Butter
Prune Juice	Dried Apricots	Brown Rice, White Rice
Kidney Beans	Whole Wheat Bread	Chickpeas

Herbs That Are Helpful
Garlic—also available in tablet form, helps prevent heart disease by lowering blood pressure
Turmeric—lowers cholesterol levels, hinders blood clotting, detoxifies liver, helps combat cancer
Ginger—acts as anti-inflammatory agent, has antibiotic properties, use fresh root when cooking
Ginkgo Biloba and Bilberry—protect cell walls from oxidative damage, enhance blood flow
Rosemary—has antiaging effects, protects cardiovascular system, fights cancer
Spirulina—blue-green algae (natural plant protein) boosts immune system, purifies
Medicinal mushrooms—Reishi, shiitake, and maitaki mushrooms contain powerful antioxidant properties
Flavonoids—are abundant in vegetables, fruits, and tea; quercetin is found in rind of citrus fruits, broccoli
Milk Thistle—helps detoxify and protect the liver from damage or overexposure to environmental toxins

Herbs
Knowledge of the healing properties of herbs, now called Earth medicine, has become increasingly easy to come by in recent years. As more and more people have become disenchanted with pharmaceutical drugs, they have sought out safer, more holistic ways of taking charge of their own health. Check out a local herbal practitioner or homeopathic or naturopathic doctor for help, and read some herb books.

Using Herbs Safely
Source: Family Circle Magazine, *Health Section*
1) Do not use herbal remedies over an extended period of time, or if you have any chronic condition, without first consulting professional guidance in herbal medicine.
2) Some herbs can be dangerous to people with preexisting conditions or health problems. Pregnant women should use caution when using any medicinal substances, including herbs. Use caution for children under two years of age—consult professional guidance. Remember herbs are to be considered as medicine.

Eight Herbs to Keep in Your House
Cascara Sagrada—is the most effective and gentle herbal laxative around. Some herbalists have found this herb to be effective in treating gallstones and liver ailments.

Chamomile—taken internally as a tea, is an effective remedy for stomach upset, indigestion, diarrhea, and menstrual cramps. Applied externally in cream form, it soothes dry or chapped skin.

Echinacea—is an all-purpose protector against colds, flu, and other infections. It is also effective for boils, tooth and gum pain, and viral skin infections such as herpes simplex. For best results, take echinacea at the first sign of illness and use until symptoms have disappeared, but no more than ten days at a time.

Garlic—is an immune-enhancing herb, effective in respiratory problems, such as asthma and bronchitis. This herb also kills bacteria, making it a useful herb against colds and intestinal problems, such as diarrhea and parasites. Recent studies show its ability to lower blood pressure and cholesterol levels.

Ginger—stimulates blood circulation, welcome news to those who shiver through winter months with cold hands and feet. It helps relieve menstrual cramps and is effective for motion sickness.

Ginseng—for centuries, has been deemed a virtual cure-all by the Chinese. This herb's powers and abilities promote mental and physical vigor, and help the body handle stress.

Goldenseal—is recommended for a wide variety of ailments, because of its tenacity in fighting infections of all kinds. It's commonly used to treat infections of the mucous membranes, including nasal passages and the upper respiratory tract, and is a proven tonic for stomach disorders and urinary tract infections.

Valerian—is used for its calming effect, such as for insomnia, because it doesn't produce side effects common to over-the-counter sleeping pills. It can also be used for headaches and intestinal cramping.

Herb Resources

The Herb Gardener by Susan McClure
Healing Herbs and Spices and Juices, Teas and Tonics by John Heinerman
Herbal Medicines Pharmacology—CD-ROM, Genusys (215) 794-7486, http://datalab.com/genusys.htm

Antioxidants/Minerals/Amino Acids

What Are Antioxidants?

Source: Prescription for Nutritional Healing—Guide to Vitamins, Minerals, Herbs and Food Supplements, *by Dr. James F. Balch and Phyllis A. Balch, CNCs*

Our bodies are faced with hundreds of thousands of free radical aggressors each day. It is a wonder we can survive this onslaught. The reason we can is our bodies have some success in forestalling free radical damage with an intricate defense system comprised of antioxidant vitamins, minerals, and enzymes. Our bodies can get out of balance from the way we live and what we are exposed to: overeating, alcohol consumption, air pollution, cigarette smoking, and excessive exercise. If any of these apply to you, are you taking enough toxin-fighting antioxidant vitamins to effectively ward off free radicals?

Free radicals are marauding molecules that wreak havoc on the cells of the body in a misguided pursuit of stability. Free radicals are unstable because they have an unpaired or "extra" electrical charge that causes them to seek out other substances in the body to bond with, in order to neutralize themselves. Free radicals are formed in our bodies as a by-product of the necessary actions of breathing oxygen and burning food for energy, and also from air pollution, tobacco smoke, ultraviolet (UV) sun rays and rancid fats. The targets of free radical attacks are often the fatty membranes that surround cells, but other body components are also damaged by free radicals.

Left unchecked, free radicals can rob our health by "rusting" our cells. Over time, this can leave us vulnerable to multitudes of health problems. Excess free radical production has been linked with more than fifty ailments, ranging from premature aging to clogged arteries, cataracts, to cancer. Helpful in reducing free radical production are vitamins C and E, and beta carotene. An antioxidant, to rich diet is one with an abundant supply of fruit and vegetables, nuts and seeds. Because we don't always eat the right foods, supplements have become popular.

The skin is one of the first indicators of free radical damage, showing premature aging. The life span of cells in the skin is very short (only a few days), so dietary deficiencies often manifest first in the skin. Antioxidants such as vitamins C and E, alpha lipoic acid, carotenoids (beta carotene), selenium and many flavonoids (vitamin-like compounds) protect the skin from this damage. Vitamin C plays a special role in maintaining healthy skin. Production of collagen (the glue-like substance that holds the skin together) is impaired by inadequate vitamin C, which is also is crucial in maintaining the connective tissue elastin.

Antioxidant Vitamin Sources

Vitamin A—for healthy mucous cells, promotes germ-killing enzymes, destroys carcinogens

Vitamin C—powerful, reduces lipid production to brain and spinal cord, crosses blood/brain barrier

Vitamin E—prevents fat and cell membrane rancidity, protects the coating around cells, improves oxygen

Gamma-Linoleic Acid, L-Cysteine, L-Glutathione, Selenium, Superoxide Dismutase.

One medium orange meets the vitamin C requirement; one medium carrot equates to the vitamin A requirement; trying to eat enough nuts and seeds to meet the vitamin E requirement, would mean you would also exceed the fat allotment that is suggested.

Enzymes

It is impossible for people to obtain great, consistent health and vitality without enzymes. Nothing in the body functions without enzymes. Though enzymes do not take the place of vitamins, minerals, herbs, proteins, carbohydrates, etc., every one of these depends on enzymes to unite and activate them. Life could not be sustained without enzymes. Made up of protein, thousands of known enzymes play roles in virtually all body activities. Found in all living plant and animal matter, enzymes are essential for maintaining function of the body's digestive system, immune system, glands, muscles, waste removal system, and tissue repair mechanisms. To ease the burden of manufacturing enzymes in the body, it is helpful to eat raw foods. Avocados, bananas, mangos and sprouts are rich in enzymes. Enzymes also utilize food ingested by the body to construct new muscle tissue, nerve cells, bone, skin, and glandular tissue. There are three types of digestive enzymes:

Amylase breaks down carbohydrates.

Protease helps digest protein.

Lipase aids in fat digestion.

Minerals

Minerals function as coenzymes enabling the body to quickly perform its activities. Minerals are needed for the proper composition of body fluids, the formation of blood and bone, and the maintenance of healthy nerve function. Minerals are naturally occurring elements found in the earth, absorbed by plants from the soil, eaten by animals, and in turn eaten by man in these plants or animals. There are two types of minerals: macrobulk (calcium, magnesium, sodium, potassium and phosphorus) and microtrace (zinc, iron, copper, manganese, chromium, selenium and iodine). Because minerals are stored primarily in the body's bone and muscle tissue, it is possible to overdose on minerals if an extremely large dose is taken. However, toxic amounts will accumulate only if massive amounts are taken for a prolonged period of time.

Listing of Minerals

Calcium, chromium, copper, germanium, iodine, iron, magnesium, manganese, molybdenum, phosphorus, potassium, selenium, silicon, sodium, sulfur, vanadium, zinc.
Selenium—found in wheat germ, whole grains, nuts, and molasses
Zinc—boosts effectiveness of our immune systems, found in legumes and fortified cereals

Amino Acids

Amino acids are the chemical units or building blocks that make up proteins. Protein could not exist without the proper combination of amino acids. It is protein that provides the structure to all living things, and participates in the vital chemical processes that enable us to sustain life. There are approximately twenty-nine commonly known amino acids that account for the hundreds of different types of proteins present in all living things. In the human body, the liver produces about eighty percent of the amino acids we need. The balance of twenty percent must be obtained from outside sources and are called essential amino acids. (Refer to information on super blue-green algae and the eighteen plus amino acids contained.)

Listing of Some Amino Acids

L-Alanine—aids in the metabolism of glucose
L-Arginine—aids in liver detoxification, causes retardation of tumors and cancer
L-Asparagine—needed to maintain balance in the central nervous system
L-Aspartic Acid—increases stamina, good for chronic fatigue
L-Carnitine—helps transport fatty acids, prevents buildup, aids in weight loss
L-Citruline—promotes energy, stimulates immune system
L-Cysteine—this sulfur containing amino acid is needed to produce glutathione, and is used by the liver and lymphocytes to detoxify chemicals and germ poison; detoxifies alcohol, tobacco smoke, and environmental pollutants, all of which are immune suppressors
L-Glutathione—protects body from harmful effects of metals, drugs, cigarette smoke and alcohol
Gamma-Linoleic Acid (GLA) — regulates T-lymphocyte function, if lacking in zinc, magnesium, and vitamins C, B, and A, conversion may be blocked; evening primrose oil and black currant seed oil are main sources of preformed GLA
Selenium—stimulates increased antibody response to germ infection
Superoxide Dismutase (SOD) — revitalizes the cells and reduces the rate of cell destruction; SOD naturally occurs in barley grass, broccoli, Brussels sprouts, cabbage, wheatgrass, and most green plants
AOX/PLX from Biotec Foods—this product contains large amounts of antioxidants to aid the body in destroying free radicals

Vegetarianism

Studies show that vegetarians as a group have less risk of heart disease, cancer of the breast, colon and prostate, diabetes, osteoporosis, diverticulitis, gallstones, and constipation. This is because as nonmeat eaters their diets are lower in fat and cholesterol. The most healthy vegetarian diets are based on a wide variety of foods including grains, nuts and seeds, soy-based foods, vegetables, fruits, and other whole foods. Vegetarians are generally leaner because of their low fat, high fiber and low calorie foods such as vegetables. There are three types of vegetarians:

1) Vegans who eat no animal or dairy products at all.
2) Lactovegetarians who eat dairy products but no eggs.
3) Lactoovovegetarians who eat dairy products and eggs but no meat, poultry or fish.

A Healthy Life Style

A healthy life style will encompass the following guidelines:
1) eat a low fat diet; especially avoid fried foods, hydrogenated oil, refined oils
2) change towards vegetarianism; eliminating the need for animal flesh is healthier
3) eat a variety of fresh raw vegetables and fruit daily
4) drink a minimum of two quarts of pure water daily, not with meals
5) avoid chemicals and preservatives like MSG, nitrites, nitrates in processed foods
6) avoid or limit empty calorie foods like soda and candy
7) avoid or limit stimulants like caffeine or sugar
8) chew food thoroughly and avoid overeating
9) eat in a relaxed atmosphere and calm state of mind
10) supplement the diet with cultures of acidophilus (i.e. yogurt with live cultures)

Nutritional Education Resources

EarthSave and Project YES
706 Frederick Street
Santa Cruz, CA 95060-2205
(502) 589-7676

Vegetarian Resource Group
P.O. Box 1463
Baltimore, MD 21203
(410) 366-8343

Basic Nutrition Guidelines

1) Upgrade the quality of food you eat:
   Processed foods deplete enzymes, vitamins and minerals; chemicals are added back for flavor. Check index for information about chemicals.
2) Read the labels before buying processed foods:
   Avoid hydrogenated oils and fats; avoid ingredients you cannot pronounce, and check the index for more information about oils.
3) Use a good water filter:
   Remove chemicals, chlorine, fluoride, and trihalomethanes, bacterial and protozoan contaminants from your water. See chapter 6 on chemicals contained in US water supplies.
4) Use an air purifier in home or office as necessary:
   One that generates ozone and negative ions is most effective.
5) Eat natural whole pure foods:
   Emphasize vegetables, fruits, grains, nuts and seeds.
6) Use fresh raw foods or organic foods:
   Food enzymes aid in digestion, help the pancreas; depletion of enzymes from exhaustion or overwork can lead to overwork of the cells of the pancreas.

7) Grow fresh herbs on your porch or deck, add to pastas/vegetables for that added zest in taste.

Foods to Avoid

Eat soybean products and peanuts in moderation. Too many legumes can create gas and discomfort. Most illnesses are accompanied by digestive problems. Avoid nuts exposed to air. Rancid nuts contain rancid oils, which can cause illness. Nuts should be raw, not roasted.

Natural Food Supplements

Found in most health food stores, supplements are high in certain nutrients and contain active ingredients that aid our digestive or metabolic processes. Be an informed consumer; read your labels.

A Listing of a Few Food Supplements

Acidophilus—assists the digestion of proteins; may help detoxify harmful substances and factors that contribute to candidiasis, which results from the recurrent consumption of antibiotics, oral contraceptives, and aspirin, a poor diet, sugar, yeast, and stress, thereby causing an imbalance in the system.

Alfalfa—one of the richest mineral foods, it has helped many arthritis sufferers;. Alfalfa, wheatgrass, barley, and spirulina, which all have chlorophyll, have been found to aid in the healing of gastritis, liver ailments, eczema, asthma, high blood pressure, anemia, constipation, body and breath odor, infections, athlete's foot, and burns.

Bee Pollen and Honey—have anti-microbial effects, are used to promote energy and healing.

Bee Propolis—collected from various plants by bees, is not made by bees; excellent aid against bacterial infections, salve for abrasions and bruises. Also for dry cough, throat problems, tonsillitis, ulcers, acne, and stimulant for the immune system.

Chlorella—has been found to protect against the effects of ultraviolet radiation.

Fiber—helps to lower the blood cholesterol level and stabilize blood sugar levels.

Pectin—slows the absorption of food after meals, is good for diabetics, removes unwanted metals and toxins, and is valuable in radiation therapy. Found in apples, carrots, beets, bananas, cabbage, the citrus family, and dried peas.

Garlic—one of most valuable foods on the planet, has been used since ancient times. Garlic lowers the blood pressure, helps inhibit platelet aggression, reduces the risk of blood clots, aids in preventing heart attacks, lowers serum cholesterol levels, and aids in digestion. It is also a potent immune system stimulant. Garlic contains an amino acid derivative. It is an anti-fungal agent effective against candidiasis, athlete's foot, and vaginal yeast infections.

Protein Combining

Complete proteins are a necessary sustenance of life. The following food combinations add up to a complete protein, although each food lacks one or more of the necessary amino acids. Only together are they a complete protein.

Beans combined with any one of the following: Cheese, corn, all nuts, rice, sesame seeds, all seeds, or wheat.

Brown rice combined with any one of the following: Beans, cheese, nuts, sesame seeds, or wheat.

Protein Misconceptions

Animal food is not the best or only source of protein available. Many plant foods, especially if eaten in combination, contain high quality proteins that can provide the amino acids (building blocks of protein) needed for nutrition. For the last several years, super blue-green algae, a protein plant food grown organically, has been on the market. (Resource: Cell Tech, see article this chapter.)

Other cultures and countries for hundreds of years have already concluded that a vegetarian diet is healthy and economical. The main foods in South America are beans and corn; in Central America, beans and corn; in the Far East and the Caribbean, beans and rice; and in India, lentils and rice.

Super Blue-Green Algae: Natural Protein Plant Food

Earth's first food, and one of the most fundamental balanced foods on the planet, is blue-green algae (a single-celled nutrient-rich aquatic organism). There are two types of blue-green algae easily available. Spirulina is cultivated and mostly found in stores, and Aphanizomenon flos-aquae (AFA) is harvested wild and delivered to you by Cell Tech (Klamath Falls, Oregon). Spirulina is a potent and powerful food for the body, but AFA has more nutrients per gram, gives more energy and also has more positive effects on the mind and brain function. We just love this algae and have met people who claim that they saw more results by taking two AFA capsules (1/2 gram) than ten capsules of spirulina.

Ninety-seven percent of AFA is assimilated, or absorbed, into the body. It has more chlorophyll than any other food known. Chlorophyll, a blood purifier, has a molecular structure almost identical to the hemoglobin in our red blood cells. Algae contains most of the vitamins, and is particularly rich in the B-vitamins, including B-12. It has seventeen different carotenoids, including a high concentration of beta-carotene, one of the most potent free-radical neutralizer/antioxidants we know. Some say it contains up to sixty-two chelated minerals and trace minerals. It has exactly the essential amino acids profile that the body needs, plus omega-3 and -6 fatty acids, more than two thousand enzymes and several different pigments that are currently being researched for their beneficial effects on many health aspects. Loaded with nutraceuticals, AFA is surely our planet's most nutrient-dense food.

Algae is low on the food chain. The higher a food is on the food chain, the more it is contaminated with pesticides, heavy metals, and man-made chemical residues. This applies to complex foods like meat and dairy products. For this reason, eat low on the food chain: eat algae.

Upper Klamath Lake in Oregon, where AFA grows wild, is a nutrient trap, surrounded by the high Cascade mountains and fed by geothermal hot springs, cold volcanic mountain streams and two pure rivers. The mineral-rich volcanic soil that washes into the lake mixes with dissolved nitrogenous matter, and a lot of sunshine (300 days per year) encourages photosynthesis, permitting the algae to bloom in abundance every year. Cell Tech's founders have been harvesting this wonder food and making it available since the late 1970s. They are former spirulina farmers who know that AFA is much superior. Cell Tech, harvests, cools and freeze dries this algae faster than anyone in the world, locking-in the highest amount of nutrients possible.

Ancient Chinese herbalists recommended taking the organism to fight vitamin deficiencies. Today Dr. Cousens, author of *Conscious Eating,* has seen spirulina help lower blood pressure, stabilize hypoglycemia, alleviate allergy symptoms, control diabetes, and combat chronic fatigue syndrome, protein deficiencies, and malnutrition. Blue-green algae has the ability to reduce nephrotoxicity (toxicity of the kidneys) by a process known as chelation, in which heavy-metal concentrations are reduced.

With all that spirulina has been shown to do, the wild AFA can do even more. Even animals do better. Dogs shed less hair and have fewer allergies. Horses win more races. Returning to human accomplishments, the greatest athlete on earth, Dan O'Brien, Olympic gold medalist in the decathlon and current record holder, is an avid AFA eater. "I really believe it gives me more energy, it prolongs my day," says O'Brien, who has been taking it for many years now.

What could you expect from eating it? AFA eaters report more energy, enthusiasm, and control over stress; better sleep, concentration, focus and memory; and fewer mood swings, sugar blues, anxiety attacks, colds, flues, allergies and joint problems. Many children with attention Deficit/Hyperactivity Disorder are doing very well on AFA and not suffering the side effects associated with the drugs normally prescribed.

AFA's positive immune system effects are proven by 1998 studies performed jointly by McGill University and the Royal Victoria Hospital in Montreal. New studies confirming many health benefits of eating AFA are being published or conducted right now (double blind studies with control groups). Call us for current results.

Like they say: "Eat algae today."

Tofu

Source: The Book of Tofu, *published by Ballantine Books*

Tofu is made from cooked soybeans. Soybeans are soaked in water, ground, cooked, filtered, curdled with a coagulant, pressed, and packed. Tofu, whether packed in water or packed in shelf-stable boxes, should be refrigerated if left out for a long period of time. Tofu is protein so when it spoils you will smell it. After opening the packaged tofu, rinse it, cover it with fresh water, and change water daily. Tofu can also be frozen for up to five months by putting it in water or simply wrapping it or putting it into a plastic container. After thawing tofu, squeeze out excess water. Frozen tofu has a yellow color and a chewier, spongelike texture. Packaged tofu is preferable to open-pickle-barrel types because of the foodborne bacteria in open warm places.

For more information contact the United Soybean Board hotline, 1-800-TALKSOY.

Pantry Checklist

Breads, Grain, and Cereals
Bagels, whole grain
Brown rice, quick cooking
Bulgar, quick cooking
Cereal, instant multigrain
Couscous/Risotto mixes
Crust, ready-made pizza
Granola/Muesli
Hummus mix
Muffin mix, multigrain
Pancake mix, multigrain
Pasta/noodles, organic
Pita bread, whole-grain
Polenta mix
Quinoa
Tabouli mix
Tortillas, corn and whole wheat

Canned and Sauce Foods
Applesauce
Bean dips and refried beans, vegetarian
Beans: black, kidney, pinto, garbanzo
Curry sauces
Enchilada sauce
Oriental sauce, non-sodium
Pasta sauce
Peaches
Pineapple juice
Pizza sauce
Salsa
Tomatoes, vegetables
Vegetarian: broth, soups, sauces

Condiments
Cooking herbs and spices
Dressings, low-fat
Lemon juice
Lime juice
Miso
Mustard
Olive oil
Vinegars, assorted

Quick Convenience Foods
Frozen foods
Fruit, without syrup
Mushrooms
Pie shells
Salad greens
Sandwich pockets
Tofu
Tomatoes, sundried
Vegetables, frozen
Vegetables without sauces: corn, peas, green beans, pepper strips, broccoli, carrots, cauliflower, potatoes, onions
Veggie burgers
Veggie hot dogs
Waffles, whole-grain

Meat Alternatives
Seitan, including fajita
Tempeh, including marinated
Tofu, including marinated and prebaked

Veggie burgers/hot dogs

Dairy and Alternatives
Nonfat and low-fat: cream cheese, cheese, soy cheese, rice/soy milk, parmesan cheese, sour cream, yogurt and soy yogurt

Startup Shopping
1) Keep your books handy, go through them ahead of time, make your lists.
2) Make up a simple shopping list to keep on hand.
3) Make a copy of acid and alkaline foods, beans (end of this chapter).
4) You may want to pot some herbs on your deck or porch, and start a small garden if possible.

Basic Pantry Needs (see list this chapter)
Grains and Breads—brown rice, oatmeal, whole grain pastas, whole grain crackers and breads
Fruits—fresh produce, preferably organic; frozen fruit; or you may want to pick your own at a local farm
Vegetables—canned tomatoes or tomato sauce, frozen vegetables or vegetable combinations
Nut and Seeds—peanut butter, sunflower and sesame seeds, and tofu
Beans—variety of canned or dried beans (red, black, garbanzo, etc.)
Seasonings—olive oil, canola oil, salsa, apple cider vinegar, herbs, spices, dips, soy sauce, all low sodium
Dairy—if you do consume dairy, choose the low-fat varieties
Eggs—organic, available at heath food stores or many grocery stores that are now stocking organic items

Supermarket Foods and Vitamins
Source: Vegetarian Times *(1996)*

Avocado—rich in folic acid, a B vitamin that helps prevent birth defects and stimulates red blood cell production. Contains large amounts of beta carotene, an antioxidant; magnesium, which helps regulate blood pressure and keeps the heart healthy, and vitamins C and E. Usually pesticide free, even when grown conventionally.

Broccoli—and other vegetables (including Brussels sprouts, cabbage, cauliflower, and dark leafy greens such as kale or mustard greens) are among nature's most perfect foods. Broccoli is full of vitamin C and beta carotene, contains antioxidants that fight cancer, cataracts and heart disease, and also strengthen the immune system. Lutein, a carotenoid found in broccoli and spinach, is especially good for combating lung cancer. Greens are an excellent source of folic acid and iron.

Brown Rice—is a great source of minerals, particularly phosphorus and potassium, B vitamins (thiamine, niacin and folacin) and vitamin E. High in fiber, which helps prevent colon cancer, and selenium, an antioxidant that boosts the immune system.

Cantaloupe—is loaded with beta carotene, which can prevent the onset of aging and help rid the body of damaging free radicals. It is low in calories and sodium. Eat when in season; cantaloupes out of season, often from out of the country, are heavily contaminated with pesticides.

Dried Beans and Peas—are great sources of folic acid, soluble fiber, and compounds called saponins, which lower blood cholesterol levels. They are low in fat and high in protein, and have been linked to reduced rates of prostate and breast cancer.

Garlic—is an herb that may help ward off colds and other infections when eaten raw. Raw or cooked, it helps prevent blood clots and heart disease by reducing cholesterol levels. Garlic also appears to increase natural killer cell activity, which enhances the immune system.

Grapefruit—like other citrus fruits, packs a generous helping of vitamin C, a powerful antioxidant that bolsters the immune system by stimulating white blood cell action. When eaten with plant foods that contain iron, the vitamin C aids in its absorption. Grapefruit is rich in soluble fiber which nourishes intestinal bacteria, lowers serum cholesterol levels and helps control blood glucose levels.

Legumes—are an excellent source of protein, carbohydrates, zinc, and iron. As for protein intakes, it equal takes four cups of green leafy vegetables or three servings of potatoes to one cup of cooked beans.

Nutritional Yeast—is rich in B vitamins, and is a good source of iron and folic acid. If you are vegan, check for vitamin B in foods, as it is essential for brain and nerve function. It is found only in animal foods and some nutritional yeast and fortified foods.

Potatoes—reward the body with potassium. If you eat the well-washed skins, they contain vitamin C and fiber. Low in calories and fat free (if you leave off the butter).

Sweet Potatoes—are rich in beta carotene and vitamins C and A, folic acid, and potassium. They are high in fiber and low in fat, sodium, and calories.

Tofu—a staple of Asian cooking, comes from the soybean. Tofu is high in protein, rich in calcium (if coagulated with calcium salts—read the label), low in calories and fat.

Wheat Germ—is loaded with iron and vitamin E, rich in folic acid and other trace minerals that boost energy and aid in the fight against heart disease.

Whole Wheat Bread—is loaded with carbohydrates and insoluble fiber, which lowers your risk of colon and rectal cancer. It also provides iron and vitamins E and B6.

Basic Herbs for the Kitchen

Basil—hints of mint, cloves, and anise
Bay Leaves—woodsy, perfumed, traces of cinnamon-like flavor
Dill—fresh, mild, faint anise taste
Mint—sweet, cool, refreshing
Oregano—strong, peppery, marigold-like
Parsley—fresh, grassy vegetable taste
Rosemary—piney, bittersweet, tea-like flavor
Sage—woodsy, pungent, faintly bitter
Tarragon—hints of licorice and vanilla
Thyme—peppery, robust, with hints of mint and lemon

Basic Spices for the Kitchen

Allspice—flavor like nutmeg, clove, cinnamon and juniper (baked squashes)
Cardamom—delicate hints of cinnamon, eucalyptus (chicken)
Celery Seed—bitter, refreshing, celery-like (potato salad)
Cilantro—also called Chinese parsley and coriander leaves
Cinnamon—sweet, warm, nutty taste (apple and pumpkin pies)
Cloves—pungent, medicinal (add to apple cider hot drink)
Coriander—lemony, fragrant (makes things taste better)
Cumin—hot, bitter, caraway-like (chili)
Fennel Seed—sweet, licorice-like (potato salad)
Ginger—sweet and biting (chicken, soups)
Nutmeg—warm, spicy, milder than cinnamon (pumpkin pies)

Paprika—hot, rich, earthy (goulash, chicken, top of deviled eggs)
Pepper—hot and biting (best if fresh ground, add after cooking)
Lemon Pepper—tart and biting all at once (fish, pasta salads, soups), add after cooking

Best Cookware
Healthiest choices for cooking listed by preference.
1) Glass   3) Stainless Steel
2) Cast Iron 4) Enamel

Be aware of what type of cooking utensils you choose, as aluminum is easily assimilated into the body. Foods cooked in aluminum can produce a chloride poison. Aluminum is deposited in the brain and nervous system and has been linked to Alzheimer's disease. Aluminum-free cookware is available.

Note: Do not use chipped or cracked dishes. Bacteria grow throughout the damaged dish and cannot be removed with cleaning.

Cooking Vegetables
Essential B vitamins are packed into vegetables, but easily lost in the process of preparing food for the table; water dissolves them, heat destroys them, and time fades them. If you must boil, add vegetables to water after the water is boiling; drain immediately after cooked. Steaming vegetables is much better, or rapidly stir-frying for retention of valuable nutrients. By cooking carefully, or serving vegetables raw, you will preserve nutrients such as the vitamins C, B, folacin, thiamin, and riboflavin.

Note: If stir-frying, add a small amount of water to the pan, then add vegetables. After steam frying, then add the oil, as the oil will change chemically if overheated. Or put water in first and then add the oil, to keep the oil for stir-frying at lower temperatures, which will not change the oil chemically.

Barbecued Meats
Source: Bottom Line *(1996)*

Eat greens with barbecued meats, if you must eat red meat. This will reduce absorption of carcinogens that are produced when the meats are cooked. The chlorophyll in vegetables such as salad greens, broccoli, and spinach seems to cut carcinogen absorption from barbecued and smoked meat, if eaten at the same time. Be sure to cook the meat thoroughly, and never eat burned food.

Organic Coffee
Available at most health food stores and some grocery stores; look for organic labeling.

Herbal Teas
Chamomile—good for relaxation and for sleep

Dandelion—good for mild constipation and stomach problems, digestive organs, and especially the liver

Fennel—seeds, leaves, and root are excellent stomach and intestinal remedies. When brewed, they arouse appetite and expel mucus accumulations

Green tea—helps restore balance and stimulates your body's natural defenses

Lemon Balm—used for colic, cramps, bronchial problems, catarrh, dyspepsia, some forms of asthma and headaches. Mint relieves cramps, coughs, poor digestion, nausea, heartburn, abdominal pains, headaches, and ailments attributed to nerves

Thyme—is ideal for calming nerves, alleviating indigestion, and clearing mucous membranes

Fat, Fiber, and Carbohydrates
Source: Eat More, Weight Less *by Dr. Dean Ornish (page 35)*

	Amount	**Fat**	**Carbohydrates**	**Fiber**
Plant Products				
apple	1 whole	0.5	21.0	2.8
baked potato	1 whole	0.2	33.6	2.7
brown rice	1/2 cup	0.9	22.5	0.3
carrots	1 cup	0.1	8.2	1.1
lentils	1 cup	0.8	39.8	5.4
lettuce	1 cup	0.1	1.3	0.9
oatmeal	1 cup	2.4	25.2	2.1
Animal Products				
butter	1 tsp	3.8	trace	0
cheeseburger	4 oz	15.0	29.0	0
chicken, fried	10 oz	52.0	26.0	0
egg, scrambled	1	1.4	1.4	0
fish, mackerel	3.5 oz	14.0	0	0
goose, roasted	1.3 lbs	75.0	0	0

Squash

Source: Super Healing Foods *by Frances Sheridan Goulart*

Squash helps protect you from bowel and bladder cancer, colon and constipation problems, and lung cancer. Squash belongs to the gourd or melon family. It comes in two categories: summer (white, yellow, bush scallop, crooked neck or straight neck zucchini) and winter (pumpkin, butternut, acorn, hubbard and spaghetti). Winter squashes top the list of the forty-five vegetables that are used in Japan, where cancer rates are low. A high intake of squash along with deep orange vegetables (carrots) provides protection from secondhand smoke. Dark yellow vegetables like winter squash are a good source of cancer-fighting nutrients such as vitamin C and beta carotene, which block the destructive activity of the free radical scavengers, as well as iron for healthy blood, fiber, complex carbohydrates, potassium and magnesium for a healthy heart.

Squash seeds are a rich source of protease trypsin inhibitors, and prevent the activation of viruses in the intestinal tract, as well as provide an abundant supply of zinc and essential fatty acids, which protect the prostate gland and reproductive organs.

Pumpkin and squash tea is a Cherokee Indian folk medicine for edema, gout, and kidney stones. In India and parts of Europe, squash pulp is used as compresses to relieve headaches, neuralgia, and burns. In Ethiopia, pumpkin and squash seeds are used as purgatives and laxatives. The Zuni Indians of Arizona use pumpkin and squash flowers to heal wounds and scars.

Quick and Healthy Vegetarian Meals

Buy organic, nonfat yogurt, rice, soy or nonfat milk, frozen vegetables or fresh organic vegetables, whole-grain cereals and pastas. Read labels carefully.

Breakfast Menus

1 multigrain muffin
1/2 cup rice/soy or nonfat milk
fresh fruit

1 cup nonfat soy or yogurt
1/4 cup muesli
seasonal fruit

3/4 cup low-fat granola
1/2 cup rice/soy or nonfat milk
1/2 cup pure fruit juice

1 whole-grain bagel
low-fat cream cheese
1/2 banana

1 pkg. instant multigrain
cereal with dried fruit
1/4 cup rice/soy or nonfat milk

1 whole-grain waffle
1/2 cup organic fruit
1/4 cup rice/soy or nonfat milk

Plain yogurt w/ prunes
chopped apple
toasted pumpkin seeds

Whole-grain toast
Miso/tahini spread
Piece of fruit

Poached egg
whole-grain toast/muffin

Oatmeal with raisins
or bananas
(optional rice milk)

Granola, low fat
vanilla yogurt
Fresh fruit

Organic wheat waffles
with fruit

Brown rice cream cereal
cooked with dried fruit

Creamy millet
with apples and honey

Baked sweet potato
with butter/date sugar

Oatmeal
chopped dates and cinnamon

B.L.T. sandwich
(whole grain bread)
tempeh bacon, lettuce

Smoothies

Add one scoop of super blue-green algae to each Smoothie:

Fruit Smoothie
1/2 cup pineapple juice
(not from concentrate)
1/4 cup nonfat/organic yogurt
1 banana
1 kiwi

Mixed Fruit Smoothie
1/2 orange, peeled
1 banana
1/2 cup frozen strawberries
1/4 cup frozen peaches
1/2 cup nonfat yogurt

Sweet & Sour Smoothie
1/2 cup fresh pineapple
1/2 banana
1/4 apple
1/2 orange, peeled
1–2 tbsp. honey (if desired)

Citrus/Carrot Smoothie
1 cup pineapple juice
1 slice lemon
1/2 cup carrots

Lunch Menus

1 organic Pizza Pocket
raw carrot sticks
piece fresh fruit

Curried Tempeh Sandwich
8 oz tempeh, cubed
3 tbsp. soy mayo
1 tbsp. mustard
Serve with: bread and mixed greens

2 tbsp. mango chutney
2 scallions, diced
1/2 tsp. curry powder

1 cup bean soup
raw jicama sticks w/lime juice
opt. piece fresh fruit

pita pocket filled w/hummus
add: lettuce, tomato,
shredded carrot
opt. piece fresh fruit

Veggie Burger
opt. whole-grain bun
add: onion, lettuce, tomato
fruit with yogurt

Natural Sweet Mush
1–1/2 cups couscous/bulgar beans
3 cups boiling water
1/4 cup chopped apricots (dried)
2 tbsp. currants
1/2 cup pine nuts or walnuts
opt. 1/2 tsp. garlic powder

Mexican Pita
portion black bean dip

1 tomato, sliced
cheddar tofu cheese
1 slice red onion/scallions
2 large lettuce leaves
pita bread

American/Mexican Pita Roll-Up
portion black beans or refried

salsa (peppers, onions, tomato)
2 scrambled eggs/opt. scallions
2 large lettuce leaves
large pita bread
(cut into 2 round pieces)

Frittata (Italian openface omelet)
3 tbsp. butter or olive oil
1 cup chopped asparagus
2 scallions, small pieces
1 cup shredded cheese
1 tsp. oregano
6 eggs (salt/pepper to taste)
Prepare in skillet/oven
 to melt cheese

Fresh Vegetables and Spread
1 clove garlic, minced
1 16-oz. can chickpeas, drained
2 tbsp. lemon juice
1–1/2 tsp curry powder
2–4 tbsp. water
(Food processor for
smooth blend)

Potato Curry (25 min
2 cloves garlic, minced
3 scallions, small pieces
3 cups vegetable stock
1 tbsp. ginger root
1 tsp chili powder
2 tsp. turmeric
1 tsp. soy sauce
4 med. red potatoes

Chinese Noodle Soup
buckwheat noodles, extra thin
6 cups vegetable broth
1 tbsp. olive oil or 1 tbsp. soy sauce
6 fresh mushrooms
1 pkg. mixed Chinese vegetables
opt. snow peas, spinach, cabbage

Miscellaneous Ideas:
Spinach salads using eggs, mushrooms, fresh vegetables
Omelets, with a variety of vegetables and/or seasonings
Sweet potatoes, fixed with seasonings and fruit
Knishes, made with variety of vegetables and cheeses
Empañadas, made with spinach and/or vegetables

Dinner Menus

American/Chinese Cuisine
1 pkg. frozen vegetables
tofu marinated in soy sauce (low sodium)
serve over cooked noodles
dessert: fresh orange slices

Vegetables/Beans/Rice Dish
2 cups fresh vegetables sauté
1 can garbanzo beans
w/bottled curry sauce
add over brown rice (quick cooking)

Eastern Indian Cuisine
8 oz pkg. soy tempeh
1/2 tbsp. fresh minced ginger
2 cloves garlic
1 tbsp. sesame oil
1/2 cup tamari, 1/4 cup water
add vegetable and seasoning
2 tbsp. arrowroot, 1/4 tsp. cayenne
dash jalapeno juice or vinegar

Veggie/Pasta Dish
organic pasta sauce
1 pkg. frozen vegetables
serve over pasta w/grated parmesan
dessert: fresh fruit

Potato/Spinach Garden Cuisine
grill/stir fry potatoes in olive oil
add fresh garlic
scallions
fresh spinach
add herbs for extra taste
pine nuts (optional)

Soup/Salad
leftover pasta, add 1 can of organic soup
1 whole grain roll
tossed green salad
dessert: fresh fruit

Natural Dressings:
Nasoya (100% dairy free,
without cholesterol)
Newman's Own

Leftovers
leftover hummus and pita bread with
grilled vegetables and couscous (quick cooking), yogurt (low fat)
dessert: piece of fruit

Chile/Potato
1 can vegetarian chile over baked potato
add cilantro and salsa
dessert: yogurt or nondairy ice cream
with fruit

Linguine and Herbs
1/2 lb. dry linguine
1 tsp. olive oil
6 cloves garlic
1 tsp. grated lemon
1/2 cup fresh parsley
fresh ground pepper or herbs

Spinach Salad
fresh spinach, scallions
fresh lettuce
leftover fresh vegetables
fresh lemon squeezed over top
opt. cheese slices, turkey
eggs, beets, add fresh herbs

Pasta

High in carbohydrates and with no cholesterol, homemade pastas are great! Pasta machines are available and becoming more popular as people experience making some unusual recipes. Remember, homemade pastas need more boiling water, usually at least four quarts.

Squash Pasta
(no eggs; can substitute peanut butter for hazelnut butter)
1 small butternut squash
1-3/4 cups all-purpose flour
1 tsp. hazelnut butter
pinch: nutmeg, garlic, black pepper

Directions:
• Cut squash into quarters, remove seeds, place in shallow baking dish with 1 to 1-1/2 cups water, cover and bake at 350° 50–60 minutes, let cool, then scrape out and mash flesh.
• In bowl or food processor, combine 3/4 cup squash with remaining ingredients to form dough.
• Turn dough out onto a floured surface and knead until smooth and pliable like firm bread dough; should be dry but not cracking.
• Place dough in bowl, cover with plastic wrap and let stand for at least 30 minutes.

- Shape and cook dough as desired, following directions for rolling and cutting pasta with your machine.

Orange Curry Pasta
(no eggs)
1 cup all-purpose flour
1/4 cup frozen orange juice concentrate, thawed
1 tbsp. curry powder
pinch: salt, pepper

Directions:
- In bowl or food processor, combine all ingredients until dough forms a ball.
- Turn dough onto floured surface, knead until smooth, pliable, dry but not cracking.
- Place in bowl, cover with plastic wrap, and let stand for 30 minutes.
- Shape and cook as desired.

Ginger Carrot Pasta
(no eggs)
2 large carrot
1 cup all-purpose flour
1 tsp. grated fresh ginger root

Directions:
- Steam carrots until tender, then puree.
- In bowl or food processor, combine 3/4 cup carrot puree with remaining ingredients to form dough.
- Follow basic directions in other recipes.

Tomato Herb Pasta
(no eggs)
1–1/2 cups all-purpose flour
2/3 cup tomato paste
1 tsp. garlic powder
2 tbsp. minced fresh parsley
2 tbsp. minced fresh basil

Directions:
- Follow basic directions in other recipes.

Emerald Mint Pasta
(no eggs)
1 cup frozen green peas, defrosted
2 tbsp. chopped fresh mint
1–1/2 cups all-purpose flour
pinch: salt and pepper

Directions:
- Place peas and mint in food processor and puree, add remaining ingredients, mix until ball of dough forms.
- Follow basic directions from other recipes.

Enjoy making up your own recipes, with your tastes and choices, then follow basic directions.

Nutrition

Evolution of Human Nutrition

Humans have had no significant biological evolution in one hundred thousand years. The vast majority of our evolution took place before the development of agriculture, so for most of that time, we have eaten wild foods. This preagriculture diet consisted of large amounts of raw fruits and vegetables, nuts and seeds, lean meat and seafood. Straying from our evolutionary hunter-gatherer diets has resulted in chronic illnesses and other physical problems. Needless to say, there is no room for refined grains, refined sugar, alcohol, processed fats or anything preserved or artificial in this diet. Dairy products were not part of our evolutionary diet and should also be avoided.

Human beings need fat in their diets, but the type and amount of fat that is consumed determines how it is used by the body. There is a crucial distinction between structural fat and storage fat. Structural fat is a major component of cell membranes, internal organs, brain and nervous tissue. Essential fatty acids (EFAs) are a vital part of structural fat, thus a dietary EFA deficiency results in the body's inability to properly synthesize it. Storage fat is largely saturated fat used by the body as "food reserve." Our ancestors needed to carry around excess food for emergencies; today, food is much more accessible. Our increasing storage fat excess is a consequence of straying from our evolutionary diet into processed foods that are loaded with sugar, refined grains, and animal storage fat, as well as hydrogenated and high-temperature–processed vegetable oils.

Vitamins, essential amino acids and EFAs may have become essential because they were abundant in our evolutionary diet, so we lost the ability to synthesize them. Our bodies learned not to waste energy making something that was readily available.

Two Classes of Foods

Group One (Proteids): Nitrogenous or albuminous. Repair and build up the physical structure. Abundant in milk, eggs, fish, other seafood, legumes, cereals, certain vegetables and meats. Protein foods, with the exception of milk and cottage cheese, are acid forming.

Group Two (Carbonaceous): Starches, sugars, and fats. Carbohydrates are foods that contain an abundance of sugar and starches and are found mainly in vegetables and fruits. They should form a large part of our daily diet, though overabundance could cause acidulation instead of neutralization. After carbohydrates are digested and assimilated, the portal vein takes them up and carries them to the liver where they are stored as glycogen and then converted into dextrose as needed by the blood. Excessive carbohydrates are consumed in the American diet, which can lead to diseases and toxicity of the liver.

Guide to Dehydrating

Dried foods have been used by many ancient cultures, including the Norsemen and Spaniards when they were traveling across the vast oceans. The Native Americans needed dried foods to help them through the harsh winters. The process of dehydrating is to heat the food to a temperature that destroys the microorganisms. Dried foods do not need refrigeration and save space. Many people have started using dehydrators in preparation for natural disasters and/or food shortages.

Some foods that do not dehydrate well are: lettuces, radishes, Brussels sprouts, guavas, quince, pomegranates and olives. Also, eggs are not recommended because of the risk of salmonella and staphylococcus contamination.

Food Cooperatives

For a co-op near you, contact the National Cooperative Business Association in Washington, D.C., (202) 638-6222; contact Northeast Co-op for co-op names in their area, or for information on how to get a co-op started, call 1-800-334-9939, ext. 366. Co-op means working together for ordering and to distribute upon delivery. Customers save money by buying foods at wholesale prices and in bulk quantities.

Cooperatives are becoming more popular due to the increasing demand for natural and organic foods. Some major co-ops have conventions in their geographic regions that have vendors displaying their product lines. This is a time to see for yourself if this is something you would be interested in.

Oils and Fats

Oils

Sources: Delicious *(June 1996) and* Virginian Pilot *(April 1995)*

The higher the polyunsaturated to saturated fat ratio, the less heart risk there is from the food. A polyunsaturate/saturate ratio greater than or equal to 1:1 is considered good and a ratio less than 1:1 is less than desirable. Some vegetable oils, such as coconut and palm, are laden with saturated fats and found mostly in processed foods. Soybean is the most commonly used oil in the U.S.A.; it is the main ingredient in generic vegetable oil. Virgin olive oils are the only unrefined oils sold to the general market that still contain phytosteroids, chlorophyll, magnesium, vitamin E, carotene and other substances present in seeds and naturally refined oils. All other mass market oils, being refined, bleached, and deodorized, are extremely nutrient poor. Their natural antioxidants, natural flavor and odor molecules, pigments, oil-soluble vitamins and plant steroids were largely removed during processing.

Saturated fat—linked to high cholesterol and health problems; carbon chains have no double bonds, solid at room temperature.

Polyunsaturated fat—found in most vegetable oils; carbon chains are completely double bonded.

Monounsaturated fat—an ingredient in olive and canola oil; carbon chains have one double bond.

Essential fatty acids (EFAs) — vital to your health. They help your immune system to function properly and help keep your weight on an even keel. The following unsaturated oils are derived from nuts, seeds and plants and are excellent sources of EFAs: Grape seed oil, flax seed oil, hemp seed oil, pumpkin seed oil, wheat germ oil, rice bran oil, black currant seed oil, borage seed oil and evening primrose oil.

Transfatty acids—disrupt the vital functions of EFAs, by interfering with enzyme systems that transform fatty acids into highly unsaturated fatty acid derivatives found concentrated in our brains, sense organs, adrenals, and testes. Ultimately this interferes with our arteries, blood pressure, regulation of kidney function, inflammation response and immune system competence. The main products we get transfatty acids from are margarine, shortening, shortening oils, all of which are made from partially hydrogenated vegetable oils; plus any products that are made with these products, such as dressings and pastry.

Hydrogenation

Source: Fats that Heal, Fats that Kill *by Udo Erasmus*

In the past eighty years Americans have been fed increasing amounts of artificially hydrogenated oils by the processed foods industry. These high-temperature–processed oils are convenient for manufacturers to use because they are stable for long periods and can sit around in warehouses and on store shelves almost indefinitely, which is good for food processors' profits. These low-cost raw materials allow margarine to be sold at lower prices. Unaware shoppers who are concerned only with money and bargains rather than health will buy the margarine.

Hydrogenation is considered the most common way of changing natural oils. This process has major effects on the body's health. Hydrogenation changes the unsaturated and essential fatty acids present in natural oils by using common catalysts such as nickel and aluminum. Remnants of these metals can remain in the products containing hydrogenated oils, and when eaten can be deposited throughout the body's organs and tissues. The presence of aluminum is particularly worrisome. Its presence in the human body is associated with Alzheimer's disease and osteoporosis and has been known to facilitate the development of cancer. A totally hydrogenated oil (now a very hard fat) has no essential fatty acid (EFA) activity; it is a dead substance.

Alternatives

Beel brand margarine contains no transfatty acids, no hydrogenated fats, and no animal fats or cholesterol. It is made from refined sunflower oil and tropical fats, so you can dip your breads into fresh unrefined olive oil, flax oil, or hemp oil. This dipping custom is of Mediterranean origin.

Frying and Deep Frying

Frying simultaneously exposes the oils used to the effects of the three major fatty acid damaging influences: light, oxygen, and heat. Under these conditions, many chemical changes can take place in oils, causing random free radical reactions to synergize with each other's destructiveness. This can impair cell respiration and other cell functions, inhibit immune functions, and lead to cancer.

Flax Seeds as Natural Oil

For better nutrients, grind the seeds because of their rough outer shell. Drink plenty of liquid because flax mucilage absorbs five times the seed's weight of water. Six tablespoons of flax seeds contain two tablespoons of natural oil. The use of freshly ground flax seeds can improve digestion, prevent and reverse constipation, stabilize blood glucose levels, improve cardiovascular health, inhibit tumor formation, and bring about many other beneficial effects. Ground flax meal sold in plastic containers is usually rancid and should be avoided. Fresh flax oil spoils when exposed to light, oxygen, and heat, and therefore care needs to be taken in the pressing process or it becomes rancid linseed oil. Fresh, it has a light nutty taste.

Food Additives

Additives MSG and NutraSweet

Source: Healthy and Natural Journal *(pages 22, 23)*

The FDA Review Panel is bogged down with "manipulating the language" in the food industry. Of particular concern are any products containing "excitotoxins," a group of compounds that can cause special neurons within the nervous system to become overexcited, to the point that cells will die. Excitotoxins include such things as monosodium glutamate (MSG), aspartame (NutraSweet), L-cysteine (found in hydrolyzed vegetable protein) and related compounds. They have been found to play a key role in degenerative nervous system diseases such as Parkinson's disease, Alzheimer's disease, Huntington's, ALS (Lou Gehrig's disease), and many others.

An imbalance of excitotoxins during critical periods of brain development can result in an abnormal formation of brain pathways ("miswiring" of the brain). This may lead to behavioral problems (hyperactivity, aggression, learning disorders, poor learning ability, and attention deficit disorders).

MSG—Some people may think they are not allergic to the MSG, but the toxic reaction occurs in everyone. Some people are just more sensitive than others, experiencing headaches, pressure in the chest, heart palpitations, numbness in the arms and face, etc. Large doses of MSG fed to research animals has led to gross obesity.

NutraSweet—This sweetener was at first rejected by the FDA as unsafe for human consumption; findings linked it with brain tumors. In a breakdown of the product NutraSweet, the product diketopiperizine (DKP) is what is causing the tumors. Usage in hot beverages or for cooking is even more hazardous.

Natural Sweeteners
Source: Delicious *(January 1996), pages 61-65*

Natural sweeteners include sucrose, glucose, fructose, maltose, dextrose, lactose, galactose, and levulose. Chemically, many kinds of sugars exist, and all nutritive sweeteners contain one or more of these sugars. Though some components of natural sugars are chemically identical to refined white sugar, it's not true that "sugar is sugar." White sugar creates a strain on our bodies. The book *Healthy Steps,* by Dr. Zehr, explains that white sugar depletes stored vitamins and minerals, and suppresses the immune system.

Healthy eating isn't deprivation: you can have your cake and eat it too, with naturally sweetened desserts. Low-tech processed natural sugars retain vitamins, minerals, and other components essential for their digestion and are metabolized more slowly than white sugar.

Some Commercially Available Natural Sweeteners
1) Pure dark maple syrup, light brown maple syrup
2) Barley malt syrup
3) Brown rice syrup
4) Mixed fruit juice concentrate
5) Dried cane juice
6) Honey
7) Date sugar
8) Granular fruit

Avoid: *Turbinado, raw* and *brown* sugars, which are essentially refined sugar; *fructose,* which is highly refined and not made from fruit; *corn syrup,* a cheap refined sweetener; *artificial sweeteners,* which are chemically derived, nonnutritive substances.

Apple Cider Vinegar
Sources: Herbal Vinegar *by Maggie Osterand and* The Vinegar Book *by Emily Thacker*

Apple cider vinegar enthusiasts can recite long lists of ailments it is reported to be able to cure or prevent. When fresh apples are allowed to ferment organically, the result is vinegar containing natural sediment with pectin, trace minerals, beneficial bacteria and enzymes. In the book resource section, *The Vinegar Book* shows 308 natural ways in which vinegar can be used, with folk remedies that show how to mix it with other kitchen staples.

Apple cider vinegar contains more than thirty important nutrients, a dozen minerals, more than half a dozen vitamins and essential acids, and several enzymes, plus a large dose of pectin for a healthy heart. Its use was described in early Assyrian medical texts, and in 400 B.C.E. Hippocrates used vinegar to treat his patients. This natural product was considered a germ killer and was one of the first medicines. It is claimed that apple cider vinegar can do the following:

1) improve metabolism
2) aid digestion
3) help slow cholesterol buildup
4) treat middle ear problems
5) fight age and liver spots
6) help gain soft and radiant skin
7) treat hair problems
8) relieve nighttime leg cramps
11) help headaches fade away
12) aid in maintaining health
13) relieve corns and calluses
14) relieve insect bites
15) remedy urinary problems
16) fight coughs and colds
17) destroy bacteria in foods
18) treat heart and circulatory problems

9) help sprained muscles
10) fight osteoporosis with calcium
19) fight high blood pressure
20) treat skin rashes and athlete's foot

Food Combining

1. Eat fruits alone.
2. Eat proteins/fats with vegetables.
3. Eat carbohydrates with vegetables and no fat.
4. Eliminate all junk food. Do not skip meals.
5. Wait three hours between meals if switching from carbohydrates to a protein/fat, or vice versa.

Definitions

Agar—a blend of seven seaweeds, used as gelatin
Falafel—garbanzo bean meal, yellow peas, onion, garlic, soy sauce powder, baking soda
Hummus—garbanzo beans pureed with garlic, lemon juice, and tamari
Kasha—buckwheat groats
Miso—aged soy or soy-grain paste containing live enzymes, which benefit intestinal flora
Seitan—wheat meat, protein substitute
Sesame tahini—nut butter from sesame seeds
Soba—buckwheat noodles
Soy milk—milk made from soybeans
Tempeh—an aged soy or soy-grain cake containing natural enzymes, which allow digestion, and vitamin B12
Tempura—veggies, tofu, tempeh, coated with batter and fried in olive oil
Tofu—soy curd, by-product of soy milk
Udon—thick noodle made of whole durum wheat

Asian Diet Pyramid (ADP)

Sources: Cornell University, Harvard School of Public Health and Oldways

The Asian diet meets every recommendation you can think of for what you need to help prevent chronic diseases. Infinitely varied and delicious, it is a nutritionist's dream of low fat, high fiber, and dairy free. The pyramid includes optional small servings of eggs, fish, poultry, and meat, but the ADP emphasizes a plant-based diet with few or no animal foods, including no dairy products.

1) Poultry, fish, soy products, tofu, and tempeh.
2) Vegetables and legumes.
3) Rice and whole grains.
4) Fruit as dessert with sweets and sugar rare treats.
5) Choice of oils, including olive oil.
6) Exercise such as a walk around the block, a trip up and down stairs, and stretching in the morning and evening.

Food Combining for Easiest Digestion

PROTEINS
Nuts (most)
Dry beans, peas
soybeans
peanuts
seeds (sunflower, sesame, pumpkin)

STARCHES
Carrots
Chestnuts
Corn
Dry Beans
peas
Potatoes
Peanuts
Winter squash
(Acorn, hubbard, butternut)
Breads
Cereals

VEGETABLES
Leafy greens
Asparagus
Bamboo shoots
Broccoli
Cabbage
Cauliflower
Celery
Cucumber
Eggplant
Green beans
Turnips
Kohlrabi
Kale
Okra
Sweet pepper
Summer squash
Zucchini squash
Yellow squash etc.

ACID FRUITS
Grapefruit
Lemon
Lime
Orange
Pineapple
Pomegranate
Sour plum
Strawberries

SUB-ACID FRUITS
Apple
Apricot
Sweet cherry
Fresh fig
Grape
Huckleberry
Mango
Papaya
Sweet Plum
Pear
Peach

SWEET FRUITS
Banana
Date
Persimmon
Raisin
Dried Fruit
(apple, fig, pear)

- Proteins ↔ Starches: POOR COMBINATION
- Proteins ↔ Vegetables: GOOD COMBINATION
- Starches ↔ Vegetables: GOOD COMBINATION
- Proteins ↔ Acid Fruits: POOR COMBINATION
- Starches ↔ Sweet Fruits: POOR COMBINATION
- Vegetables ↔ Sub-Acid Fruits: POOR COMBINATION
- Acid Fruits ↔ Sub-Acid Fruits: FAIR COMBINATION
- Sub-Acid Fruits ↔ Sweet Fruits: FAIR COMBINATION

Mediterranean Diet Pyramid

Source: Health News Naturally

The Mediterranean Diet Pyramid (MDP) recommends a diet based largely on grains, vegetables, and fruits, and differs from the American Food Pyramid (AFP) and other pyramids in the following ways:

1) The MDP recommends using olive oil. It is a monounsaturated fat that is linked neither to cancer nor to heart disease. The AFP doesn't distinguish between types of fats.
2) Health supportive plant protein (beans, legumes and nuts) can be eaten on a daily basis; eggs and fish a few times a week. The AFP doesn't distinguish between vegetable and animal protein.
3) The MDP recommends daily servings of cheese or yogurt, but in small amounts; the AFP recommends two to three servings of milk, yogurt and cheese.
4) The MFP recommends drinking only a small amount of alcohol; the AFP states that drinking has no health benefits.

Mediterranean Diet Pyramid

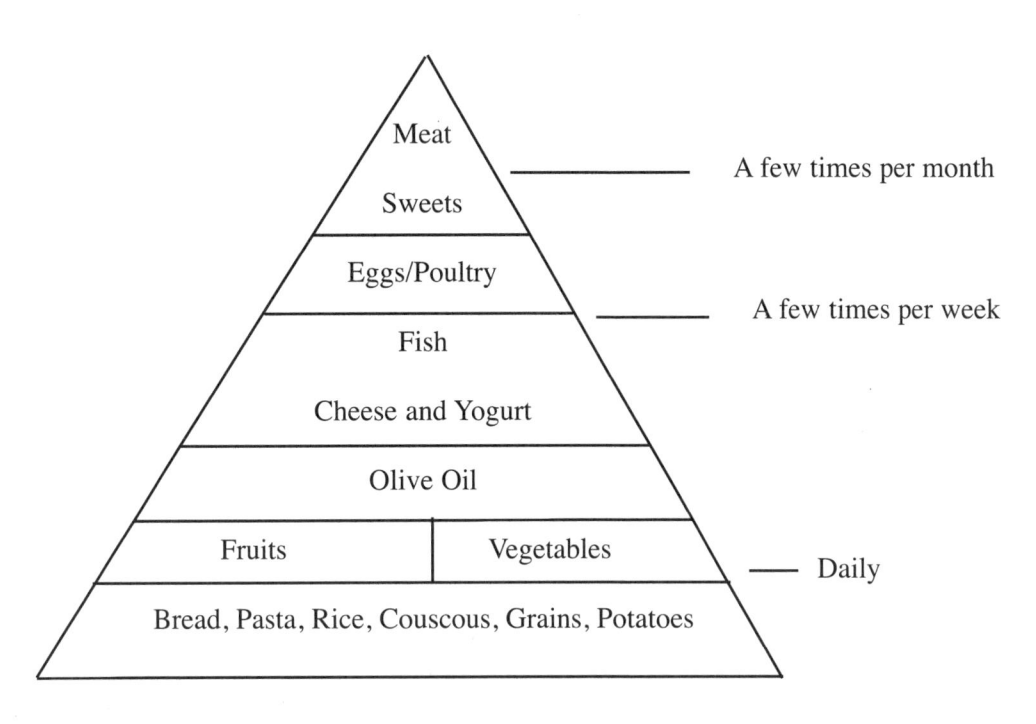

```
              /\
             /  \
            /Meat\            ———— A few times per month
           /------\
          /Sweets  \
         /----------\
        /Eggs/Poultry\
       /--------------\         ———— A few times per week
      /     Fish       \
     /------------------\
    / Cheese and Yogurt  \
   /----------------------\
  /      Olive Oil         \
 /--------------------------\
/  Fruits   |   Vegetables   \   ——— Daily
/-----------------------------\
/Bread, Pasta, Rice, Couscous, Grains, Potatoes\
--------------------------------
```

Acid- and Alkaline-Forming Foods

Note: Just because a food is acidic is no indication it will remain acidic in the body; it can turn alkaline. Honey or raw sugar produces alkaline ash because a high concentrate of sugar becomes acid forming. One should eat eighty percent alkaline to twenty percent acid for best health. *Citrus fruits should be eaten with citrus fruits, melons should be eaten with melons; all other fruits may be combined with other fruits, but not with other foods.

Alkaline Fruits
apples
apricots
avocados
bananas
berries, all
cantaloupe
cherries
currants
dates
figs
grapes
grapefruit*
kumquats*
lemons,* ripe
limes*
mangos
melons, all
nectarines
olives
oranges
papayas
passion fruit
peaches
pears
persimmons
pineapple
plums
pomegranates
prunes
raisins
tangerines*
tomatoes

Acid Fruits
canned fruits, all
cranberries, dried/sulfurized
olives, pickled
preserves, all

Alkaline Vegetables
alfalfa sprouts
artichokes
asparagus
bamboo shoots
beans, green, lima, or string
beets
broccoli
cabbages
carrots
cauliflower
celery
chard
coconut
corn
cucumber
dill
eggplant

endive
escarole
garlic
horseradish
kale
leeks
lettuce
mushrooms
okra
onions
parsley
parsnips
peppers-bell
potatoes
pumpkin
radishes
romaine lettuce
rutabagas
sauerkraut
soybeans
spinach
sprouts
squash
sweet potatoes
turnips
water chestnuts
watercress
yams

Acid Vegetables
asparagus tips
beans, dried
Brussels sprouts
garbanzos
lentils
rhubarb

Alkaline Dairy
acidophilus milk
buttermilk
milk, raw
whey
yogurt

Acid Dairy
butter
cheese, all
cottage cheese
cream
custards
margarine
milk, boiled, dried,
 cooked, malted

Alkaline Misc.
coffee substitute
honey
kelp

tea, herbal

Acid Misc.
cocoa
coffee
condiments, all
dressings
eggs
flavorings
mayonnaise
tapioca
teas
vinegar

alcoholic drinks
drugs
lack of sleep
tobacco

Acid-Flesh Foods
all meats
fowl, fish
jello, gelatin
shellfish

Alkaline Nuts
almonds
chestnuts, roasted
coconut, fresh

Acid Nuts
nuts, except above
coconut, dried

Mineral-Rich Foods

High In Copper
almonds
apples
asparagus
avocado
bananas
beans, dried
beef
beef liver
cabbage
carrots
cheese, American
chicken
citrus fruits

corn
dried prunes
eggs
grapes
kale
lima beans, dried
lobster
mushrooms
oats
oysters
peas, dried
pecans
pork chops
rye, whole

shrimp
spinach
sweet potatoes
turkey
walnuts
wheat, flour
white bread

High in Calcium
broccoli
canned sardines, salmon
egg yolk
kale
milk/dairy products

mustard greens
shellfish
soybeans
turnip greens
vegetables, green

High in Iron
apricots, dried
beans, dried
cocoa
egg yolk
fruits, dried
grain cereals
lean meats

legumes, all
liver sausage
molasses, dark
nuts
peaches
shellfish/seafoods
soybeans
vegetables, green leafy
wheat germ

High in Manganese
bananas
barley
beans, dried
beets
brown rice
carrots, raw
citrus fruits
cocoa
kale
lettuce
lima beans
liver
nuts: almonds, Brazil,
    cashews,
hazelnuts, peanuts,
    walnuts
oatmeal
peaches
peas, dried
potatoes
poultry, roasted
prunes, dried
rye bread, whole grain
snap beans
soy flour
spinach
sweet potatoes
tomatoes, raw
wheat
wheat flour
white flour

white rice
whole corn

High in Zinc
applesauce, canned
barley
beets
cabbage
carrots
cherries, canned
clams
corn, whole
cow's milk
eggs
herring
lettuce
maple syrup
oatmeal
oysters
peanut butter
pears, canned
peas
rice
rice cereal
rye bread
spinach
wheat bran
wheat bread
yeast, dry

High in Phosphorus
apricots, dried
beans, raw, dried
blackberries
blueberries
bran flakes
Brussels sprouts
buttermilk
cauliflower
chocolate
corn bread
cooked meats

cow's milk
currants, red
dandelion greens
dark rye flour
goat's milk
mustard greens
puffed wheat
raspberries, red
roasted nuts
seafood
swiss cheese
turnip greens
wheat flakes

High in Potassium
artichokes
asparagus
avocados
bananas
beet greens
beets, raw
broccoli
brown sugar
cabbage, raw
carrots, raw
catsup
cherries
citrus fruits, all
citrus juices, all
dried fruit: dates, figs,
    prunes, raisins
kale
lentils
molasses
okra
peas
parsley
parsnips, raw
potatoes, raw
pumpkin
radishes
soybeans

spinach
sweet corn
turnips, raw
wheat bread
wheat germ
wild rice

High in Sodium
asparagus
bacon
beans, baked
bologna
butter
buttermilk
canned: fish, crab
carrots
cheddar cheese
chipped beef
corned beef
cottage cheese
cream cheese
cured ham
flakes: rye, bran, corn, rice
    and wheat
French dressing
graham crackers
hot dogs
lima beans
liverwurst
milk, evaporated
mushrooms
olives
peas
popped corn
potato chips
pretzels
rye and wheat bread
saltines
sauerkraut
spinach
tomato catsup
white bread

Love is a fruit in season at all times,
And within reach of every hand.
Anyone may gather it and no limit is set upon it.

Mother Teresa

Book Resources

Ayurveda and Aromatherapy (essential oils) by Drs. Light and Bryan Miller
Cunningham's Encyclopedia of Magical Herbs by Scott Cunningham
Diet for a New America by John Robbins
Diet for a Poisoned Planet by David Steinman
Diet for a Small Planet by Frances Moore Lappe
Eat Great, Lose Weight (food combining) by Suzanne Sommers
Encyclopedia of Fruits, Vegetables and Herbs by John Heinerman
Fats that Heal, Fats that Kill by Udo Erasmus
Food for Life by Dr. Neal Barnard
Fresh Herb Extracts and Homeopathic Medicines by Dr. Jan de Vries
Health Through God's Pharmacy by Maria Treben
Healthy Steps by Dr. Albert Zehr (vitamin charts this chapter)
Herbal Vinegar by Maggie Oster
Herbally Yours by Penny C. Royal
Herbs, How to Grow and Use Them by Jacqueline Heriteau
Magic and Medicine of Plants by Reader's Digest
The Mediterranean Diet Cookbook by Nancy H. Jenkins
Prescription for Nutritional Healing by Drs. James and Phyllis Balch
Rodale's Illustrated Encyclopedia of Herbs
The Good Herb (recipes and remedies from nature) by Judith Benn Hurley
Today's Herbal Health by Louise Tenney
The Vinegar Book and *The Garlic Book* by Emily Thacker
Vegetarian Times Cookbook by editor of Vegetarian Times 1-800-793-9161

Recipe Books

1,000 Vegetarian Recipes by Carol Gelles
Eat Great—Lose Weight by Suzanne Sommers
Encyclopedia of Fruits, Vegetables and Herbs by John Heinerman
Moosewood Cookbook and *Enchanted Broccoli Forest Cookbook* by Mollie Katzen
The Natural Health Cookbook by Dana Jacobs and Editors of Natural Health Magazine

Magazines for Better Health

Better Nutrition (770) 955-2500
Delicious (303) 939-8440
Energy Times 1-800-937-0500
Healthy News Naturally
Herbalgram Journal of American Botanical Council for Herb Research (512) 331-8868
The Herb Companion 1-800-456-5835
Veggie Life and *Vegetarian Times*

Resources

Hanna's (Kroeger) Herb Shop, 5684 Valmont, Boulder, CO 80301 (herbs and seminars), 1-800-206-6722
The Herb Research Foundation (will provide information packets on specific herbs, $7.00 each), 1007 Pearl Street, Suite 200, Boulder, CO 80302, (303) 449-2265
North American Vegetarian Society (518) 568-7970

Product Resources

Cell Tech 1-888-748-4849, reference #268719 (for information about blue-green algae)
Corganics (wheatgrass, produce) 1-800-872-8571
Eden Foods (tomato products), Clinton, MI, 1-800-248-0320
Frontier Foods (herbs, coffee, teas), Norway, IA, 1-800-786-1388
Garden Valley Naturals (pasta sauce), Burlingame, CA 94011, (650) 579-5565
MexiSnax, Inc. (snack chips), (510) 786-2751
Millina's Finest (pasta sauce), PO Box 550, Aptos, CA 95001-0550
Muir Glen (pasta sauce), PO Box 11498, Sacramento, CA 95812
New Age Foods (herbs/balancer called electrilizer), 1122 Pearl Street, Boulder, CO 80302
Outrageous Fruit and Grains (breakfast cereals) 1-800-378-6476

Sources: Organic Seed Catalogs

Frog Pond Organic Farm (herb plants) (607) 527-3308
Goodwin Creek Gardens, PO Box 83, Williams, OR 97544, (541) 846-7357
Greenfield Herb Garden (plants and books) (219) 768-7110
Herbalist Catalog (500 different herbs) PO Box 5, Dept. VLTP, Hammond, IN 46325
Johnny's Selected Seeds, 123 Foss Hill Road, Albion, ME 04910-9731, (207) 437-4301
Monticello Seeds, PO Box 316, Dept. AD, Charlottesville, VA 22902
Seeds of Change (organically grown open pollinated seeds) 1-800-95-SEEDS
Shepherd's Garden Seeds, 6116 Highway 9, Felton, CA 95018, (860) 482-3638
The Herbfarm, Box AC22, 32804 Issaquah Fall City Road, Fall City, WA 98024, (206) 784-2222
The Herb Garden, PO Box 773H, Pilot Mountain, NC 27041
Vermont Bean Seed Company, 64 Garden Lane, Fair Haven, VT 05743

Chapter Four

Natural Earth Healing—
Physical Body

Aromatherapy and Natural Body Products

The essences of aromatic plants have been recognized for more than six thousand years. Modern aromatherapy can be traced to Germany in the sixteenth century. It was most likely brought to Europe with the invading Romans (who were supporters of the baths), although this therapy was practiced by the ancient Egyptians and Greeks, and has been a foundation in traditional Chinese and Eastern Indian Ayurvedic medicine for thousands of years. The French used these medicinal remedies during World War II, and their medical field is still using them today.

Used for healing, cleansing, preservative, and mood enhancing properties, aromatherapy harnesses the potent pure essences of plants, flowers, and resins to work on the most powerful of the senses, smell and touch, to restore the harmony to body and mind. The tools of aromatherapy are natural, botanical essences and vegetable oils in varying combinations and amounts delivered through massage, baths, inhalants, compresses, antiseptic creams to induce relaxation, increase energy, reduce the effects of stress, and restore balance. These essences have also been used by psychotherapists to help people open up to their past life traumas.

Popular Essences

Chamomile—Gentle, calming, and soothing. Chamomile eases depression, stress, anger, irritability, and hypersensitivity. It promotes a sense of inner peace when one is feeling overwhelmed, aids digestion, induces peaceful sleep, and can be used for children. Use: Massage, bath, hair, and skin.

Clary Sage—Earthy, dreamy and yet pungent, Clary Sage is an antidepressant that brings tranquillity and balance to the mind and emotions by calming anxiety or panic. It relaxes muscles, strengthens the kidneys, promotes hair growth, regenerates skin cells, and is excellent for skin care. Use: Massage, bath, skin, and hair care. Note: Do not use during pregnancy.

Eucalyptus—Invigorating, balancing, penetrating, eucalyptus helps open and clear the energetic pathways of the mind and body. It purifies and clears negative energy from one's aura and can be used in a spray bottle in the home or in a steamer for respiratory problems, and to control insects and airborne bacteria. Eucalyptus has antiseptic and antibiotic properties. Works with the heart chakra to balance grief and sorrows. Use: Massage, bath and sauna, steam inhalation, chest rub, and spray mist.

Lavender—The most popular essence, lavender was used in Egyptian times to rub the body before

burying. Gentle and versatile, it works with intuitiveness and activates the crown chakra and inner guidance. Lavender brings about clarity and peace of mind. It is useful for respiratory problems, blood pressure, insomnia, depression, stress, worry, shock, impatience, sore throats, burns, wounds, and headaches. It strengthens the immune system, speeds healing, and regenerates skin cells. Use: Massage, bath, steam inhalation, chest rub, sauna, skin and hair, and for foot reflexology.
- Rose—Elegant and romantic, rose is a symbol of love. This oil awakens, inspires, and brightens the heart. Rose helps activate the sacral, heart, and crown chakras, uniting the physical and spiritual as one. It enhances creativity and evokes an appreciation of beauty. Use: Massage, bath, and skin care, spray mist.
- Tea Tree—The single most effective, nontoxic, antibacterial and anti-fungal essential oil, tea tree oil may be applied directly to skin, liberally. Useful for the immune system, it speeds healing of burns, wounds, infection, tooth and gum infections, insect bites and stings, cold sores, dandruff, acne and rashes. Use it in a steamer for respiratory systems, flu, cold and bronchitis. Use: Massage, bath, steam inhalation, chest and skin application. Tea tree oil is as effective as benzoyl peroxide but significantly less drying.

Body Oils
Source: Delicious *(March 1996)*

Conventional Body Oil (ingredients mineral oil and fragrance)

Mineral oil—A mixture of refined liquid hydrocarbons derived from petroleum, mineral oil is colorless, transparent and odorless. It stays on top of the skin and leaves a shiny protective surface; when heated, it smells of petroleum.

Fragrance—Synthetic fragrances used in cosmetics can have as many as two hundred ingredients. There's no way to know what the chemicals are, since the labels will simply say "fragrance." Some of the problems caused by these chemicals are headaches, dizziness, rash, hyperpigmentation, coughing, and skin irritation.

Natural Body Oil (ingredients peanut oil, birch leaves, chamomile flowers, calendula extracts, and natural fragrances, such as lemon oil)

Peanut oil—Excellent for sun-protection products, peanut oil natural skin softener and emollient.

Birch leaves—Taken from the silver birch tree, birch leaves enhance skin-cleaning properties of products and promote an even distribution of active ingredients, and possess antiseptic and astringent properties.

Chamomile—This well-known medicinal plant with skin-calming properties is used for the care of delicate, sensitive skin.

Calendula extract—With its calming, anti-inflammatory effect and promotion of cell formation, calendula is used for sensitive skin and for skin in need of regeneration.

Lemon Oil—An antiseptic and antibacterial, it performs a tonic action on the lymphatic system.

Homeopathic First Aid Kit (for strains or sprains, stings, burns, and bruises when hiking)
Arnica montana—for strains and sprains
Belladonna—for infected wounds
Bryonia alba—for all-over aches
Calendula—for cuts and lacerations

Hypericum perforatum—for crushing-type injuries to fingertips or toes
Rhus veneata—for poison ivy and poison oak
Ruta graveolens—for shin splints
Symphytum—for bone injuries

Aromatherapy for Flying
Source: Delicious *(February 1996), page 37*
Here are some hints for dealing with relaxation, stress, and skin problems when you fly.
1) Drink plenty of water; avoid alcoholic beverages, which dehydrate you.
2) Smooth on body lotion from head to toe.
3) Never wear makeup, as the pigments can dry your skin.
4) Use alcohol-free styling gel or hair spray to prevent drying.
5) For overseas flights, pack cotton pads presoaked in chamomile tea for relaxing eye cover and to prevent eye puffiness.

Calming Herbs—Valerian, passionflower, chamomile, hyssop, lavender, St. John's Wort, skullcap
Stimulating Herbs—Peppermint, wormwood, and mugwort
Nausea—Basil, cardamom, fennel, lavender, peppermint, rose, sandalwood
Mental Fatigue—Basil, cardamom, peppermint, rosemary
Anxiety—Bergamot, chamomile, cypress, geranium, jasmine, lavender, patchouli, ylang ylang
Insomnia—Basil, camphor chamomile, lavender, marjoram, rose, sandalwood, ylang ylang
Rejuvenation—Frankincense, jasmine, lavender, myrrh, patchouli, rose

Natural Soap Labels
Source: Delicious *magazine*
Here's a list of terms and ingredients you might see on a natural soap label, and what they mean.
Aloe vera gel—An effective healer, it soothes, oxygenates, helps tighten pores, holds oxygen to skin.
Castile oil—Olive oil.
Citric acid—It is added to soap to make it more compatible with skin pH levels. In clay form, it helps to draw excess oils and toxins out of the skin.
Essential oils—These are added to soap to make it fragrant and to balance, soothe and heal skin. Those most often used are: *Calendula,* soothing and helps treat acne; *Chamomile,* for sensitive skin, soothing, healing and moisturizing; *Eucalyptus,* antiseptic, antibacterial and cooling, its sedative effects soothe the skin; *Lavender,* an antiseptic and antibiotic that helps promote healing; *Rosemary,* stimulates circulation; *Tea Tree,* antiseptic and helps clear blemishes. For normal/dry skin, use soaps with essential oils (Jasmine, Rose, or Neroli); for oily skin use Lavender, Bergamot or Geranium.
Glycerin—A sweet, syrupy alcohol obtained during saponification of fats, it helps soften skin and contributes to longevity of bar soaps.
Iron oxide—This naturally occurring compound of iron and oxygen, found in a wide range of colors from black to yellow; is used as a natural colorant.
Lecithin—A vegetable extract high in natural fatty acids that helps condition skin.
Milling—A soapmaking process involving grinding soap after it's made, then pressing it into cakes. The more times soap is milled, the denser it becomes.
Oatmeal—A gentle skin exfoliant.
Saponified—An alkaline substance, such as lye, has been added to a fat or vegetable oil to make soap.

Sea mud and seaweed—Detoxifiers that provide minerals to skin.

Vegetable oils—Along with alkali, these oils are the basic ingredients in soap. All vegetable oils are emollients, with not much difference in reference to effects on the skin. *Almond oil,* high in oleic, linoleic and other fatty acids, ideal for dry skin; *Apricot oil,* softens skin; *Avocado oil,* good source of vitamins A, D, and E; *Carrot oil,* rich in beta carotene and vitamins A and E; *Jojoba oil,* acts as a humectant when used in soaps; *Kukui oil,* natural moisturizer obtained from Hawaiian kukui nut; *Olive oil,* a mild and soothing emollient.

Natural Soaps

Source: Better Nutrition *magazine (November 1995), pages 72-75*

Listed below are some types of all-natural soaps to look for:

Avocado and Lemon grass Soap—Avocado oil is a rich moisturizer; lemon grass helps keep the natural moisture level balanced.

Basic Castile Soap—The Castilla region of Spain is know for its fine soaps prepared from olive oil.

Carrot and Oatmeal Soap—Carrot oil is rich in retinal, an effective skin softener; oatmeal is ideal for combination skin.

Coconut Oil Soap—Coconut oil one of the most commonly used ingredients in commercial soap; it is an all-vegetable soap and is very mild.

Oatmeal Soap—Oatmeal is added to soaps to give them extra texture, which is helpful in removing surface dirt impurities.

Olive and Aloe—Olive oil has been traced back six thousand years to Syria. Its skin-friendly components include vitamin E, provitamin A, saturated fatty acids (oleic), and unsaturated fatty acids (linoleic). Aloe vera promotes healing and soothes the skin.

Glycerine Soap—Glycerine is found naturally in many plants, and it is also a by-product of soap making.

Honey and Rosemary Clay Soap—These ingredients are said to draw toxins out of the skin and aid in healing minor skin blemishes.

Tea Tree Oil Soap—With its penetrating vegetable oils, this soap keeps the skin clean and healthy.

Skin Care for Babies

Source: Delicious *(September 1996)*

Babies don't produce oil from their sebaceous glands until several weeks after their birth. This is why babies often appear to have dry or flaky skin. The mother's body furnishes the baby with a natural moisturizer called vernix, which serves as a barrier between the baby's skin and the amniotic fluids. If the baby is overdue there will be little vernix, and the baby's skin may look wrinkled or prunish, like from staying in the bath too long.

Natural products for babies are all natural, just like the baby. The most popular herbs in these products are calendula, chamomile, and aloe. These herbs are nourishing, soothing, and gentle, and promote skin healing. For diaper rashes, you will commonly see vitamins E and A added. When mixed into creams, lotions, and oils, naturally scented essential oils derived from herbal extracts, such as rose oil, bergamot, and geranium, are soothing additions to skin care products for our little ones.

Bathe babies only a couple of times a week for the first couple of weeks, and use only water to avoid dryness. Use only natural products on the baby, avoiding products that are perfumed and full of synthetic chemicals.

Cradle cap is addressed by using virgin olive oil and rubbing gently into the scalp, then using a fine-toothed comb on the hair. If dryness of the baby's skin and scalp continues, look to the mother's intake of essential fatty acids. If this is a nursing mother, she is not getting enough omega–3 or omega–6 essential fatty acids. Next, supplement the diet with the right oils. Remove all saturated fats from her diet and supplement with flaxseed, evening primrose, cod liver, or black currant oil.

Skin reactions are mostly from food allergies. Ideally, babies shouldn't eat food other than breast milk for six months until their digestive systems are more developed. If there is continued redness of cheeks, diaper rash, constipation, or eczema, the child is probably allergic to some food. Common food allergies are to wheat, dairy products and eggs.

Diaper rash is usually a yeast overgrowth. This can be given to the baby from the mother and vice versa. A good bacterial supplement is acidophilus and/or bifidus, to use rather than taking antibiotics, which starts a breakdown of the immune system. White vinegar has anti-fungal properties. Use a ratio of one part of vinegar to six parts of water, and follow up with a cream that has calendula or comfrey, but not tea tree, which is too strong. Cornstarch can aggravate yeast if you are using it to help keep the bottom dry. Use a bentonite clay powder instead, but beware of talc, which has molecules similar to asbestos. Healing herbs are powdered rose buds, powdered slippery elm bark, or ground myrrh.

Natural Baby Products
Aubrey Organics—A producer of natural baby products (shampoo, bath soap, and body lotion), which are made with herbal extracts, oils, and natural soaps, and do not contain any harsh synthetics or chemicals.
Diapers—One of the worst offenders has been the disposable diaper, which is made with plastic, synthetic fibers, cellulose, and other environmentally damaging materials. These diapers do not break down in our landfills. There are, however, biodegradable diapers and all-cotton reusable diapers. For your baby's sake and their future, start saving the earth.

Support During Pregnancy
Source: Ayurveda and Aromatherapy *by Drs. Light and Bryan Miller*

Stretch marks are small tears in the skin surface. You can see them at first as red or purplish marks, which eventually fade to a color lighter than your skin. They are caused by rapid weight gain (you don't have to be pregnant to get them). You can assist the body during this process by keeping the skin supple and elastic. True essential oils can minimize the scarring of the skin. Massage or oil the body with essential oils once a day, especially the stomach, breasts, and thighs. The best oils for this condition are frankincense, tangerine, rose, chamomile, sage, rosewood, and neroli.

Skin Care Techniques
Source: Better Nutrition *(February 1996)*
Body Wash—New, all-natural body washes rinse off easier than soap and help hydrate and soothe skin while they clean. Natural ingredients like lavender and peppermint are excellent. Natural humectants hold in antiaging moisture.
Hot Water—Causes blood to rush to the skin's surface and can cause damage to the skin, and make the body perspire, which can lead to dry skin.
Scrubs—Some scrubs are made with shells and this could widen pores. Use scrubs gently.
Astringents—Can inflame skin; some actually dehydrate and age skin, further enlarging pores. Instead, find a natural or nonalcoholic astringent.

Natural Skin Aids—A natural product called jojoba oil cleanses pores. This oil from the bean of a desert bush helps destroy sebum (a mixture of fat and wax produced by the oil glands), which clogs pores.

Facial Lotions, Creams and Toners

Essential oils possess a number of therapeutic qualities. Lavender, neroli, patchouli, and others have the ability to rejuvenate the skin. Many of the essential oils are antiseptic and fight infectious germs. Sensitive skin responds well to rose and neroli, which are anti-inflammatory. Sandalwood and cypress help treat broken veins. Carrier oils, such as avocado and wheat germ, with their high vitamin content, make useful additions to help mature, cracked or dry skin.

Alphahydroxy Acids (AHAs)—New Skin Care

Source: Heritage Store Newsletter *(August 1996)*

In times past, ladies of the French court applied wine to their faces as a beauty treatment, and in the Near East they were using milk baths for that silky soft feeling.

Alpha and beta hydroxyl acids are derived from apples, ginger, oranges, grapefruit, sugarcane, or willow bark. It has been shown that they will gradually peel off the top layers of dead skin and minimize wrinkles. For treating aging skin, this is not a chemical but a natural nontoxic acid. There are five basic types: malic acid from apples, citric acid from citrus, glycolic acid from sugar cane, lactic acid from milk, and tartaric acid from old wine.

AHAs work to loosen the bond, the cellular glue, that holds old dead cells together in the skin's uppermost layers, where visible aging takes place. Borlind of Germany buffers the acids and encases them in liposomes, rendering them safe even for sensitive skin, and making them highly effective due to the liposome action. Reviva Labs adjusts the pH of their cream to facilitate effectiveness; they also use only glycolic acid polymers, which are molecular strands that release slowly into the skin's surface, maximizing the positive effects of the acids.

Choose carefully if you are unfamiliar with these products. The concentration of AHAs in a skin-care product is important, as most people cannot tolerate more than a forty-six percent concentration on a daily basis. If you have sensitive skin, you may need a product with a lower percentage, around twenty-four percent hydroxyl acids. Products made with glycolic acid are more effective at exfoliating (sloughing off dead cells to renew skin) while those made with lactic acid are more moisturizing.

Deodorants: Conventional vs. Natural Deodorant

Source: Delicious *(January 1996), page 41*

Today's harsh chemical deodorants absorb rapidly into your underarm lymph nodes. Most deodorants on the market today are metal based. There are better choices available.

Conventional Deodorant Ingredients

Aluminum zirconium tetrachlorohydrex glycerine—These aluminum salts are used to combat body odors caused by bacterial action on moisture, and are used to impede the body from sweating. Some scientists believe aluminum compounds may cause Alzheimer's disease.

PEG-7 glyceryl cocoate—A fatty acid combined with glycerine and one or two drops of fragrance.

Dipropylene glycol—A clear viscous liquid. It is the most common moisture-carrying vehicle in cosmetics other than water, but is being replaced in cosmetics by safer glycols.

Octoxynol-16—A wax-like emulsifier derived from phenol and obtained from coal tar. It is an agent used to blend nonmixable liquids, dispersing agents, and detergents used in hand creams, lotions, and lipsticks.

Isopropyl myristate—A fatty compound derived from alcohol and myristic acid, it causes blackheads. Scientists are concerned that with usage over a long period of time (e.g., in sun block), it will allow significant absorption of NDRLA (an impurity).

Natural Herbal Spice Deodorant Ingredients
Purified Water
Witch Hazel—A distillate skin freshener, it is made from leaves or twigs of Hamamelis Virginians; the extract is useful in cosmetics for its toning properties.
Vegetable emulsifying wax—Three fatty alcohols (myristyl, cetyl, and stearyl) derived from coconut oil.
Citric acid—Natural pH (a measure of acidity or alkalinity of a solution) adjuster in cosmetics.
Azalene—An anti-inflammatory agent derived from chamomile and yarrow (herbs) that gives cosmetic products a deep blue color.
Clove oil—Derived from cloves, this oil is analgesic, antiseptic and an anti-irritant.

Arm and Hammer Baking Soda
Source: Baking Soda: Over 500 Uses You Probably Never Thought Of

Put water on your armpits and pat with baking soda. This natural deodorant will last most of the day. It allows your body to sweat naturally, without inhibiting the toxicity from expelling itself, which is its natural course. You will not have a foul odor! A new product on the market is a baking soda deodorant.

Baths
Source: Better Nutrition *(November 1995)*

Baths soothe, calm, and revitalize our mind and body. They clean away dirt, pollution, perspiration and oil, plus bacteria that multiply around body fluids and cause odors. Stick to your natural soaps or a hypoallergenic soap. Natural bath oils added to the water, after you have soaked for at least fifteen minutes, help the body to retain moisture. Use natural oils, i.e., jojoba, lavender, rose, jasmine, and chamomile. For bathing, use warm water, rather than hot water, and use a soft towel (cotton or terry) to pat dry, rather than rub vigorously.

There are also baths for sore muscles (Epsom salts) and detoxifying (Epsom salts with sea salt). You can also use 1/2 cup Clorox in bath water without soap for metal detoxification.

Hair and Scalp
Source: Better Nutrition *(March 1996)*

Our hair is a great indicator of our general health. Other indicators are complexion, fingernails, and the clearness of the eyes. Our hair is a form of outer body protection that contains a protein known as keratin. It gets its nourishment from the foods we eat, and responds quickly to lack of nutrients, and to absorption of specific foods. If your parents had strong hair, most likely you will too. Other factors affecting healthy hair are stress, sleep disorders, and lack of protein. Our hair also needs an internal source of oil and moisture. When you are not feeling good, shampooing your hair and massaging your scalp starts the energy flowing from head meridian points; this in turn starts an internal healing process.

Hair's Worst Enemies
1) Too much sun.
2) Chemicals, such as rinses, bleach, and tints.
3) Nylon brushes, which split hair ends and damage over time.
4) Too many carbohydrates, i.e., processed cereals, cake, soda, and sugar.

Ingredients to Look for in Shampoo and Conditioners

Vinegar—To overcome most dandruff and scalp itch, massage diluted or undiluted apple cider vinegar into scalp. To create an aromatic vinegar, add lavender water.

Oil—This is an excellent hair aid. Castor oil strengthens the hair, as does olive oil or flaxseed oil. Massage the warm oil into your hair, then cover your hair with a plastic cap to keep the heat in and allow the oil to penetrate into the hair. Be sure to use a natural shampoo to wash.

Hair or Scalp Problems

Dandruff, dry hair, oily hair, or even lice respond well to specific blends of essential oils such as thyme, sage, and lavender diluted in a carrier oil, such as wheat germ oil. There are also completely natural remedies available.

Gray Hair

The genes that are inherited strongly influence the distribution of an individual's hair—its thickness, quality, color, rate of growth, and whether the hair is curly or straight. One of the reasons hair turns gray is a copper deficiency, which prevents the formation of Tyrosinase, thereby interrupting the pigmentation process. The possible reason that pantothenic acid has been reported to reverse graying is that this nutrient has some function in bonding copper to Tyrosinase. Zinc deficiency can also cause a loss of pigmentation. Edgar Cayce, in readings 2582-2 and 349-25, recommends putting some Irish potato peelings in just enough water to cover, then drinking the broth three times per week to help defer premature graying.

Hair Spray

One serious environmental issue has been to stop the use of aerosol sprays, in beauty and other products, which contain chlorofluorocarbons (CFCs) or man-made gases. These gases form an invisible shield in the atmosphere endangering our natural ozone layer, which protects all living things on Earth. Some states have regulations banning the sale of products containing CFCs. Many products are now sold in pump sprays. Watch for Earth-friendly products. Look for the label that states it is a biodegradable product. But to be on the safe side, if it's an aerosol, don't buy it.

There are now many companies that sell ecologically safe cosmetics and body products that are formulated with one hundred percent natural ingredients. Read the ingredients on the container. There are now natural toothbrushes and hairbrushes with all-natural bristles, alcohol-free mouthwashes, and deodorants without aluminum.

Hair, Skin, Nails, and Nutrition

Source: Energy Times *(March 1996)*

If the body is deprived of proper nourishment, it will affect the hair, skin, and nails. Watch for dry, scaly skin, brittle nails, and dull thinning hair as signs that your diet needs to be evaluated. Drink eight glasses of water for maintaining skin moisture and normal oil secretion for skin, hair, and nails.

Vitamin A—Sloughs off dry skin cells, stimulates the growth of new healthy cells, protects against dryness, premature aging, acne, dandruff, itchy scalp, and dry, splitting nails. Sources: Carrots, squash, sweet potatoes, cantaloupe, beet greens, broccoli, spinach, apricots, fish, and liver.

Vitamin B6 — (pyridoxine) Is necessary for collagen and elastin to help the skin stay smooth, and protect against hair loss. Sources: Soybeans, kale, spinach, bananas, lentils, liver, and salmon.

Vitamin B2 — (riboflavin) A lack may cause gum problems and erosion and cracks at the corners of the mouth. Sources: Cottage cheese, broccoli, low fat milk, yeast, and mushrooms.

Vitamin B3 — (niacin) Maintains the nervous system and the gastrointestinal tract. A lack causes scaling and brownish skin around the neck and on the backs of hands and feet. Sources: Lean meat, fish, soybeans, cottage cheese, beans, peas, yeast and peanut butter.

Vitamin B12 — (cyanocobalamin) A lack causes pale skin and dandruff. Found in cottage cheese, milk, eggs, cheese, liver, and kidneys. (pantothenic acid) Prevents premature aging, and protects against cellular damage caused by sunlight. Sources: Broccoli, soybeans, lentils, yeast, peas, milk, rice, yeast, wheat berries, eggs, and liver.

Vitamin C—Supplies oxygen to capillaries that carry blood to the follicles. This helps keep skin and hair healthy. C is essential to the production of collagen, the glue that holds the cells together. Sources: Orange juice, citrus fruits, cantaloupe, leafy green vegetables, broccoli, and Brussels Sprouts.

Vitamin E — (tocopherol) Increases the oxygen intake of cells, which speeds healing and regeneration. Sources: Corn, brown rice, beet greens, spinach, almonds, and blackberries.

Vitamin F — (unsaturated fatty acids) Maintains skin, hair moisture and radiance by maintaining the cells' proper metabolism rate. Strict fat-free diets may have a lack of fatty acids, which can result in dry, scaly skin, thinning hair and brittle nails. Sources: Seeds, wheat germ, butter, safflower oil, whole grains, lecithin, fish liver oil, and avocados.

Biotin—Wards off split ends, helps make the hair grow faster, strengthens weak nails, and protects against dry skin. Sources: Cauliflower, soybeans, lentils, liver, yeast, cereals, eggs, and peanut butter.

Folic Acid—A lack of folic acid can cause pale skin and premature graying. Source: Garbanzo beans, kidney beans, asparagus, spinach, yeast, liver, romaine lettuce, and orange juice.

Iodine—Protects against rough and wrinkled skin, helps keep hair strong. Sources: Fish and seaweed.

Iron—Is the most important since it promotes healthy red blood cells, good skin color, and strong nails. A deficiency results in darkened under-eye circles, brittle nails, and dull thinning hair. Sources: Prune juice, beans and lentils, spinach, eggs, liver, and blackstrap molasses.

Protein—Maintains the elasticity and structure of the skin, regulates skin pigments, and nourishes healthy hair, which is ninety-seven percent protein and three percent water. Sources: Cheese, fish, beans, nuts, seeds, and super blue-green algae, which is a protein plant food.

Selenium—Keeps skin elastic and young looking. Sources: Seafood, whole grains, eggs, onions, garlic, brewer's yeast, and Brazil nuts.

Silicon—Keeps skin glossy and smooth, strengthens hair. Sources: Apples, avocados, and honey.

Zinc—Has enzymes necessary for wound healing. Sources: Beans, rice bran, soy products, whole grains, yeast, fish, pumpkin seeds, and green peas.

Fiber—Keeps skin clear and healthy, aids digestion and elimination. Sources: Raw fruits and vegetables.

Beauty Enhancement Using Essential Oils

The following two pages are reprinted with permission by Drs. Light and Bryan Miller, authors of Ayurveda and Aromatherapy, and cofounders of Earth Essential Oils.

Essential Oils penetrate deep into the layers of the skin, affecting not just the surface of the skin, but deep within the whole person physically and psychologically. Due to their nourishing, cleansing, and detoxifying qualities, these oils tighten the skin, increase the blood circulation, calm the nervous system and support the skin's functions. As a rule essential oils should always be diluted, whether into a steam bath, a compress, bath oil, body or skin lotions, or massage oil.

The following is a list to help you choose the appropriate essential oil for your skin type. They may be used alone or mixed into a combination with other essential oils.

Normal Skin—Chamomile, geranium, jasmine, neroli, rose, ylang ylang.
Irritated, Troubled Skin—Cedarwood, eucalyptus, peppermint, rosemary.
Oily Skin—Bergamot, camphor, cedarwood, cypress, geranium, juniper berry, lavender, lemon, vetiver.
Dry Skin—Chamomile, clary sage, geranium, lavender, jasmine, neroli, orange, patchouli, rose, vetiver.
Rough, Broken Skin—Chamomile, lavender, rose, sandalwood.
Broken Veins—Chamomile, lavender, neroli, rose, rosewood.
Edemas—Chamomile, birch, clary sage, fennel, juniper berry, cypress, orange, neroli, peppermint.
Acne—Camphor, bergamot, cypress, cedarwood, chamomile, eucalyptus, geranium, lavender, lemon, thyme, sandalwood, peppermint, rosemary.
Sensitive Skin—Chamomile, geranium, jasmine, neroli, rose, rosewood.
Inflamed Skin—Chamomile, clary sage, geranium, jasmine, neroli, sandalwood.
Mature, Aging Skin—Blue chamomile, clary sage, cypress, frankincense, lavender, fennel, neroli, orange, rose, rosewood, sandalwood, vetiver, ylang ylang.
Cellulite—Birch, cypress, juniper berry, lemon, orange, rosemary.
Psoriasis—Bergamot, lavender, neroli, cajeput.

Essential Bath—One of the most soothing and effective ways to use essential oils is to add fifteen to twenty drops to 104°F bath water. Add: rose, cypress, ylang ylang, clary sage, chamomile, lavender, or juniper berry. Each makes a wonderful relaxing bath individually or as a blend. Especially helpful before or after the female cycle. You can also add specific steeped herbs (strained) to the bath.

Essential Facial—Purchase a complexion brush and brush your face (dry) daily. Wash your face with warm water. Use no soap. Pick essential oils according to your skin type and condition (see above). Put thirty drops total into one ounce calendula or jojoba oil and massage into the face with a circular motion, allow skin to absorb.

Clay Mask—Purchase cosmetic grade clay (Indian Earth or Aziec Earth). Mix two tablespoons of clay with juice of one lemon, stir until paste is thick, apply and allow to dry. Wash with hot wash cloth or warm water. Rinse with cool water. Mask should be followed by an essential facial.

Facial Steams—Make a strong tea with your favorite herbs (sage, rose petals, chamomile, lavender, rosemary, lemon grass, peppermint, and marigold flowers) by steeping in covered pot for fifteen minutes. Remove cover and carefully allow the steam to bathe your face. Not recommended for very dry skin.

Hydrolates — (essential waters) Add twenty drops of essential oils according to your skin type and special conditions into spray bottle along with four ounces of distilled water. Spray three to four times per day on your face in a light mist, especially on hot days. Hydrolates can also be purchased premixed.

Essential Oils Added to Body Products
Shampoo—five to ten drops per pint
Conditioner—five to ten drops per pint
Shower Gel—ten to fifteen drops
After Shave Lotion—ten to fifteen drops

Tea—one to three drops per cup
Food—one drop to replace, not add to one teaspoon of powdered herb in a recipe
Perfume—best diluted with oils of calendula, jojoba, almond, or grape seed
Salve—mix approximately ten drops of three or four essential oils to a base of either almond, calendula, or coconut in a small two- to four-ounce brown bottle, let cool, apply to problem area

Earth's Essential Oils
Camphor—Acne, facial wash, cleanser.
Cypress—Astringent, antiseptic, diuretic, oily skin, acne, varicose veins.
Cedar—Astringent, cleanser, antiseptic, oily skin.
Chamomile—Anti-inflammatory, dry skin, inflamed skin, irritated skin, sunburn, eczema, sensitive skin.
Clary Sage—Antiseptic, infections, boils.
Champa—Dry skin, diuretic.
Bergamot—Antiseptic, astringent, cleanser, acne, eczema, herpes, infections, varicose veins, psoriasis.
Birch—Skin sores, inflammations, chronic skin problems, firms and tightens skin.
Eucalyptus—Antiseptic, regenerative, skin blemishes, acne, skin ulcer.
Frankincense—Wrinkles, mature sensitive skin.
Jasmine—Antiseptic, perfumery, dermatitis, eczema, dry, irritated or inflamed skin, stress related skin disorders.
Juniper berries—Diuretic, acne.
Lavender—Deodorizing, circulatory stimulant, detoxifying, tonic, fluid retention, dry skin, all types skin.
Lemon—Antiseptic, detoxifying, oily skin, swollen infected skin, broken veins.
Marjoram—Sensitive skin, varicose veins, broken capillaries.
Neroli—All skin types, sensitive and inflamed skin, aging skin, broken veins.
Orange—Cellulite, dry skin, aging skin, rough skin, poor circulation to skin.
Palmarosa—Sensitive skin, wrinkles, cellular stimulant.
Patchouli—Wrinkles, inflamed skin, fluid retention.
Peppermint—Antiseptic, strengthens skin's normal defenses, cellular stimulant, acne, swollen and blemished skin.
Rosemary—Antiseptic, blemished skin, oily skin.
Rose—Astringent, tonic, cleanser, all skin types—especially dry, wrinkles, skin allergies, baby skin care.
Rosewood—Cellular stimulant.
Sandalwood—Antiseptic, tonic, dry skin, acne, itching skin.
Thyme—Antibacterial, infections.
Ylang Ylang—Oily skin, stressed skin.

Natural Room Freshener
Environmental fragrancing with essential oils instead of synthetics is more effective, fun, and non-allergenic. Add twenty drops of a combination of lemon, bergamot, orange, lavender or lemon grass to plain, filtered water in a spray bottle and spritz the room.

Natural Product Resources

Aubrey Organics (Silken Earth natural cosmetics, hair and baby products), 1-800-AUBREY H
Borglind of Germany, available through many health food stores
Burt's Bees, Inc., 8221A Brownleigh Dr., Raleigh, NC 27612, (919) 510-8720
Earth Science (skin care), 23705 Via Del Rio, Yorbia Linda, CA 92687, 1-800-222-6720
Earth Essential Oils, call 941-316-0920.
Frontier (herbs, bath and aromatherapy products), PO Box 299, Norway, IA 52318, 1-800-786-1388
Kiss My Face (herbal soaps, lotion, lipstick), PO Box 224, Gardiner, NY 12525, 1-800-262-KISS
Living Earth Crafts (OASIS massage oil and beauty products), 1-800-358-8929
Nature's Care, #6 Charles Park, Guilderland, NY 12084, (518) 464-6002
Nature's Plus by Natural Organics, Inc., 548 Broadhollow Rd., Melville, NY 11747
NeemAura Naturals, 4605 NW 6th St., Suite H, Gainsville, FL 32609, (352) 375-2503
Orjene Natural Cosmetics, 543 48th Ave., Long Island City NY 11101, 1-800-88ORJEN
Simmons Pure Soaps (natural products), 42295 Hwy. 36, Bridgeville, CA 95526, 1-800-428-0412
Pro Life Massage Oil, 1-800-900-7873, or Jason Massage Products, 1-800-JASON-05

Book References

Aromatherapy for Common Ailments by Shirley Price
Ayurveda and Aromatherapy by Drs. Light and Bryan Miller
A Consumer's Dictionary of Cosmetic Ingredients by Ruth Winter
Blended Beauty, Botanical Secrets for Body and Soul by Philip B.
Essential Oils that Build Natural Defenses, the Science of Aromatherapy by Dr. William H. Lee
The Complete Herbal Guide to Natural Health and Beauty by Dian Dincin Buchman
The Green Witch Herbal by Barbara Griggs
The Illustrated Encyclopedia of Essential Oils by Julia Lawless
Feather River Co. Cosmetic Ingredient Glossary (Feather River)
Natural Organic Hair and Skin Care by Aubrey (Organica Press)
Natural and Synthetic Chemicals in Cosmetics by Aubrey (Organica Press)

Organizations

National Association of Holistic Aromatherapy, Box 17622, Boulder, CO 80308
The American Alliance of Aromatherapy, Box 750428, Petaluma, CA 94975
Transitions for Health (mail order catalog of natural health products for menopausal women) 621 Southwest Alder, Suite 900, Portland, OR 97206, 1-800-888-6814

Chapter Five

Ayurveda—Wisdom of the Ancients

Ayurveda is the most ancient healing system of India; people have been following it for at least five thousand years. It seems that Ayurveda and Chinese traditional medicine have an even older common root system than what was previously known. The holy men known as the Rishis compiled the ancient Hindu philosophical and spiritual texts called the Vedas. This is a remarkable system of knowledge, comprised of the science of life as revealed to the Rishis through what we today call "divine inspiration."

Ayu means life, *Veda* means knowledge. So Ayurveda (pronounced "ah-your-vay-dah") stands for the knowledge of how to live, or health. It has many common links to indigenous peoples' medicine: a marked emphasis on prevention, an unquestioned acceptance of the mind/body/spirit unit of each human being, and an understanding of our connection to the all and to our environment.

The four main branches of the Vedic sciences are:

1) Self-knowledge.
2) Yoga: Right path, emphases all aspects of living healthily and harmoniously in the world.
3) Medic astrology.
4) Ayurveda: The science that deals with physical healing, diet, herbs, and bodywork massage. This was originally intended to support the body, so that the spiritual development could be pursued unhindered by health concerns. Its methods are noninvasive and nontoxic, and heavily dependent on the individual's willingness to participate voluntarily in a healthier way of life. Along with the eight branches of traditional medicine, India's hospitals and more than a quarter of a million practitioners promote this healing tradition. Dr. Deepak Chopra has been instrumental in promoting healthy living. Dr. Chopra is an author, and lectures throughout the world.

Ayurveda is based on a concept of vital energy called "prana," which is the primal energy that enlivens the body and mind. The Chinese call this "chi energy." It is this unseen power that is the basis of all life and healing, and is considered to have the qualities of a nutrient that can be taken into the body through the breath. Breathing exercises hold an important role in health promotions according to Ayurveda.

The Five Elements

The heart of Ayurveda is the concept that all of existence comprises five basic elements: earth, air, fire, water, and ether, a belief that is similar to the Native Americans' four directions, with the center/heart being spirit or ether. Ayurveda uses this as the basis for treatment, which includes aromatherapy, Indian music (called gandarvaveda) a form of self-massage, and incorporating the six tastes daily in one's diet. These terms represent principles of action and interaction that guide and shape all existence on the material world plane and in life's processes. All five elements work together as one. These elements are present in all matter in the universe. This energy flows from Cosmic Consciousness, Divine Creator, or the One. The actions of these elements serve as the basis for understanding our health, illness, and individual constitution, and how to restore and maintain harmony in the body.

In simple terms, Ayurvedic philosophy sees the cosmos (humans are a part of) as divisible into three basic broad principles known as "dosha": Vata (Vahtah), Pitta (Pitah), and Kapha (Kafah). Together they determine our personal metabolism and our psychophysiological, or mind/body, type. The unique pattern that they take in each of us at conception is called our "prakriti." There are seven general patterns possible, with subtle variations. The prakriti for each person is diagnosed and described according to which dosha are naturally predominant, and which are the least dominant, in a person's function.

Ayurveda Breakdown

Dosha theory: A medical concept developed in the five-thousand-year-old tradition of Ayurveda is the creative struggle mankind faces to stay healthy. The dosha theory emphasizes Vata, Pitta, and Kapha, which are believed to be essential to human existence on the spiritual, physical, emotional, and intellectual levels. Within the unique imprint of these three elements is a peculiar form of genetic coding. To learn about your dosha imprint is like getting to know your genetic makeup. A self-diagnosis of our health can be done by a self-analysis of ourselves in our daily routines, in a conscientious and intelligent way, using our senses of sight and smell. Checking your tongue (and how this relates back to major body organs and your urine along with the charts and information pertaining to the three dosha). This information will help you understand which one or two dosha predominate in you.

Vata—Incorporates the elements ether and air, has to do with movement, and is the lightest of the dosha. Vata represents easy movement at all levels and in all ways. It governs the cells, the circulation of fluids and materials through the cells and through the body, and the activity of organs and muscles as they perform their functions. It also guides the motor and sensory functions of a person as they move through the world, and the movements of thoughts through the mind. Vata-predominant people tend to be active, alert, and restless. They need to be involved; movement and activity are needed to feel a sense of harmony. They have a lot of energy, although they are not always focused with that energy. They are often fiddling or doodling, and can't sit still. They are likely to spend money easily, and prefer to be self-employed rather than work for someone. They are unpredictable, thin, hungry anytime, enthusiastic, have light-boned builds, cool dry skin, cramps, and constipation, are irregular sleepers, moody, and hyperactive, hate the cold and love the sun, and are not always practical. Vata disperses.

Pitta—Transforms and incorporates the elements fire and water, and has to do with all metabolism or digestion and the transformation of food into energy, which ultimately goes into the tissues of the body and governs the body's temperature. Pitta-predominant people are often involved in transformation types of activity, taking one thing and changing it into something else. They may also have fiery qualities in their personality, such as a lot of anger, irritability, aggressiveness or competitiveness. These people are inclined to budget their money and transform it into useful things, such as stock market investments, in order to improve their standard of living. They are predictable, medium set, confident, courageous, aggressive, intense, efficient, orderly, intelligent, insightful and ambitious, leaders and planners, regular sleepers; they have athletic builds, warm wet skin, heartburn, ulcers, hemorrhoids; they tire easily in excessive heat, hate to miss a meal, eat a lot and love spicy, oily foods, and enjoy physical and mental challenges. Pitta transforms.

Kapha—Incorporates the elements water and earth, and has to do with stability. It is the densest element. It provides the physical structure and contents of the body, and is the bodily tissue, fluid and substance. It brings about the healing of wounds, fills spaces, and brings physical strength and resiliency to the body. Kapha people tend to be heavy, slow moving, and solid and have great muscular strength. They are usually stable and grounded, with a steady and tranquil personality. They tend to hold onto money and are likely to be wealthy because of their tendency to accumulate. They don't like to move around much, and tend to make good middle managers. Relaxed and heavyset, they have square powerful builds, exotic heavy features and lustrous hair, oily cool skin, allergies, and high cholesterol. They are forgiving, tolerant, and tend to procrastinate. They're graceful, relaxed, compassionate, loyal and calm, they like to sleep a lot, are reliable workers, enjoy gourmet foods and make money easily. Kapha accumulates.

Ayurveda physicians identify the person's constitution (or dosha) by measuring the pulse and examining the tongue and skin. Pulse diagnosis is an essential diagnostic tool; it is done with three fingers.

Each of us has some unique blend of these three principles in our basic physioemotional makeup. In addition, the balance that we have of these three in our systems at any given time depends upon the choices we have made in living. To help maintain inner balance, meditation is a method that allows us to stay centered during the day.

Health Imbalances

Ayurveda health is considered a balance and harmony among all of these forces, within the person and between the person and their environment. The optimal state is one in which the person is living in accordance with their prakriti at conception. In other words, their life style and current state of health reflect alignment with their unique constitution. Illness occurs when a person falls out of alignment with this inborn pattern. Imbalances can be caused by chronic stress, eating certain foods, environmental toxins, inadequate rest, and other factors. In keeping with the Ayurveda focus on the mind/body connection, repressed emotions are considered an important cause for imbalance.

Diseases are classified according to whether their origins are spiritual, physical or psychological, where they manifest in the body, and what dosha they represent. Since we each have all three dosha, we can have disorders caused by imbalances in any one or all three of them. However, most problems are associated with our predominant dosha.

Another important concept is elimination of waste materials from the body. A great deal of attention is given to detoxification and elimination of "ama" through the three malas: sweat, urine, and feces. Production and elimination are considered absolutely essential to health.

Vata people are most likely to have conditions such as intestinal gas, lower back pain, sciatica, arthritis, paralysis, neuralgia and nervous system diseases.
Pitta people are most likely to have gallbladder, liver and bile disorders, hyperacidity, peptic ulcers, gastritis, inflammatory diseases, and skin disorders such as hives and rash.
Kapha people are most likely to have tonsillitis, bronchitis, sinusitis, and lung congestion.

Food and the Six Tastes

The therapy of the Ayurveda diet is oriented towards rebalancing the dosha. Thus, there are specific diets for reducing or pacifying each dosha, depending upon which one is out of balance. The tastes of the foods are a key in Ayurveda, because they provide clues to which foods are helpful and which are harmful. Dietary guidelines are based upon one's body type or current imbalance. When we have a preference for certain tastes, this usually indicates that those tastes are needed to balance our predominant dosha. Extreme cravings or addictions to tastes could indicate an underlying imbalance that will be further aggravated by those tastes.

1) sour (yogurt, lemon, cheese)
2) sweet (sugar, milk, butter, rice, breads, pasta)
3) salty (salt)
4) bitter (green leafy vegetables, turmeric)
5) pungent (spicy foods, ginger, hot peppers, cumin)
6) astringent (beans, lentils, pomegranate)

Ayurvedic Body Style Massage Blends

Vata—Base oil of sesame or avocado with herbs: ashwagandha, brahmi, and comfrey; and essential oils of clary sage, jasmine and sandalwood.

Pitta—Base oil of sunflower or safflower with herbs: amalaki, coriander, and majishta; and essential oils of gardenia, lemon grass and vetiver.

Kapha—Base oil of olive or almond with herbs: bibtaki, fenugreek, and neem; and essential oils of cedar, frankincense, and patchouli.

Aromatherapy

Can be used by anyone. Self-massage is recommended to get in touch with ourselves in a touch-starved society. Gandarvaveda music helps restore balance and there are specific versions for times of day and for the three main versions, Vata, Pitta, or Kapha. There are special aromatherapy misting machines or diffusers to fill your home with the pure fresh fragrance of essential oils.

Ayurveda Skin Care

The first step is to clean the body's organs through proper digestion and elimination (see the section on detoxification). The state of our digestion is linked to our skin problems. Embryonically, the lining of the digestive system is similar to the skin. It develops from the same cells as the outer layer of the body.

Guidelines for digestion include:
1) Never eat when angry, upset, exhausted, bored or in depression.
2) Bathe before eating; if not practical, wash your hands and face, and brush your hair.
3) Eat either alone or with people who relax you.
4) Eat in surroundings that are quiet, peaceful, and colorful; play music and perhaps light some candles.
5) Environmentally, facing east maximizes the energy for digestion.
6) Observe regular meal times, leave three to six hours between meals and to allow the digestion system to rest.
7) For proper nutrition, foods should be organic, in season and fit a person's personality (dosha).
8) Exercise helps improve blood circulation and is an important part of your life style.

After life style adjustments, the following Ayurveda skin product herbs are mixed for your specific dosha: burdock root, dandelion, red clover, yarrow, turmeric, heart-leafed moonseed and sandalwood. Ayurveda medicine always combines the herbs, and they must be mixed in proper amounts. There

AYURVEDA DOSHA CHART

Instructions: Check each box that pertains to you, basing your choice on what is most consistent over a long period of time. This is to find your basic constitution. Complete the form again based on your current state. This will tell you where you may have an imbalance that should be corrected, and guide you towards the proper diet. ©1994 reprinted with permission by Usha and Dr. Vasant Lad, authors of *Ayurvedic Cooking for Self-Healing*.

Guideline for Determining Your Constitution

Observations	V P K	Vata	Pitta	Kapha
Body size	O O O	Slim	Medium	Large
Body weight	O O O	Low	Medium	Overweight
Chin	O O O	Thin, angular	Tapering	Rounded, double
Cheeks	O O O	Wrinkled, sunken	Smooth flat	Rounded, plump
Eyes	O O O	Small, sunken, dry, active black brown,	Sharp, bright, gray, green, nervous yellow/red, sensitive to light	Big, beautiful, blue, calm, loving
Nose	O O O	Uneven shaper deviated septum	Long pointed, red nose-tip	Short rounded, button nose
Lips	O O O	Dry, cracked, black/brown	Red, inflamed, yellowish	Smooth, oily, palm whitish
Teeth	O O O	Stickout, big, roomy, thin gums	Mcdium, soft, tender gums	Healthy, white strong gums
Skin	O O O	Thin, dry, cold, rough,	Smooth, oily, warm, rosy	Thick, oily, cool, white, pale
Hair	O O O	Dry brown, black, knotted, bridle, scarce	Straight, oily, blond, W. red, bald	Thick, curly, oily, wavy, luxuriant
Nails	O O O	Dry, rough, brittle, break easily	Sharp, flexible, pink, lustrous	Thick, oily, smooth, polished
Neck	O O O	Thin, tall	Medium	Big, folded
Chest	O O O	Flat, sunken	Moderate	Expanded, round
Belly	O O O	Thin, flat, sunken	Moderate	Big pot-bellied
Belly-Button	O O O	Small, irregular, herniated	Oval, superficial	Big, deep, round, stretched
Hips	O O O	Slender, thin	Moderate	Heavy, big
Joints	O O O	Cold, cracking	Moderate	Large, lubricated
Appetite	O O O	Irregular, scanty	Strong unbearable	Slow but steady
Digestion	O O O	Irregular, forms gas	Quick, causes burning	Prolonged, forms mucous
Taste	O O O	Sweet, sour, salty	Sweet, bitter, astringent	Bitter, pungent, astringent
Thirst	O O O	Changeable	Surplus	Sparse
Elimination	O O O	Constipation	Loose	Thick, oily, sluggish
Physical Activity	O O O	Hyperactive	Moderate	Slow
Mental Activity	O O O	Hyperactive	Moderate	Dull, slow
Emotions	O O O	Anxiety, few, uncertainty	Anger, hate, jealousy	Calm, greedy, attachment
Faith	O O O	Variable	Extremist	Consistent
Intellect	O O O	Quick but faulty response	Accurate response	Slow, exact
Recollection	O O O	Recent good, remote poor	Distinct	Slow and sustained
Dreams	O O O	Quick. active, many, fearful	Fiery, war, violence	Lakes, snow, romantic
Sleep	O O O	Scanty broken up, sleeplessness	Little but sound	Deep, prolonged
Speech	O O O	Rapid, unclear	Sharp, penetrating	Slow, monotonous
Financial	O O O	Poor, spends on trifles	Spends money on luxuries	Rich, good money preserver

are now premixed products on the market. In the book *Ayurveda Beauty Care,* there are remedies that can be mixed in your own kitchen, with recipes for cleansing, herbal steams, scrubs, masks, toning and full-body massage oil. There are also Ayurveda cookbooks available, in the natural product section of your local bookstores.

Ayurveda Vitamins and Minerals

The following pages are printed with permission of Dr. Light Miller (ND), author of Ayurveda and Aromatherapy *and co-founder of Earth Essential Oils – Florida. Call (941) 316-0920) to order oils and for workshop and seminar schedules.*

Vitamin A and Beta Carotene
Vata: Fish oils, carrots, spinach, red pepper, winter squash, sweet potatoes, yams, mangos.
Pitta: Kale, collard greens, turmeric, lemon grass, mangos, cabbage, raspberry leaves, dandelion, mints, cilantro, lamb, spirulina, dark leafy greens.
Kapha: Lemon grass, parsley, spinach, mangos, nettles, mints, soaked seaweed, dry paprika, sage, cayenne, chickweed, kelp, turmeric.

Vitamin B1 (Thiamine)
Metabolism.

Note on B vitamins: It is best to take all B vitamins together in a complex; isolated B vitamins create deficiency of other Bs. They are depleted by smoking or second hand smoke, medication, and antibiotics.
Vata: Asparagus, shatavari (asparagus), citrus, garlic, blackstrap molasses, seaweed (nori, kelp), catnip, watercress.
Pitta: Cauliflower, kale, barley grass, seaweed, asparagus, dandelion, red clover, raspberry leaf, catnip.
Kapha: Cauliflower, kale, citrus, spirulina, garlic, ghee, asparagus, brewer's yeast, dandelion, red clover, raspberry leaf, watercress.

Depleted by alcohol, coffee, and sugar.

Vitamin B2
Emotional Balance, Blood
Vata: Raspberry leaves, catnip, hops, dulse, currants, watercress, rose hips, ginseng, mushrooms, organ meats, blackstrap molasses, parsley, fenugreek.
Pitta: Brussels Sprouts, red clover, raspberry leaves, alfalfa, yarrow, sago palm, steamed onions, legumes, dandelion, yellow dock.
Kapha: Nettles, red clover, peppermint, rose hips, beans, beet greens, asparagus, shatavari, legumes, parsley, dandelion, fenugreek, yellow dock.

Depleted by hot flashes, crying jags, antibiotics, and tranquilizers.

Vitamin B3 (Niacin)
Vata: Peanuts, rice bran, potatoes, burdock root, hops.
Pitta: Milk, rice bran, potatoes, burdock root, hops, raspberry leaves.
Kapha: Potatoes, burdock root, hops, raspberry leaves.

Vitamin B4 (Choline)
Vata: Egg yolk, organ meats, wheat germ.
Pitta: Soybeans.
Kapha: Brewer's yeast, soybeans.

Vitamin B5 (Pantothenic Acid)
Muscle spasms, allergies, adrenal insufficiency, assists the body in producing cortisone.
Vata: Rice bran, organ meats, egg yolk.
Pitta: Green vegetables, legumes, soybeans.
Kapha: Green vegetables, legumes, soybeans.
Depleted by stress, overwork, and not enough self-care.

Vitamin B6 (Pyridoxine)
Immune system, skin, herpes sores, cancer preventative.
Vata: Fish, turnips, cooked spinach, green pepper, organ meats, blackstrap molasses, wheat germ.
Pitta: Broccoli, kale
Kapha: Fish, spinach.
Produced by healthy intestines.
Depleted by constipation, fasting, oral contraceptives, radiation, and heart problems.

Vitamin B7 (Biotine)
Consult Ayurveda diet/dosha type.
Vata: Liver, sardines, whole grains.
Pitta: Unpolished rice, legumes, whole grains.
Kapha: Citrus, whole grains.

Vitamin B7 (Inositol)
Consult Ayurveda diet/dosha type.
Vata: Blackstrap molasses, whole grains.
Pitta: Milk, whole grains.
Kapha: Citrus, whole grains.

Vitamin B12
Vata: Pork, cheese, lamb, banana, kelp, comfrey, catnip, seaweeds (kelp, dulse).
Pitta: Freshwater fish, milk, banana, alfalfa, catnip, miso.
Kapha: Kelp, peanuts, alfalfa, miso.

Vitamin B13 (Pangamic Acid)
Consult Ayurveda diet/dosha type.
Vata: Brown rice, laetril (apple seeds), grape seeds, nuts/seeds, wheatgrass, pink lentils (well cooked).
Pitta: Sunflower seeds, laetril (apple seeds), grape seeds, legumes, nuts/seeds, wheatgrass.
Kapha: Brewer's yeast, pumpkin seeds, sesame seeds, laetril (apple seeds), grape seeds, lentils, legumes.

Vitamin B (Niacin)
Anxiety, depression.
Vata: Hops, slippery elm, asparagus, bee pollen, licorice, rice syrup.
Pitta: Slippery elm, spirulina, echinacea, cabbage, red clover, licorice, nettles, rice syrup.
Kapha: Spirulina, bee pollen, nettles, parsley.

Vitamin C
Strong bones, circulation, night sweats, infections, immune builder, adrenal builder, menopause.
Vata: Acerola, tamarind, lemon saffron, strawberries, rose hips, comfrey, primrose oil.
Pitta: Yellow dock, dandelion, raspberries, red clover, alfalfa, rose hips, green pepper, saffron, kale, sago palm, cabbage, primrose oil.
Kapha: Red clover, alfalfa, yellow dock, raspberries, rose hips, spinach, beet greens, parsley, strawberries, cayenne, cabbage, primrose oil.

Depleted by aspirins, pain reliever, coffee, stress, smoking, baking soda, fevers, and pain killers.

Bioflavonoids
Varicose veins, circulation.
Vata: Apricots, blackstrap molasses, citrus pulp, rind amlal or amalaki, plum, rose hips, tomatoes, black currants.
Pitta: Buckwheat, grapefruit, bulgar, broccoli, papaya, algae, shepherd's purse, chervil, elderberries, horsetail, apricot, sweet pepper, violet leaf.
Kapha: Buckwheat, greens, blue-green algae, rose hips, pepper, prune, lemon, parsley, violet leaf, tamarind, horsetail, citrus (consult Ayurveda diet/dosha type).

Depleted by poor diet, lack of exercise, pregnancy, losing and gaining weight, antibiotics, aspirin and pain relievers, sulfa, mental/physical stress, inhalation of petroleum fumes, and genetics.

Vitamin D
Strong bones, cancer prevention, balances glucose.
Vata: Ghee, eggs, cod, liver, shrimp, tuna, mackerel, sardines, sunflower seeds.
Pitta: Trout, egg white, ghee, butter, sunflower seeds, alfalfa, nettles, raspberry leaves, red clover.
Kapha: Ghee, trout, sunlight, alfalfa, nettles, raspberry leaves, red clover.

Depleted by mineral oil.

Vitamin E
Night sweats, cancer, wrinkles, arthritic joints, aging process. Consult Ayurveda diet/dosha type.
Vata: Brown rice, oats, shatavari, cold pressed oils, organ meats, blackstrap molasses, sweet potato, watercress, rose hips, nuts.
Pitta: Alfalfa, rose hips, buckwheat, sunflower oil, sweet potato, dandelion, cold pressed oils.
Kapha: Wheat, corn, rye, almond oil, cold pressed oils, watercress, dandelion.

Vitamin F
Consult Ayurveda diet/dosha type.
Vata: Ghee, sunflower seeds, vegetable oils.
Pitta: Butter, ghee, sunflower seeds, vegetable oils.
Kapha: Ghee, vegetable oils.

Vitamin K
Consult Ayurveda diet/dosha type.
Vata: Safflower oil, blackstrap molasses, kelp, green leafy vegetables.
Pitta: Safflower oil, cauliflower, alfalfa, nettles, green leafy vegetables.
Kapha: Cauliflower, alfalfa, nettles, kelp, green leafy vegetables.
Depleted by frozen foods, rancid fats, radiation, sulfate drugs, and sulfates in food.

Vitamin O
Vata: Pinto beans, all legumes, soybeans.
Kapha: Pinto beans, all legumes, soybeans.

Vitamin T
Consult Ayurveda diet/dosha type.
Vata: Sesame seeds, egg yolk, raw seeds.
Pitta: Butter, raw seeds.
Kapha: Raw seeds.

Vitamin U
Vata: Fermented vegetables.
Pitta: Raw cabbage, leafy green vegetables.
Kapha: Raw cabbage, sauerkraut, leafy green vegetables.

Folic Acid
Healthy bones, calm nerves, flexibility of tissues, adrenal insufficiency.
Vata: Catnip, comfrey, dark green vegetables, root vegetables, salmon, parsley, sage.
Pitta: Greens, plantain, chickweed, peppermint, kale, broccoli, milk, nettles, alfalfa.
Kapha: Nettles, alfalfa, parsley, sage, chickweed, broccoli, kale, beet greens, dark green vegetables, oysters, root vegetables, catnip.

PABA
Vata: Organ meats, wheat germ oil, yogurt, molasses.
Pitta: Green leafy vegetables.
Kapha: Green leafy vegetables.

Arsenic: Asparagus (VK), celery (VPK), salmon (V)

Boron: All sweet and sour fruit (V), purslane (V), dandelion (P), yellow dock (P), chickweed (PK), astringent fruit (P), bitter herbs (K)

Barium: Organic fruit (VPK), vegetables (VPK), nuts (V), chickweed (PK), purslane (VP), nettles (PK), dandelion root (V-PK+), dandelion leaf (PK), yellow dock (PK-V+)

Bromine: Melons (VP), cucumber (VP), alfalfa (PK), turnips (PK), seafood (VK)

Calcium:	Raw egg yolk (V), shellfish (V), milk (P), cheese (V), greens (PK), apricots (VPK), figs (VP), cabbage (PK), bran (VK), alfalfa (PK), red clover (PK), comfrey (VK), nettles (PK), shepherd's purse (PK-V+), horsetail (PK-V+), coltsfoot (K), chamomile (VPK), plantain (PK), borage (VPK), chicory (PK-V-), dandelion (P), kelp (VP), dulse (VK) Depleted by enemas, lack of exercise, coffee, sugar, alcohol, and cortisone.
Chlorine:	Goat and cow milk (P), salt (V), fish (VK), cheese (V), cream cheese (P), coconut (VP), beets (VK), radishes (VP-K+), avocado (VK), kelp (V-PK+)
Chromium:	Corn oil (VK), clams (VK), whole grain cereals (VP), brewer's yeast (VP+/K+), barley grass (PK), bee pollen (PK-V+), red clover (PK), catnip (PK-V+), sarsaparilla (PV-K+)
Cobalt:	Organ meat (V), seafood (V), clams (V), poultry (P), milk (P), green leafy vegetables (PVK), fruits (PVK)
Copper:	Organ meat (V), seafood (V), nuts (V), legumes (PK), molasses (V), raisins, soaked (P), whole grain cereals (VPK—check dosha), watercress (VK), spinach (PV-K+), garlic (K), kale (PK-V+), cabbage (PK-V+), chickweed (PK), chard (PV)
Fluorine:	Cauliflower (PK-V+), cabbage (PK), cheese (V), raw goat milk (P), egg yolk (V), Brussels sprouts (PK)
Fluoride:	Tea (V), seafood (VK), watercress (VK), spinach (K), garlic (K)
Iodine:	Seaweed (VP), seaweed, soaked (P), kelp (V), seafood (V), carrots (VK), pears (PK), onions (PK), tomatoes (V), pineapple (VK), parsley (KP-V+), sarsaparilla (PK), dulse (VP), mushrooms (PV), Irish moss (V-PK+)
Iron:	Organ meat (VP), eggs (V), fish (VK), poultry (VPK), blackstrap molasses (V), apricots (VP), potato peelings (PK), nettles (PK-V+), dandelion (PK), alfalfa (PK-V+), fennel (PKV), yellow dock (PK-V+), comfrey (VP-K+), chickweed (PK), mullein (PK-V+), sorrel (VK-P+), watercress (VK) Depleted by black tea and high protein diet.
Magnesium:	Nuts (V), figs (V), green vegetables (PK), seafood (V), molasses (V), yellow corn (VP), coconut (PK), apples (PK), watercress (VK), alfalfa (PK-V+), oatstraw (VK), clover (VPK), nettles (PK-V+), burdock (PK), carrots (VK), horsetail (PK), raspberry (VP), sage (PK) Depleted by chemical drugs.
Manganese:	Beets (V), peas (PK), citrus (VK), rice bran (VP), green vegetables (PK), kelp (V-PK+), nuts (V), pineapple (V)

Molybdenum: Legumes (PK), whole grain cereals (VPK), milk (P), dark green vegetables (PK), liver (VP)

Nickel: All vegetables (VPK), all herbs (VPK), alfalfa (PK), oatstraw (PK-V+), fenugreek (VK-P+), red clover (PK)

Phosphorus: Milk (P), cheese (V), meat (V), fish (P), fowl (P), egg yolk (V), beans (PK), peas (PK), caraway seed (KV-P+), parsley (KV-P+), comfrey (PV-K+), watercress (KV-P+), nettles (PK-V+), chickweed (PK-V+), alfalfa (PK-V+), marigold (PK-V+), dandelion (PK-V+), licorice (VP-K+), lentils, well cooked (V), grains (check dosha)
Depleted by sugar, mental stress, and high fat.

Potassium: Lean meats (PK), dried fruits (K), dried soaked fruits (VP), vegetables (PVK), nuts (V), seeds (V), alfalfa (PK-V+), comfrey (PV-K+), coltsfoot (PK-V+), watercress (KV-P+), borage (PK-V+), chicory (PK-V+), eyebright (PK-V+), mint (PK-V+), kelp (V-KP+), plantain (PK-V+), parsley (KV-P+), dulse (V), grains (check dosha)
Depleted by excess urination, excess perspiration, and salt intake.

Selenium: Tuna (V), herring (VP), brewer's yeast (VK), wheat germ/bran (V), broccoli (PK), whole grains (check dosha)

Silicon: Apples (PK), kelp (V-KP+), grapes (VP), beets (V), almonds (VK), seeds (V), parsnips (VPK), tomatoes (V-PK+), spinach (PK), horsetail (PK-V+), dandelion (PK-V+), nettles (PK), leeks (VPK), strawberries (VK), sweet onions, well-cooked (VP), grains (check dosha)

Sodium: Watermelon (V-PK+), romaine (PK-V+), celery (VPK), kelp (V-PK+), sea salt (V), asparagus (VPK), okra (VP), carrots (VK), coconut (PK)

Sulfur: Eggs (V-PK+), ocean fish (V), freshwater fish (PK), cabbage (PK), Brussels sprouts (PK), horseradish (KV-P+), shrimp (VK), chestnuts (PK), nettles (PK-V+), plantain (PK-V+), parsley (KV-P+), kale (PK), coltsfoot (PK-V+), mullein (PK-V+), sage (KV-P+), shepherd's purse (PK-V+), cabbage family (PK), meat (consult dosha)

Tin: Plants and animals

Vanadium: Herring (V), sardines (V), vegetables grown in vanadium rich soil

Zinc: Sunflower seeds (VP), seafood (V), organ meats (V), mushrooms (VP), soybeans (PK), brewer's yeast (K), watercress (VK-P+), pumpkin seeds (VK)
Depleted by air pollution, alcohol, and pregnancy.

Book Resources

Ayurveda and Aromatherapy by Drs. Light and Bryan Miller
Ayurveda Beauty Care by Melanie Sachs
Ayurveda Cooking for Self-Healing by Usha and Dr. Vasant Lad
Ayurveda Healing: A Comprehensive Guide by David Frawley
Perfect Health: The Complete Mind/Body Guide by Dr. Deepak Chopra
Ayurveda, the Science of Self-Healing by Dr. Vasant Lad
Yoga on Herbs by Drs. David Frawley and Vasant Lad

Chapter Six

Natural Earth Healing—Environmental

Everyday Personal Products Chemically Influenced
Source: Connecting Link Magazine, *Issue 28, page 86*

Scientists and professionals, through numerous articles, are warning the public of the harmful ingredients in shampoos, conditioners, toothpaste, skin lotions, cosmetics, baby wipes, etc. There is excellent information out there. Before buying products, check to see if any of the following ingredients are listed:

Nitrates and Dioxins are serious carcinogens, and both are found in shampoos.

Sodium Laurel Sulfate (SLS) is found in most shampoos, bubble baths and shower gels; it is also found in toothpastes, even the ones in health food stores. This is what industrial chemists use to clean garage floors and degrease engines; it is also found in car wash soap. This chemical cleans by corrosion. When SLS gets down into the hair follicle, it literally corrodes it and plugs it up; its use can lead to baldness.

Propylene Glycol is a humectant used by the cosmetic industry, which is also found in antifreeze and brake fluid. Because of the effects of cleaning them by corrosion, our skin and hair can't hold onto moisture and start to dry out. Propylene glycol mixes well with the above degreaser, SLS, and water, giving you a smooth, greasy feeling. When applied, it holds in the moisture by "greasing your skin." However, it also keeps the skin from breathing and prevents toxins from escaping through the skin (skin is the main eliminator of toxins in our body). This could lead to liver and kidney damage. If you purchase Propylene Glycol from a supplier, he is required to furnish you with an MSDS (Material Safety Data Sheet), stating "Avoid skin contact."

Mineral Oil is distilled from crude oil petroleum and suffocates the skin.

Glycerin draws moisture from the inside out.

Collagen and elastin are of high molecular weight and also suffocate the skin. They are derived from animal skins and ground-up chicken feet.

Soaps from animal fats and lye create a great environment for bacteria to feed and grow in.

Fluoride in toothpaste has been fought against by scientists for years. Native Americans and Hawaiians did not use fluoride and did not have cavities, which are diet influenced.

Talcum powder has been made with asbestos; check out your brand.

Chemical Ingredients to Avoid in Cosmetics, Shampoos, Conditioners, Fragrances, Etc.

First learn to read the labels.

Propylene Glycol	Nitrates	Dioxins
Petrolatum (mineral oil)	Sodium Laurel Sulfate	Synthetic Colors
Stearalkonium Chlorine	Triethanolamine	Synthetic Fragrances
Prowl	Butyl	Ethyl Paraben
Methyl	Imidazolidinyl Urea	Diazolidinyl Urea
Copolymer		

Lead-Free Faucets

Source: Bottom Line *(1996)*

NSF International, a standards-setting group, now certifies individual faucet models for compliance with safety standards for lead, cadmium, mercury and other toxic substances. Standards were developed by the plumbing industry, the public health profession and the U.S. Environmental Protection Agency.

The test involved holding water in faucets for specified periods over nineteen days. The water was then tested to determine if it had picked up any of the potentially dangerous , which are sometimes used in the faucets themselves.

For a list of NSF-approved models call 1-800-673-8010 (main testing laboratory).

National Science Foundation Website: www.nsf.org (information for consumers).

Environmental Protection Agency 1-800-426-4791 (safe drinking water hotline).

Water

Sources: Nebraska Environmental Training Center and Nebraska Rural Water Association. Longevity (March 1994) has a listing of how your state stacks up in violations of "water treatment."

Article upon article is being written about aluminum and fluoride in our drinking water. Contact the Clean Water Network, 1350 New York Avenue NW, Washington, DC 20005, (202) 289-2395 with any questions.

Why does the United States still favor water fluoridation? Water is the most essential commodity we have.

So, What Chemicals Are in Your Water?

Source: Better Nutrition *(February 1996)*

Environmentally concerned communities are upset that our government is fluoridating all of the water supplies in our country, especially when twelve Nobel Prize winners have termed the process "worthless." Many foreign countries have discontinued fluoridation of water, including Austria, Belgium, Chile, Denmark, Egypt, France, Germany, Greece, Holland, India, Italy, Luxembourg, Norway, Spain, and Sweden. The United States is one of the few countries still promoting this technique, which has been considered ineffective against tooth decay. Fluoride, put into use fifty years ago, has been linked with many of our leading known diseases. In a study of effects of various pollutants on abnormal plant development, fluoride was shown to be more toxic than lead, and only slightly less toxic than arsenic. Among the seventeen elements studied, cadmium, lead, aluminum, and fluoride were the most toxic.

Uses of Chemicals for Water Treatment

Coagulation
Alum
Ammonium alum
Bentonite clay
Ferric sulfate
Ferric chloride
Ferrous sulfate
Sodium aluminate
Magnesium carbonate
Sodium silicate
Polyelectrolytes

Dechlorination
Activated carbon
Sodium pyrosulfite
Sodium thiosulfate
Sulfur dioxide
Sodium sulfite

Fluoridation, or Prophylaxis
Fluorosilicic acid
Hydrofluoric acid
Sodium fluoride
Sodium silicofluoride

Softening
Calcium hydroxide
Calcium oxide
Sodium carbonate
Sodium chloride

Taste and Odor Control
Activated carbon
Chlorine
Chlorine dioxide
Copper sulfate
Ozone
Potassium permanganate
Sodium bisulfite
Sodium chlorite

Disinfection
Ammonium chloride
Ammonium aluminum sulfate
Ammonium sulfate
Anhydrous ammonia
Ammonium hydroxide
Calcium hypochlorite
Chlorine
Sodium dichloroisocyanurate (swimming pools only)
Chlorine dioxide
Ozone
Sodium chlorite
Sodium hypochlorite

Scale/Corrosion Control
Disodium phosphate
Sodium polyphosphate, glassy
Sodium hydroxide
Sodium silicate
Sodium sulfite
Sulfuric acid
Tetrasodium pyrophosphate
Trisodium phosphate
Sodium carbonate

In America we have not been accustomed to worrying about our water, but that has changed. More and more people have started to drink bottled water or have some type of water filter for their homes. Turning on the tap and expecting clean, detoxified water is now a thing of the past.

Source: Delicious *(October 1996), page 18*

California recently passed a law mandating statewide fluoridation of the public water supply, despite the fact that health professionals, including doctors and dentists, have long decried the addition of fluoride, which comes from industrial waste from fertilizer and aluminum production, to drinking water. Scientific studies show no evidence that fluoride helps prevent tooth decay, and the belief that there is little risk to humans ingesting this toxic substance may be in error. Studies on humans implicated fluoride as a cause of increased rates of hip fracture, bone cancer, Down's syndrome, goiter, lower fertility, and lower IQ.

Fluoride cannot be removed from your household drinking water by simple carbon filters, only by expensive deionization or reverse osmosis systems.

Water Pollution

Source: The Healthy Home (1989), by Linda Mason Hunter. Attic to basement guide to toxin free living

No state or country is immune from water pollution. The EPA reports that twenty-five states have groundwater contamination by pesticides; twenty-eight states have contamination by metals; forty states have contamination from organic chemicals; and forty-three states have contamination from inorganic chemicals.

- Researchers state that the thirty-seven million people living around the Great Lakes generally have twenty percent higher levels of toxic chemicals in their bodies than other North Americans.
- In Newark, New Jersey, seventy-five percent of the city's water pipes are composed of lead.
- New Orleans draws its water from the Mississippi River, which is the final repository for the wastes of hundreds of industrial companies that line the river's bank.
- In San Francisco, asbestos in the water is sometimes found at more than one hundred times the acceptable level.
- In 1986 in Tucson, Arizona, part of the city's residents were discovered to have been drinking water containing dangerously high levels of trichloroethylene (TCE), an industrial solvent, which had contaminated the water in the 1950s.
- More than 2.5 million steel tanks containing fuel for automobiles are buried underground. Estimates are that more than half a million of these tanks are already leaking into groundwater. According to the American Petroleum Institute, 350,000 older tanks will be leaking by the end of the century.
- Nine out of ten toxic chemical dumps are located directly above underground water supplies.

Bottled Water

Source: Delicious *(October 1996), page 16*

New rules have been set down by the Food and Drug Administration (FDA) for uniform national standards in labeling and identifying the different types of bottled water. To receive a free brochure on FDA Standards of Identity and general information about bottled water, call 1-800-WATER11.

Artesian water—from a well that taps a confined aquifer (water from an underground layer of rock or sand).
Distilled water—free of bacteria and cryptococci, has had lead and copper removed, tastes flat, allow to oxygenate.
Mineral water—contains not less than 250 parts per million total dissolved solids; no minerals can be added to this product.
Purified water—produced by distillation, deionization, reverse osmosis or other suitable processes.
Sparkling water—after treatment, including possible replacement of carbon dioxide, water contains the same amount of carbon dioxide it had at emergence from the source. (Soda water, seltzer, and tonic water are not considered bottled waters.)
Spring water—from an underground formation that flows naturally to the surface of the earth.
Well water—obtained from a human-made hole in the ground that taps an aquifer.

Air Quality

Source: Sunday World Herald *(January 1995)*

The US Environmental Protection Agency has concluded that the level of indoor pollutants is two to five times greater than outdoor levels. During winter months, a time when homes are sealed tighter, this quality drops even lower. This results in increases in dust mites, pet dander, leaf dust, pollen, cooking smoke, and soot from fireplaces, aggravating allergies.

Asbestos concern—for a free copy of EPA certified asbestos detection agencies, write to Asbestos List, US Consumer Product Safety Commission, Washington, DC 20207, or call the Toxic Substances Control Hotline at (202) 554-1404 or the EPA at 1-800-368-5888.

Indoor air pollution examples—Biological contaminants: pollen spores, debris from microscopic dust mites, bacteria, viruses, house dust, human and animal dander. Gas and smoke: tobacco, cooking soot and soot from wood burning stoves; gas appliances may emit carbon monoxide if not vented properly. Chemical vapors and fumes: from carpet, furniture, drapes, processed building materials, cleaning products, personal care products, and chemicals from hobbies, such as painting, woodworking, and photography.

Ways to Improve Indoor Air Quality

1) Remove source of pollution, don't allow smoking in the home. Dedicate an area outside.
2) Ventilation helps dilute indoor pollution; open windows or doors, or buy energy ventilation system.
3) Clean indoor air with high efficiency filters or air cleaner, or a portable room air filter; there are many on the market. The FDA lists some air purifiers, e.g., Alpine and Bionaire.
4) Check light switches, since old ones used mercury (see following pages for more details).

Bedroom—Put several layers of cheesecloth over heating vents in winter, use washable curtains or shades, and always wash bed linens in hot water, since this helps kill bacteria. Encase pillows and mattresses in airtight covers to keep molds and mites away from face. Keep pets out of the bedroom; animal skin dander and bird feathers give off particles that can cause allergies.

Living Room—Hardwood flooring, vinyl, or tile is good. Dust mites thrive in carpets, so shampoo carpets with an allergy-control solution that kills dust mites. It is best to shampoo at least once a year rather than spraying carpet with chemical products for long-lasting wear. Use a vacuum cleaner equipped with air filters and double-lined collection bags.

Bathroom—Use unscented bathroom cleaners (bleach, baking soda, or vinegar). Use an exhaust fan to get rid of shower steam, which increases mold and fungus growth causing possible allergies.

Kitchen—Clean the bottom and back of the refrigerator at least three times a year. Use bleach, baking soda and vinegar for cleaning the kitchen. Borax or baking soda is good for dishwasher soap.

Basement—Change furnace filters monthly. Use high-efficiency particulate air filters to cut down on the dust being circulated with the heat. Cleaning heat ducts annually removes mold.

Wintertime—The risk of carbon monoxide (CO) poisoning increases when windows are closed or sealed. It can lead to fatalities. This odorless gas is produced by faulty heating/venting systems, and malfunctioning appliances powered by oil, natural gas, coal, and wood. Do not run automobiles in an attached garage.

Self-defense—Leave one window ajar at night, have your heating system inspected annually, and install a CO alarm ($50–$100) near your bedroom. Be careful about leaving a fireplace to burn all night without supervision.

Clearing up Harmful ElectroMagnetic Rays (EMRs)

Sources: Earth Star Journal *4, no. 89;* Inner Self Magazine *8, no. 11; Clarus Systems Group*

The common use of something as simple as electricity, the power source that courses through the walls of nearly every American home, may be a health threat. In the last fifty years, man has created an environment of artificial electromagnetic fields, which virtually replace the subtle energies of the natural environment. Scientists estimate that an average person is exposed daily to one hundred million times the electromagnetic radiation that his grandparents were exposed to. This is disruptive to the body's own natural energy field (prana, chi, ki) within which millions of subtle electrical impulses balance and regulate the activity of every living cell. Our energy field is the foundation of health and wellness.

The problem centers on extremely low frequency (ELF) waves, non-ionizing electromagnetic radiation that most closely resembles the body's own micropulsations. It is an invisible form of energy generated by high voltage, alternating current (AC) power lines. Nikola Tesla invented direct current (DC), which is used mostly outside the United States and does not seem to have the same effects on humans as AC. Rays are emitted through every conceivable gadget we use, exposing us on all levels to EMRs. Tesla was far advanced in his scientific findings; his research could have benefited all people through the adoption of his designs directed towards free electricity. Politics overrode his findings, and AC was the elected choice to use throughout this country. (See more on Tesla, this section.)

Electromagnetic radiation fields (EMFs) are generated by all electrical appliances: hair dryers, computers, television, electric blankets, microwaves, clocks, fish aquariums, radios, stereos, VCRs, washers, dryers and…!

People in electronics, computer users, and others have been aware of the problems connected with indispensable pieces of technology. Continuous exposure to EMRs from all electrical devices, computers, power lines, and broadcast signals results in thousands of EMFS frequency wave forms containing many millions of electrostatically charged particles (nonbinary photons) disruptively passing through every human cell each second of the day.

Modern electronics developed a simple solution to this problem. New products by Clarus engineering strengthen and activate the essential energies of vitality, which clears up the chaotic EMR fields in our environment. A simple unit plugs into any ordinary electrical outlet, and works by organizing random photon waves that exist in an electromagnetic field, much like a magnet aligns iron fillings. The result is a smoothing out of the turbulence, so that cellular stress is reduced. This effect creates a more balanced life because it helps fortify our natural immunities to these man-made electromagnetic fields, especially that radiation produced by computers, televisions and cordless telephones. Man functions,better when his mode of feeling is peaceful, and his environment is not bombarding him with stress in a subtle unseen way.

For more information, contact Clarus Systems, 1120 Calle Cordillera, San Clemente, CA 92673, 1-800-4CLARUS

The Art and Science of Holistic Interactions between Life and Our Living Environment
Source: BauBiologie Institute and Ecology, Clearwater, FL, (727) 461-4371,
Website: www.bau-biologieusa.com, e-mail: baubiologie@earthlink.net.

Building materials impact the varied spaces we live, work, and exist in. What types of construction materials have been placed in your home? Many building materials are still using hazardous chemicals, such as mercury, formaldehyde, aluminum wiring, plastic piping, etc. Ninety percent of our time is spent indoors, and approximately eighty percent of today's building materials consist of artificial things. There are fifty thousand different chemicals in modern technology. Some are suspected to be dangerous and their effects to our health are unknown. However, we do know there has been an increase in illnesses over the last seventy-five years, during which we have moved away from the organic, into a chemically based society of technology.

The basis of organizations like BauBiologie is to inform, educate, and train people. We are just now becoming aware of the health hazards that exist in our homes and workplaces. Up-to-date materials are available, the average person just doesn't know about them. Ignorance can lead to poor health and eventually to the demise of our planet. If you are interested in learning about your own environment, there are correspondence courses available. Cable television is now showing new materials available in the building trades. Learn to look differently at your sacred space.

Air—There are different ways to look at how air is utilized throughout the home, and designs that will not expose you to organic compounds, combustion gases, asbestos, vinyl, pesticides, formaldehyde, etc.
Water—The very source of our existence. Learn about different water systems, water contaminants, inorganic contaminants, microbiological contaminants, etc.
Building Materials—Examine each item from windows to floors, to walls and so on.
Energy—There are different layouts to best utilize the energy within the house, so as not to expose yourself to harmful electromagnetic radiation fields that surround you in the walls, ceilings, etc.

Products and Objects to Have around the House
(See Environmental Products and Books at the end of this chapter.)
- Baking soda for teeth, deodorizing, refrigerator, cleaning, laundry, dishwasher.
- Borax for laundry and general cleaning (1/2 cup to 1 gallon water); also for liquid hand cleaner.
- Bleach to wipe things down (wear rubber gloves).
- White vinegar (two teaspoons diluted in a quart of warm water) for cleaning glass. Use a soft cotton cloth.
- Wooden spoons; wipe down with baking soda before rinsing with water.
- Wax/parchment paper; avoid storing, warming up foods in plastic, foam, or aluminum foil.
- Natural sea salt for flavoring rather than regular salt. Fresh garlic is excellent too.
- Powdered vitamin C to add to mayonnaise or catsup. Acts as a preservative and helps to kill parasites.
- Cotton liners for bed pillows and mattresses; help with dust mites. White is recommended because colors can come from uncertain dyes or from uncertain sources. Use natural fibers for throw pillows, etc.
- Fire extinguisher; keep handy and be aware of its expiration date.
- Lemon and limes to help get rid of bugs (more in this chapter).

- Carbon monoxide alarm.
- Weather scanner.
- Smoke detector.
- Plants to help filter and clean the air you breathe.
- Natural unbleached paper coffee filters.
- Natural incense without chemicals is available; also sage for spiritual cleansing of the house.
- Wind chimes create an atmosphere of lightness in a house (Source: Feng Shui or Sacred Space).
- Natural air sprays or spritzers. See Aromatherapy section.
- Books to add an element of restfulness to a room.
- Colorful surroundings, noncluttered and dust-free, make a peaceful home.
- Water purifier; reverse osmosis is the best. Air filters remove pollen, molds, and some chemicals.

Be Aware of Dangers in Household Products
- Do not use floor waxes, because very toxic/chemicals can be absorbed by bare feet, animals too.
- Avoid aluminum cookware, food foil liners, body deodorants, dental amalgams.
- No aerosol cans for anything; many contain hazardous chemicals that pollute air and water.
- Throw away old foods, as they become very toxic when sitting in refrigerator.
- Keep shoe polishes in airtight containers.
- Keep paints, lamp fluids in area that is well ventilated, like an outside shed, deck or porch.
- Shoes off at the door. You are dragging in junk (bacteria, etc.) from wherever you have walked.
- Alarm clocks, television, radios, computers, some telephones, fish aquariums, etc. emit electromagnetic radiation (EMR). (See Clarus, this section, about neutralizing.) You may also call the product manufacturer with questions about your particular product.
- Belts on washer and dryer: be sure they are made in the United States, as foreign belts are made with asbestos. When running, they can emit asbestos into the air. Many major brands use belts from out of the country, so call and check about your brand, and ask where the belts were made.
- Hang dry cleaning outside, to air out odors from the chemical process.
- Sunlight is excellent to kill contact germs.
- Microwave ovens won't kill harmful salmonella and other bacteria. Microwaving pizza doesn't kill bacteria in the cheese. Radiation rays from microwaves have been linked to cataracts.
- Check labels on cosmetics, food, shampoo, conditioner, lotion, fragrances, and cleaning products for chemicals that are harmful. Try to use natural products only.
- Deadly E. coli bacteria have been found in meat packages. Be sure to cook meats until well done.
- Sunscreens: check out chemical ingredients, or be old fashioned and enjoy the sunshine. Natural sunscreens are available. If you're exposed to too much sun, wear a hat and long sleeves. Wearing sunglasses all the time can cause eye deficiencies.
- Talcum powder, for the last twenty-five years, has been noted to contain asbestos. Most doctors stopped using it in surgical gloves five years ago. Talc has been linked to genital cancer. Check powder ingredients.
- Pesticide residues are on fruits and vegetables. Wax coatings (apples, cucumbers, peppers) often contain fungicides, which are toxic and cannot be removed except by peeling. Look for foods labeled organic or pesticide free. Rinse leafy lettuces or spinach with a couple of drops of bleach in water, and scrub vegetables with brush. Rinse thoroughly.
- Synthetic fireplace logs are basically made from wood pulp and chips, contain highly flammable

resins and alcohol, and are imbued with chemicals that give off bright colors. Traces of these chemicals persist in the air and cling to fibers, such as curtains, carpeting, and upholstery.
- Ironing board covers are mostly made with fabric containing asbestos, especially harmful if old or torn. One hundred percent cotton covers are available, but hard to find.
- Potholders with silver are sometimes made with asbestos materials, harmful when handling hot pots or pans. Potholders also need to be washed or replaced frequently, as they gather bacteria when dirty.
- Plastic dish drains collect bacteria. It is better to use a fresh towel each time.
- When buying property, have it checked for radon levels. There are now many areas in the US that have radon pockets. Check library for books on the subject.
- Irons that have the safety feature of turning off automatically by themselves may use mercury.
- Cigarette smoking for a long period of time may show up in lung tissue. Some filters are made with asbestos fibers, which are indestructible. Some filters contain arsenic.
- Fluorescent bulbs use droplets of mercury that vaporize during lamp operation, but are self-contained in the tube. Bulbs are now no longer being manufactured using mercury, but millions of older bulbs are still on the market. It is the breakage of the bulbs in disposal that is hazardous. Full spectrum bulbs act as normal sunlight and emit a natural range of colors.
- Thermostats use a mercury tube switch. Digital thermostats are mercury free but use batteries. Carrier has developed a new digital programmable and nonprogrammable thermostat that is mercury and battery free, and will hold its program if the electricity goes out.
- Old "no click" sound or "silent" electrical switches were manufactured using mercury. These were discontinued about five years ago. Do not confuse with quiet switches using silver alloy.

Beware of improper disposal of all batteries, fluorescent lights, thermostats, old electrical switches, etc. that contain mercury, although encapsulated when manufactured. Breakage and breakdown of these products has allowed mercury seepage into landfills, and into our water supply!

Hazardous Household Products
Source: The Healthy Home *by Linda Mason Hunter*

Laundry detergents—Contain liver-damaging chemicals and bleaches that irritate the lungs and skin.

Drain, toilet, oven cleaners—Contain sodium hydroxide (lye), a powdered toxin and mucous membrane irritant.

Carpet shampoos—Contain a respiratory irritant. Outbreaks of flu-like symptoms have been reported after carpet cleaning in offices, motels, and schools.

Ammonia—Is a powerful toxin; if mixed with chlorine bleach, it produces deadly chlorine gas.

Aerosol sprays and paint strippers—Contain methylene chloride, a suspected carcinogen.

Glue, liquid spot remover, paint, and varnish—Frequently contain toluene, a toxin that can cause fatigue, muscle weakness, and confusion. When vapors are inhaled, they can cause central nervous system depression, psychosis, and liver and kidney damage.

Stopping Household Pests Safely

Ants—Know what kind you are dealing with first. If they are the tiny reddish-brown variety, tempt them with a mixture of mint-apple jelly and boric acid, which they will take back to the nest. For other ants, trace their trail to the point of entry. Caulk any openings, keep food off counters, and clean up pet dishes. Add lemon, lime, or pepper juice to water and spray the area.

Fleas—Feed your dog garlic daily. If pet is already infested, put two cut-up lemons into two cups of boiling water, let mixture stand overnight, dab the liquid on pet and let dry. Bathing washes off fleas.

Mice—Produce litters every fifty days; mousetrap is best, but do not touch, as they carry diseases.

Moths—Keep cleaned clothing put away in plastic or cloth liners. Mothballs or moth flakes will kill them. Place in tissue paper to keep from harming fabrics. Cedar closet is great.

Pantry Pests—Moths and beetles enter house through boxed grocery items. to kill them, dispose of all food that is infested, and put everything else in the freezer for a day to kill any eggs. Thoroughly clean pantry shelves with bleach to prevent re-infestation. Store food in plastic or glass containers.

Roaches—Sprinkle boric acid powder, a natural element that is toxic to insects and harmful to humans and pets in large doses. Apply along baseboards and under sinks. The powder sticks to their leg hairs and when they groom, they should be goners.

Spiders—Feed on small insects. Keep house dusted and vacuumed thoroughly and regularly.

Garbage Production

A family of four produces one hundred pounds of trash weekly. Please recycle! You can even recycle clothing. Someone may need it, and clothing takes up lots of landfill space.

The Environmental Protection Agency (EPA) can be reached at 1-800-368-5888. For free advice or information, write to them at 401 M Street, Washington, DC 20460.

World Health and Toxicity

Source: Earth Change Reports *(1993)*

New diseases have hit the world population, beginning in late 1993, especially affecting the lymphatic system and parasympathetic systems. The cause? One or more of the following: toxicity due to environmental pollution of water and foods, diet, and inability to adjust to new planetary energies.

Pesticides

Source: Vegetarian Times *(June 1996), pages 20 and 22*

The common pesticide chlorpyrifos (brand name Dursban) is used to exterminate pests on crops, other insects, and especially termites. Eighty-two percent trace amounts have been found in adult urine. Eighteen percent of Americans have a container around the house. This product has been linked to severe birth defects, but there hasn't been enough evidence for the federal agency to take action.

Top Ten Toxins in the House

Source: Energy Times *(1996)*

1) Formaldehyde in building materials, fabrics, pillowcases, upholstery, drapes and carpets.
2) Synthetic upholstery and fabrics containing toxic chemicals like 4-phenylcylohexene, moth-proofing pesticides, or flame-proofing chemicals.
3) Toxic paints and paint strippers containing heavy metals and volatile organic compounds. Those manufactured before 1978 may contain deadly lead.
4) Tetrachloroethylene used in dry cleaning solvents.
5) Tobacco smoke containing formaldehyde, hydrogen, cyanide, arsenic, benzene, and other toxic chemicals.
6) Cleansing products containing harsh ingredients like ethanol, ammonia, and artificial colors and fragrances that are inadvertently inhaled or absorbed through the skin. Instead, use vinegar, borax, or baking soda.

7) Toxic pesticides and herbicides. Americans spend 2.5 billion dollars on chemicals for their lawns. Many of these products contain highly toxic chemicals. Instead, plant marigolds to discourage pests, release a cup of ladybugs (from nurseries) and introduce toads into your garden.
8) Plastics containing chemicals that mimic estrogenic compounds. Scientists believe these may be responsible for male infertility, and prostate and breast cancers.
9) Radon, a silent killer, an odorless, colorless and tasteless gas. You can have your home checked.
10) Molds and their spores, living organisms that thrive in moist, damp places, and can cause sinus and digestive problems. Helpful—sunlight, fresh air, a humidifier, and cleaning your air/heating vents.

Tesla the Inventor

Source: High Voltage Press, *4326 SE Woodstock #489, Portland, OR 97206*

Nikola Tesla once said, "Electric power is everywhere present in unlimited quantities and can drive the world's machinery without the need for coal, oil, gas, or any other fuels" from *The Buried Secrets of Tesla*. In 1891, Tesla invented the Tesla coil, which can boost power from a wall socket or battery to millions of high frequency volts. Learn how to build your own from everyday stuff. Light your home at a fraction of the usual cost, disinfect water, or build a powerful radio transmitter.

These inventions could have advanced mankind towards an environmentally healthy planet. These inventions have been suppressed in the United States! Imagine utilities and heat being offered at a fraction of the cost with far less damage to the environment.

The International Tesla Museum is located in Colorado Springs, Colorado.

Earth First—Everything We Do Has Consequences!

- Assess how any product affects the environment. It is recycled, recyclable, organic, biodegradable, reusable, durable, or packaged in wasteful way; less toxic alternative, and is it made by a company with a good environmental record?
- Do you really need the product?
- Determine whether the company that makes/sells the product reflects your political and social values. Does it treat workers fairly and pay them well; does it support worthwhile projects in the community? Where are the products made; is the company a cooperative/employee-owned business or local business?
- Try to boycott products from manufacturers that are known polluters.

Environmental Shopping

- Choose soap or paper products that have no artificial scent, color, or harmful chemicals.
- Choose organic shaving cream over those containing ammonia and ethanol, or use pure soap.
- Choose botanical shampoos or make your own.
- Avoid CFCs in aerosol products and polystyrene cups, plates, and egg cartons.
- Avoid products with excessive packaging; preferably buy a recyclable package.
- Diapers—use cloth ones.
- Reuse containers and products as much as possible.
- Avoid disposable products, such as razors.
- Buy products that are in recyclable containers.

- For menstrual pads, some companies use dioxin, a harmful chemical used for bleaching paper products

Telephone Books

Most telephone companies are recycling old telephone books. BellSouth has used these books to make envelopes that the company then uses for billing. In 1993, the program salvaged more than eight thousand tons of phone books that were earmarked for landfills and saved $300,000 in envelope costs. Check your local area for where they collect your telephone books.

Plastic Bags—What to Do with Them

The company Phoenix Recycling, Inc., pays schools a dollar a pound for clean plastic grocery bags, which are then recycled into trash bags and resold. Since 1991, they have recovered more than fifteen million grocery bags, and paid out $160,000 to participating schools. A good fundraiser.

Paper, Not Plastic

Thousands of animals are killed each year by plastic bottles and plastic rings. Now International Paper Company has developed a paper version of the plastic yoke. The paper holders are recyclable and break down easily in landfills and water. Vote to support this issue.

Source: The Healthy Home *by Linda Mason Hunter*

Plastics do not break down, and when burned, plastics form some of the most toxic gases known (dioxin and hydrochloric acid) which hang in the air for days. Aluminum is not biodegradable at all, and plastic toys will be around forever. Four billion dollars a year go to collect and dispose of trash. Out of sight out of mind?

When Earth sits alone, all that will be left is 300,000 toxic dump sites, aluminum, plastic, and cockroaches!

Environment on the Web

EnviroLink: E-mail—admin@envirolink.org; World Wide Web—http://www.envirolink.org
EcoNet: E-mail—econet@econet.org; Web—http://www.econet.org (some costs); 415-442-0107

Book Resources

Beyond 40 Percent (record-setting recycling and composting programs), Institute of Self-Reliance
Enduring Seeds (Native American agriculture and wild plants) by Gary Paul Nabhan
    (more seed listings in chapter 3)
Excitotoxins: The Taste that Kills by Dr. Blaylock
Greening International Law (laws designed to control the environment), edited by Phippe Sands
Garage Primer, Plastic Waste Primer, Nuclear Waste Primer available through League of Women Voters
    Education, 202-429-1965; $13.50 each
Grandmother's Home Remedies by Dr. Myles H. Bader
Medicine from the Earth (guide to healing plants) by William A. Thomson
Making Peace with the Planet (stop wasting precious nonrenewable resources) by Barry Commoner
Preventing Industrial Toxic Hazards (guide for communities) by Marion Wise and Lauren Kenworthy

The Big Family Guide to All the Minerals by Frank Murray
The Earth Manual (how to work on wild land without taming it) by Malcolm Margolin
The Global Ecology Handbook (what you can do about environmental crisis), Beacon Press
The Healthy Home (attic to basement guide) by Linda Mason Hunter
The Truth About Where You Live (atlas for action on toxins and mortality) by Benjamin A. Goldman
Rubbish (archaeology of garbage) by William Rathje and Cullen Murphy
Salvaging the Land of Plenty (garbage and the American dream) by Jennifer Seymour Whitaker
Soil and Water Quality by National Research Council Committee
Switched-On Living: Ways to Use the Mind/Body Connection to Energize Your Life by J. Teplitz, PhD
Toxic Trade Update (quarterly in English, French, Spanish), provided by Greenpeace
Your Body's Many Cries for Water by F. Batmanghelid, MD

Environmental Product Resources

Air Therapy (100 percent natural purifying mists) 1-800-292-6339
Allergy Free Inc. (allergy free filters) 1-800-ALLERGY
Alpine Air Purifiers 1-800-989-2299
Bear and Company (planetary ecology and books) 1-800-WEBEARS
Bronson Vitamins and Herbals (natural vitamins/herbs) 1-800-235-3200
Cloth Bag Company (100 percent cotton for groceries) 1249 Pitte Road, Atlanta, GA (770) 393-0058
Diamond Organics (organic fruits and vegetables delivered) 1-888-674-2642)
Ear Candles, AP Enterprises 1-800-309-EARS
Earth Changes Reports (world information and maps on Earth changes) 1-800-628-7493
Earth First Newspaper, PO Box 1415, Eugene, OR 97440, (541) 344-8004
Earth Friendly Products, 1-800-335-ECOS
Earth Tones (100 percent profit to environmental groups, long distance service) 1-800-EARTH56
Environmental Magazine, Subscription 6 issues/$20.00 - PO Box 699, Mount Morris, IL 61054-7589
Fisher-Henney (100 percent cotton apparel) 1-800-3HENNEY
Great Smokies Diagnostic Lab (stool, detoxification, intestinal) Web: www.gsdl.com, (704) 252-9833
Huggins Diagnostic Lab (blood work for metals present and materials usable-dental) (719) 548-1600
Living Free Paper Co (100 percent tree free) 1430 Willamette St. #367, Eugene, OR 97401, 1-800-309-2974
National Arbor Day Foundation (plant trees for America) order ten Colorado spruces for $10 donation to: #100 Arbor Avenue, Nebraska City, NE 68410
Natracare (100 percent cotton tampon with cotton over-wrap, no synthetics or additives), available in U.S.A.
Reflections Organic (100 percent cotton clothing) 1-800-852-9273
Seed Catalogs (listings for organic places to buy seeds), see chapter 3
Sinan Co. (natural construction, redecorating supplies) PO Box 857, Davis, CA 95617, (530) 753-3104
Tools for Exploration (full-spectrum fluorescent lights) 1-800-456-9887
Wright's (silver cream for silver) PO Box 566, Keene, NH 03431, 1-800-922-2625

Chapter Seven

Toxic-Free Health

Parasites, Candida, and Dental Amalgams

How could something so simple become so complicated?

This chapter will help you understand the basics, first, about how chemical cleaning products, body products, foods, drinks, drinking water, and metal dental fillings have slowly crept into our busy life style; second, about how we have allowed this to go on in our society, without questioning; third, we are probably the most influential country on this planet, and we, as consumers can demand changes. Fourth, will you take the time to write a letter, or refuse to buy products that harm you? Will you boycott the bad guys?

Today, many people want to take charge of their health, now thought of as self-health. Gone are the days when you visited your dentist or doctor, and did only what they told you without asking questions! Our planet is "shrinking" on the level of networking, information, space, food, and natural resources. What affects each one of us has an impact upon your family, your neighbors, your town, your country and other countries. To take charge, we must create a healthy environment by promoting products that will not harm the water and soil, products that will create natural resources for inexpensive heat and electricity. We need to treat our bodies with respect. A body free of viruses, bacteria, and parasites is a happy body. There are many books and much information available to us. We must take control of our lives because if we don't, no one else will.

What is this leading up to? Some simple things we can do to help our body feel better and get healthy! It is like comparing our body to the automobile we drive. We wouldn't put sand in the gas tank. We put in good fuel, add oil, check the battery, give it a wash job, vacuum it out, and keep it in good working order. Why don't we do the same for the body we live in?

Everything we eat, drink, and touch is absorbed into our bodies; most products have "chemical" agents.

- The things we eat, the products we put into our body, are the fuel to keep the body energized.
- Many foods we eat are not energized foods, but ones that produce sluggish energy or no energy.
- Fast foods are not cooked well; foods are cooked with old oils; oversalted, chemically imbued products have preservatives for long shelf life; and what grade of meat do we buy?
- Drinking water is highly chemical. The United States has refused to resolve this because you're talking major work across the lands. The water mains of many cities are contaminated with lead,

copper, and fluoride (a known poison). Fluoride is a hazardous waste product that couldn't be dumped legally, yet we put it in the very water we drink.
- We are using cleaning products for house, office, and automobile that are also highly chemical. These solvents, absorbed into the human body, produce adverse affects.
- Body products, including shampoos, soaps, deodorants, creams, perfumes, and lipsticks, are highly chemical. These chemicals are also absorbed into the body.
- Fiberglass from furnace filters, molds, dust, toxic fumes from paints, solvents in the garage or basement, yard fertilizers, and insect sprays permeate our air.
- Cigarettes have toxic-treated paper for preserving freshness, pesticides used on the growing tobacco, and arsenic in the filter area. Alcohol contains a toxic chemical preservative.
- Many use and abuse prescription drugs.
- Metal fillings and root canals have mercury and various unhealthy metals. Mercury is a hazardous waste material, a poison. There are laws in many states about removal of this hazardous waste material. Talk about a Catch-22, and our mouths are housing the landfill!

What happens when we do all or some of the above?

When we expose ourselves to all of the above, without eating proper nutritious foods, or we don't get enough sleep, don't take any vitamins, or get any exercise, we start on the road of immune system breakdown. This leads to two major basic problems.

1) Our body cannot defend itself against the parasites we are exposed to called flukes.
2) Candida (yeast infection) thrives in the body, producing ill effects in many of the body's systems.

There is a cure!

Research into Parasites

Source: The Cure for All Cancers *by Dr. Hulda Regehr Clark*

Studies show that the pesticides used to protect our farms and the solvents they contain leach back into the products grown. That means that all vegetables, wheat, oats, potatoes, and tobacco, and other food products grown in these fields, are chemically exposed. From these products are made pet foods, human foods, and food for cattle, turkey, and chickens. This has produced a biological reservoir of solvents in these animals —which we as humans eat. What are the types of chemical solvents? Isopropyl alcohol, benzene, methanol, xylene, and toluene are some of the residues our foods and body products contain. Animals and plants are naturally infested with parasites called flukes. Flukes in inactive cyst forms are routinely passed on to human beings. Instead of passing harmlessly through our body, they are induced by the solvents to hatch, grow, and reproduce. What does this mean. These different solvents can accumulate in preferentially different organs.

Isopropyl alcohol—accumulates in the liver, which means that a parasitic worm can start there as a baby and literally grow up and produce and produce and produce, continuing its full life cycle in that organ. This establishes the cancerous process, namely the production of the mitotic stimulant orthophospho-tyrosine. This organ appears to be chosen on the basis of metal concentration. Metals in the liver come from the fillings you have in your mouth, and heavy metals present in our polluted environment. Again, all of this is based on how many toxins we have in our body from foods, and how many fillings we have in our mouth. You will also discover just how many products on the market contain isopropyl alcohol when you start reading labels.

Benzene—accumulates in the thymus gland, which can lead to a full life cycle there by flukes. This can help the AIDS (acquired immune deficiency syndrome) virus establish itself due to interference with thymus functions, such as the production of T-cells. When using what is called a parasite flush with herbs, the virus disappears within twenty-four hours after the last fluke has been destroyed.

Undercooked Meats

Metacercaria parasites come from eating animal flesh infested with this parasitic fluke and their eggs. If we enjoy a rare steak that is infested, we are then ingesting the fluke eggs and all stages of their development. They attach themselves to the lining of our intestines, grow larger, and produce more eggs. Then propyl alcohol from the use of normal body products, allows the stages to start developing in the liver. That is why those quick burgers or a spatula that turns those burgers can stay infected with raw meat juice. Even your hands can pick up parasites when you are making meat loaf or meatballs.

Flukes

The early stages of intestinal flukes are found in blood, breast milk, saliva, semen, and urine. This can be seen directly in these body fluids using a low power microscope. You can transmit parasites then, by kissing on the mouth, breast feeding, and sexual encounters. The recipient would only develop cancer if their body was overly toxic, with excess isopropyl alcohol in their organs, or if an accumulation of toxins had created immune deficiency syndrome. You can see some flukes with the naked eye.

When eating out, it's best to have seafood or fowl. Cook all meats—chicken, turkey, fish, beef, and pork—until they fall off the bone. Be cautious about eating deli meats. Consider becoming vegetarian soon!

Studies Show

A cure is black walnut hulls, cloves, wormwood (see section Herbs to Kill Parasites). Also beneficial is removal of chemical solvents from our home—more details in this section.

What Do We Do?

Removal of Toxic Conditions

Removal of all solvents from our life style and destruction of all fluke stages, as well as elimination of undercooked beef, turkey and chicken in the diet, results in quick recovery. Most diseases, even cancer and AIDS could be eradicated in a very short time by clearing our food animals and household pets of fluke parasites, by monitoring all the food we eat, and by eliminating our need for certain cleaning solvents.

Stopping the consumption of aflatoxin and other mycotoxins must also be done. Stay clean by staying away from fast foods and delicatessen meats, or you could immediately reinfect yourself.

I went through my house and eliminated all the junk under my kitchen sink.

Remember you can use bleach, borax, Arm and Hammer washing powder, and other natural products for cleaning. Borax mixed with water makes a great hand soap for pump dispensers.

I cleaned out under my bathroom sink.

I almost cried when ridding myself of chemical shampoos, soap, deodorant, hair gel, makeup, perfume, etc. On the bright side, I won't have so much to clean around. It has helped me get organized.

I removed hazardous materials from my attached garage.
You can put into your outside shed all your paints, oils, shoe polish, etc. Or, if the items are small, store them in plastic containers. These items should not be in the garage where your furnace is; this allows toxic fumes into the house. Definitely do not store gasoline and lawnmower in attached garage.

Closet space.
I put candles, ink pads, glue, art supplies, extra pens and pencils, etc. into sealed plastic storage boxes.

Pet food.
Store in garbage can or large plastic kitchen basket.

Laundry area.
I removed dryer fabric sheets, washing powder, and rinse containers. I replaced them with Arm and Hammer, bleach, and sea salt products. Check your machine belts for United States manufacture (see environmental tips).

Pantry.
I now read labels. I shop more carefully and buy organic fresh vegetables and fruit. I have enjoyed picking up a couple of interesting cookbooks with vegetarian recipes.

Water filter.
I bought a Brita (water pitcher to sit on kitchen counter). I use this water for drinking, cooking, and making an organic cup of coffee. If you can afford a larger filter system, reverse osmosis is best.

Metal removal.
I personally found several wonderful dentists. One removed all my mercury fillings, and another my root canals. I also chose to change my eating habits, and ordered reliable vitamins and herbs.

Parasite Remedies

Source: The Cure for All Cancers *by Dr. Clark—book has recipes for natural household cleaners*

Warning: Do not substitute drugs for herbs. Pharmaceutical parasiticides can be toxic and dangerous. Other cultures knew that humans have parasites. The Native American peoples from the Arctic to Antarctic knew that humans have parasites, just like the animals. They had frequent purging that included vomiting and diarrhea to rid themselves of these slimy invaders. Do you remember when you were young, being fed sulfur, molasses, or castor oil? This helped rid our bodies of these worms. With time and our hectic lifestyles, we forgot these old remedies and started taking prescriptions.

Studies have shown that eczema is due to roundworms. Seizures are caused by a single roundworm getting into the brain. Schizophrenia and depression are caused by parasites/flukes in the brain. Asthma is parasites in the lungs, diabetes the pancreatic fluke of cattle. Migraines are caused by threadworms, and heart disease by the dog heartworm.

By doing four simple things we can rid ourselves of parasites:
1) Kill all stages of the parasites
2) Stop using any products with propyl alcohol
3) Flush the metals out of your body
4) Flush the toxins out of your body

Detailed Instructions on Herbs to Kill Parasites

Source: The Cure for All Cancers *by Dr. Clark, pages 21–22*

Using the following three herbs together will solve the parasite problem. The black walnut hull and the wormwood kill the adults and the developmental stages of more than one hundred parasites. Cloves kill the eggs.

1) Black walnut hulls tincture—from black walnut trees, only the green hull works, only buy if tincture is green, not black
2) Wormwood—read label for way it is processed; check resource listing in Dr. Clark's book
3) Whole cloves—grocery store, do not buy already ground cloves, it will not work, as the parasitic killing properties will have been lost. I bought mine and ground them up in a coffee grinder then put them into vegetable capsules, size 00, that I bought from a health food store. Store in closed bottle.

Nonessential Items that Could Prove Helpful

Parasites produce a great deal of ammonia as their waste product. This is their urine, and it is set free in our bodies by parasites in large amounts. Ammonia is very toxic, especially to our brains, and can cause some sleep problems. "Parasite" comes from the Greek word meaning "one who eats off the table of another." A parasite survives by hijacking another organism, robbing it of nutrients, and leaving behind toxic waste. Parasitic infection spreads from garden soil, through puddles, through all foods and water, and can be transferred from pet to owner, from children to adults. Signs of infection include a runny nose, nighttime restlessness, and blisters on the lower lip inside the mouth. Infected individuals may feel bloated, tired, and hungry. They may have allergies, anemia, lethargy, fuzzy thinking, headaches, roller coaster blood sugar levels, and nighttime teeth grinding. Our environment and our life styles have allowed parasitic infections to get out of hand. Many health care professionals do not address the concept that people can be ill from the effects of parasites.

Candida Yeast Syndrome (Fungus)

Sources: Healthy Steps *by Dr. Albert Zehr and* Better Nutrition *(January 1996)*

Several things we eat and do on a daily basis affect our health. See the following:

White Sugar—Our body was not made with the capacity to deal with refined carbohydrates or sugar. You will find that sugar is added to the many processed foods on the market. Our body handles the normal sugar intake from fruits.

White Salt—Salt in the old days, was used to preserve meat products. Salt is sodium chloride. Too much salt is harmful to the heart, affects the blood pressure, places great stress on our kidneys, and replaces the calcium and potassium in our body. Too much salt in the diet can lead to heart disease and osteoporosis.

White Flour—White flour is a grain (usually wheat) that has been stripped of its fiber, which our bowel need. It loses its life germ and endosperm, which contain the vitamins, minerals, and protein. It creates lifeless bread, but it is a good wallpaper paste. I use it for craft projects that need a glue consistency.

Milk—Only humans drink the milk of another species. Pasteurization destroys two-thirds of the vitamins and minerals and ninety percent of the enzymes, and causes alteration to the fatty acids and protein our body needs. Any antibiotics, medications, steroids, or chemical based feeds given to the cattle are passed on in their milk. Associated with mucus-type health problems, allergies, and asthma.

Coffee—Contains caffeine, which can affect your blood pressure, increase your pulse rate, stimulate the kidneys, and temporarily relieve fatigue or depression. Use in moderation. Check out organic coffee. Cigarette studies have shown that smoking impairs both thyroid hormone secretion and thyroid hormone action. A reduced production of thyroid hormone leads to manifestation of thyroid insufficiency, including low metabolic rate, tendency to gain weight, sleepiness, skin dryness and loss of hair. One component of tobacco smoke is cyanide. Smoking increases the risk of cancer, heart disease, stroke, bronchitis and other degenerative diseases.

If you suffer from acne, allergies, anxiety, asthma, constipation, depression, fatigue, headaches, coughs, depression, irritability and premenstrual syndrome, you may be a victim of the Yeast Syndrome. This specific form of yeast is usually found in the digestive tract, bronchial tubes, and vagina, spreading as our immune system starts failing. Our immune system fails due to chemicals in water, foods, cleaning and body products, and air pollution; too many prescription antibiotics; and stress in our daily life.

Our body's white cells or T-cells are the most important factors in our immune system. The T-cells are formed from white blood cells by the hormones from the thymus. They control certain blood cells by commanding them to destroy bacteria and kill foreign invaders.

The yeast converts itself into fungal form that is rooted into the walls of the intestines. Natural sources of caprylic acid, garlic and acidophilus are the most beneficial, along with vitamins C, A, and E, for fighting infection. A complete program and instructions are available on pages 61 to 72 of *Healthy Steps* by Dr. Zehr. You can also check your health food store for other books on the Yeast Syndrome.

Recap:
1) Understand how the parasites affect your body
2) The immune system starts breaking down so your body cannot fight against any other invaders
3) Then the parasites and fungus take over the body's blood and organs
4) Disease is close by

Simple Solution:
1) Start on the parasite treatment and follow through
2) Acidophilus
3) Garlic, vitamins C, A, E
4) Eat healthy
5) Get rid of the pollutants in your home
6) Follow an exercise program

Dental Amalgams—Mercury Removal
Article in Extraordinary Science *(April/May/June 1994) by Thomas Levy, MD, FACC)*

The American Biological Medical Foundation, the Environmental Dental Association, the Foundation for Toxic Free Dentistry, the International Academy of Oral Medicine, Toxicology, the Toxic Elements Research Foundation, and the Huggins Diagnostic Laboratory have alerted thousands of people about the relationship between their health and amalgam fillings, which contain mercury. I am grateful to every dentist that has stepped forward and made a statement about the amalgams.

The books mentioned in the resource section have researched facts, including personal stories from before and after amalgam removal, and what to look for in your own health. I personally applaud Dr. Huggins for his dentistry methods of mercury removal, and for the technology procedures used in my own blood workup. The Compatibility Report, of approximately thirty pages, showed what metal activity was present in my blood, and what type of products could be used in the future for fillings, crowns, cements, bonding agents, and so forth.

Since June of 1995, Europe has taken a decisive stand in banning the further use of mercury amalgam dental fillings. Sweden has concluded that more than 250,000 Swedes had immune and other health disorders, felt to be directly related to their amalgams. The purpose of banning the mercury fillings was to protect the people and the environment. Germany is right behind them.

In the early 1800s the National Association of Dental Surgeons actually advocated the elimination of mercury amalgams. But their cheapness kept many dentists using amalgam materials, in spite of their toxicity. This association was disbanded several decades later. When the American Dental Association (ADA) came into being, they proclaimed amalgams' safety.

Leakage or release of mercury vapors was proved conclusively by Vimy and Lorscheider in 1985. They demonstrated that the air inside a mouth with amalgam fillings continually contained elemental mercury vapor. Also, the dynamics of chewing increased this vapor level substantially. They further concluded that the amount of mercury released daily in patients with twelve or more amalgams either exceeded or comprised a major percentage of the maximal permissible dose of mercury from all environmental sources, as established by the World Health Organization (WHO) in 1972. It is also highly debatable whether a poisonous heavy metal as toxic as mercury should have a politically derived permissible dose.

Mercury is the most toxic nonradioactive heavy metal known to man. Its effects are enormously widespread and leave no part of the body untouched. Exposure to mercury through numerous industrial and commercial uses accounts for significant accumulation in our bodies.

Mercury vapor is almost completely inhaled. Little of it is lost outside of the mouth. This allows for a rapid and complete absorption across the alveolar membrane to the lungs. Mercury easily crosses the blood/brain barrier (the brain/nervous system's natural defense against many toxic substances), subsequently binding very strongly to the sulfur-containing proteins of the nervous tissue.

This same affinity for binding sulfur allows mercury deposits in virtually all of the body's other tissues and organs. Sudden fits of uncontrolled anger, bad temper, severe depression, loss of coordination, and loss of motor control are some of the most common manifestations of chronic mercury poisoning.

Official American Dental Association Stand

Source: American Dental Association (ADA) Code of Professional Conducts, which states: "Based on available scientific data, the ADA has determined through the adoption of Resolution 42H1986 that the removal of amalgam restoration from the nonallergic patient for the alleged purpose of removing toxic substances from the body, when such treatment is performed solely at the recommendation or suggestion of the dentist, is improper and unethical."

In other words, the ADA is telling the dentists in America that they do not have the right to counsel their patients regarding the poisonous effects of mercury, unless, of course, they don't mind losing their licenses to practice dentistry. More than one-third of the dentists in a survey published in December 1989 by *Dentist Magazine,* believe that all silver-colored (mercury) alloy fillings should be removed and replaced with composites. What the ADA's true intent is, is hard to fathom, but it is hard to believe that patient welfare is high on their agenda.

CBS's *60 Minutes* segment on the Amalgam issue was aired in December 1990. The Washington State Dental Association promptly informed its members that patients did not have a right to know that their "silver-colored fillings" contained mercury. This segment received the highest viewer response ever, but it has never been repeated. Rumor has it that it was too political. Is there another unknown agenda here? Greed?

Mouth Wired

The brain and central nervous system (CNS) are strongly affected by the electrical current present in all mouths containing metal. This phenomenon is called oral galvanism. These currents can be measured with a probe and microammeter. Amalgams, metallic crowns and braces generally register from 1 to 100 microamperes of current in a positive or negative polarity. The natural currents found in the brain are in the range of 7 to 9 nanoamperes, making the mouth currents from one hundred to ten thousand times more powerful. The base of the brain is only roughly one inch away from the upper teeth.

Dr. Huggins's success rate of sixty percent in 1979 came when he realized the importance of sequential removal of the amalgams, according to the amount of current measured on each tooth. Removal of the highest negative current came first. Realization also came about the importance of proper nutrition and supplementation of vitamins and minerals specifically based on each patient's laboratory profile. In the late 1980s, Huggins saw the importance of chronic dental infections, as seen in virtually all root canals and cavitations. With these teeth removed and the sites properly cleaned came the success of health.

Dr. Huggins applied research done by Weston A. Price in the 1920s. Unfortunately, even now only a tiny percentage of dentists are aware of or concerned about its clinical application. Even the Multiple Sclerosis (MS) Society has actively campaigned against looking into the mercury issue, sending out letters stating that they have "thoroughly checked" the literature, and found no correlation between amalgams and MS. Once again, we can only wonder what their real agenda is!

In a twenty-year period of seeing thousands of patients, Dr. Huggins noticed MS patients are becoming younger, and the disease is progressing more rapidly. Around the same time this was observed, the high-copper amalgam (an amalgam with greater amounts of copper) began to be utilized. This amalgam was found to release fifty times more mercury than the previous conventional amalgam. Amazingly, high-copper amalgams had actually been outlawed several decades ago, due to their severe cytotoxicity (ability to kill cells in the body). Why are they back and being used today?

Mercury Vapor

When test animals inhaled mercury vapor, the residual mercury was greatest in the kidneys, followed by brain, heart, intestine, and liver in decreasing order. Additional target sites include the testes, ovaries, and pancreas, as well as the thyroid, adrenal, and pituitary glands.

In the pancreas there are groups of cells called the Islets of Langerhans, which function to secrete the body's insulin and therefore regulate the blood sugar. Mercury has an affinity for these cells and appears to directly affect the sugar metabolism in some patients.

Deadly Alternatives

Nickel is rapidly gaining a toxic reputation. Most partial dentures are made of nickel, and approximately eighty percent of crowns utilize nickel. It is often the base onto which the porcelain crown is fired. Nickel compounds have been implicated as human respiratory carcinogens in studies of nickel refinery workers. It is now indicated that there is a relationship between nickel crowns and breast cancer in women. Nickel is also linked to the death of lymphocytes (white blood cells important in immune process).

Cast glass crowns and inlays are some of the latest dental materials; however, be aware that this "glass" generally contains more than twenty-five percent aluminum as aluminum oxide. About eighty percent of patients with such dental work show laboratory findings consistent with a drop in immune function.

Serum Compatibility Testing

There are one thousand different metal alloys from which to choose. Dr. Hal Huggins found that the only safe and scientific way to choose among them was to check the immune reactivity of the patient's blood serum against all the commonly used dental materials. Laboratory profiling allows for an intelligent selection of the least reactive dental materials in a given patient.

Some Scientific Facts
- Mercury is a poison and mercury vapor is the most dangerous form.
- Dental amalgam fillings are approximately fifty percent mercury. One average filling contains about 780 milligrams of mercury, which exceeds the USEPA intake standard for a period of one hundred years.
- Mercury is not locked into the amalgam fillings, and leakage from fillings occurs constantly when we eat and brush our teeth, or from heat. This is called mercury vapor leakage.
- Mercury vapor enters the human body and its cells, and penetrates the blood/brain barrier. We breathe 17,280 times a day; it takes 3070 days to eliminate one-half of each dosage of mercury.
- Mercury studies show it is damaging to the brain, the nervous system, the thyroid, pituitary, and adrenal glands, the heart and the lungs. Mercury is a suppressor of our immune system.
- Human autopsy studies show that through dental amalgams, mercury enters the body and builds up with time.
- The American Dental Association, OSHA, and EPA have declared leftover scrap dental amalgams to be a toxic hazard to dental personnel, dental offices, and the environment, and they must be disposed of as a hazardous material. But they put them in our mouths!

Book Resources on Amalgam Toxicity

Defense against Mystery Syndromes (reveals mystery of "silver" fillings), DAMS Group
How to Save Your Teeth (toxic free preventive dentistry) by Dr. David Kennedy
It's All in Your Head (the link between mercury amalgams and illness) by Dr. Hal Huggins
Toxic Metal Syndrome (how metal poisoning can affect your brain) by Drs. Casdorph and Walker
Toxic Teeth: A Guide to Mercury Exposure from "Silver Fillings" by Dr. Murray J. Vimy, Canada
What Your Doctor Won't Tell You by June Helmlick

My Personal Story

by S. Jeanne Gunn

I have had twelve amalgam fillings for the last forty years, and in the last ten years have ended up with five root canals. I had always thought myself to be healthy, with few colds or childhood diseases ,and thought I had good teeth. I ate what was considered nutritious food and stayed active. In the last four years, I had been environmentally exposed to toxins in the home and on the job. My leg had been swelling up on a daily basis, I was tired all the time, I became aware of sinus problems, and I incurred my fifth abscessed tooth, along with heart pains. This put a real scare into me.

I was then reacquainted with the dangers of mercury amalgam fillings. Reacquainted, I say, because I had previously asked my dentist to remove any old or cracked fillings, and replace them with the new white composite fillings. My dentist told me that the white fillings would not last, and that he would not recommend it. He said there was nothing to the story about mercury affecting my health. I bought the story. Big mistake! When my fifth tooth erupted, which would normally require a root canal procedure, I knew I had to make some new educated choices. Why? For one thing, this tooth was the third tooth in a row, and it had been bothering me for three years. I kept asking my dentist about this, but received no answer. It was like I didn't know anything. Another root canal was not the answer.

A friend who reads and researches everything was aware of what amalgam fillings really are! Well, everything fell into place. We made arrangements to have our blood work sent off to the Huggins Lab in Colorado. We flew to another state to find a dentist who was familiar with removal of mercury amalgam fillings. Dentists who recognize the need for eliminating mercury fillings are afraid and threatened by the ADA, the FBI, and the IRS.

My procedures took three, three-hour sessions. The dentist was a wonderful, very spiritual, loving person. Everything was explained and a genuine concern was expressed about the decision required. Removed were all of the mercury amalgams and all of my five root canals. Studies show root canals affect the immune system. The tooth sites must be thoroughly cleaned, with the periodontal membrane removed and the decayed bone cleaned out, or the autoimmune cells will remain active and the bone does not completely fill in. Not all dentists do this procedure in tooth removal.

I had a different dentist for the root canal removal. That office had a three-hour time slot open up five minutes before I walked in the door. They said I could have this time frame. I said, "Let me go outside and pray for a few minutes. This is really a traumatic decision for me." Outside, I took a deep breath, asked for spiritual guidance about the decision, and then went back inside, saying, "Yes."

A root canal is the center of a tooth that houses arteries, veins, lymphatic vessels and nerves and gives a tooth its life. When a tooth dies, the putrefied contents are removed and replaced by sterile materials that fill up the space. In study cases by Dr. Weston Price, it was found that ninety-nine percent of these treated teeth remain sterile for only three days. This gives time for bacteria to reside in the three miles of tubules within a single rooted tooth. White blood cells cannot reach the area, but the holes permit nutrients for the bacteria to slip through. The bacteria cannot get out of the tooth, but their toxic by-products can!

I am in the process of detoxifying myself from forty years of mercury and metal poisoning. I am taking vitamins, herbs, and blue-green algae, letting go of my chemically influenced household products, and using essential oils. The reclaiming of health does not happen overnight. Making these choices requires long-term commitment and follow-through. Chelation can cleanse heavy metals from the blood; that's next.

I am anxious for everyone to know about mercury dental amalgams, demand safer dental care, and demand that our government stop allowing large political organizations to use humans for dumping sites of poisonous and toxic materials.

Appendix A has a dental chart showing the connection between teeth and the body's organs. This may help you recognize existing conditions within your own body. Once root canals are removed, the immune system and the organs have an opportunity to start healing, hopefully leading to recovery.

Chronic Fatigue Syndrome
(Dedicated to two people who did not understand why they were always tired)

This story revolves around the lives of two different people from two different walks of life. One is a man who is a carpenter and in the construction business; the other is a young housewife who runs a small business from home and has two active dogs.

At the young age of thirty-five the construction worker became seriously ill. Daily he would become fatigued and nauseated after working only three or four hours. As with most of us, he tried to figure out why he didn't feel good, and examined his diet. But needing to work to support his family, he carried on the best he could. When exposed to any glues, sealers, stains or paints, he realized he was worse off than just being fatigued. After a couple of years, he was forced to leave his job.

His upper body, face, neck, chest and arms had become swollen and inflamed, and his skin itched constantly, almost as if he had chicken pox or a case of poison ivy. In the morning, his eyes were swollen and almost glued shut. At night, the itching was worse, and sleep was sometimes impossible, though it came with a short nap here or there and was very sporadic. With days and nights like this, he slipped into being irritable and depressed.

At a younger age, this man had had skin rashes and chronic allergies. Specialists and dermatologists gave him cortisone, antihistamines, and nerve pills, all with little or no effect. So now, at this later time of his life, he reached out to a different direction for help, a homeopathic clinic. They diagnosed him with problems that are really the aftereffects of what happens to the body's immune system when the body goes into overload. By this time he had Candida and Epstein-Barr virus which relate to fatigue. Recommended remedies were too expensive for someone out of work and responsible for a family.

However, he did start using some natural alternative therapies to fight the virus. This helped and he was able to go back to work part-time. Continuing to take the herbs and vitamins, he was able to work on and off for several months. He also became very diet conscious, eating no sugar or white flour, little dairy or meat, and no chemical additives. Alcohol was totally out of the question, because one beer set him back three or four days.

The following summer, while he was working on a large housing project, his problems continued, but were controlled by the taking of mega doses of vitamins and herbs. Sweating brought on rashes, itching, and burning, and the fatigue put him into bed every weekend to recuperate, just so he could go back to work on Monday. The last project was the staining of a house. So that he would not be overly exposed to the chemicals in the stain, he hired someone to do the job for him. However, he did get exposed and spent the next month in bed.

It was totally exhausting just to get up and have a shower. Some days he could work for only three or four hours, but he struggled. Besides the exhaustion, he still itched and had pain in his liver and kidneys, head, joints, and muscles. This went on without any relief in sight, and wondering what to do, almost pushed him over the edge.

Then one night on television, *60 Minutes* aired a show about mercury poisoning. The symptoms matched his and he immediately contacted a dentist who specialized in mercury removal. The dentist told him it was one of the worst cases he had seen and suggested a mercury detoxification program. This needed to be done before any work could be done in his mouth.

After each of the quadrants of fillings was removed, he spent three or four days recovering and detoxifying. People detoxify differently; some sweat and really have a body odor; some itch and get rashes, headaches, fatigue and nausea.

Six months later, he had the stamina he had been missing for years.

Fatigue and poor health had plagued the young housewife for several years. In her younger years she just pushed on ahead and did not stop. She had a small vegetarian catering business, and so she had enjoyed a healthy diet. She had traveled to Israel and worked there for a year, and had lived simply without very much stress. Later she started a house cleaning business and was then exposed to unsafe amounts of chemicals in the cleaning products. Because of her health, she made a career change.

Getting married and moving into a bachelor's apartment, and acquiring two dogs, sent her mind and body spinning into reaction. She wanted to make the new home a place to be proud of, and one that their friends would enjoy visiting. The chronic fatigue took over again. Tired almost every morning, she found it almost too much just to take the dogs for a walk. Finding enough energy to clean, do laundry, cook, and just exist was almost too much for her. It took almost three years to finish the apartment.

She had an abscess and root canal, and this was the turning point. She had become so familiar with how her body felt, that she knew something was just not right after the root canal. She wanted the root canal removed, but the dentist argued about how stupid that was. Within sixty days she went in for an emergency appendectomy. She started investigating, bought some books, and then the answer came. Mercury poisoning.

We made the choice to have our amalgams removed. Mercury detoxification was next. It takes months, sometimes years, for the body to detoxify from the effects of mercury poisoning.

When your body has been poisoned by mercury, your immune system starts breaking down and your body starts failing in different areas, depending upon which teeth/body organ (see chart, Appendix A) this relates to. That is why some people have chronic fatigue, headaches, backaches, kidney or liver problems, or the body overloads into gradual failure and major disease. Utilizing alcohol is the body's way of trying to leach mercury from the system, a self-defense mechanism. This causes the body to be constantly in a mercury poison mode, and side effects could lead into alcoholism. The body wants the alcohol to help let go of the mercury.

Day after day of overloading the body's organs with foods that react with mercury, such as hot liquids, acid foods, dairy, and meat, causes mercury vapor and the leaching of this poison into the body's systems. Our immune system can only handle so much. Our body is not meant to be overtaxed with as many chemicals and toxins as we are exposed to from our environment.

Chapter Eight

Body Awareness and Detoxification

We Are Made Up of Mind, Body, Spirit

By neglecting our body, we are limiting our receptivity to the influence of spirit, we are closing down one-third of a part of our being, although the effects of neglectfulness may not show up immediately. In fact, think it through: without the body, we cannot fulfill our soul's purpose.

When not properly cared for, the physical body, existing from the vital life force, must devote more of its attention to tasks related to basic survival, for example, maintaining the endocrine and lymphatic systems, repairing damage to tissues and muscles, protecting itself from endogenous toxic influences.

The process of gaining spiritual awareness entails subtle changes in the molecular vibrational rate of each cell of the body. So, under-nourished cells or biochemically unbalanced tissues are limited in their vibratory rate when unable to receive, or withstand, the higher intensity vibrations that accompany the influence of a spiritual vibration. It is our receptivity to spiritual influences that allows us the avenue to cocreate with spirit, and in so doing, to serve our purpose and humanity.

Learning to live with a body means respecting a sacred creation, and is probably one of our major spiritual lessons of earthly existence. It means loving the body for the opportunity it gives us to carry out our purpose. Only on this Earth plane do we have the opportunity of expressing this unique existence. Part of this lesson is learning the fine line of balance between the care of the body, our thinking mind, and our spiritual endeavors.

Bodywork and Fitness

What kind of exercise, bodywork, play, physical activity, do we involve ourselves in? Just how much do we know about our body, the "thing" we just happen to live in? And more than just knowing, it means respecting that knowing, and loving yourself enough to take action and provide for that need. The basic and essential ways to learn about caring for the body are through understanding diet, nutritional values, exercise, and how your body systems function, and getting in touch with your own spiritual being.

We replenish the cells of our body completely every seven years. This renewal can only come from the substances we eat and our environment, which can lead to a biochemical imbalance at the cellular level. Without proper nutrition our cells do not have adequate or appropriate substances (amino acids, carbohydrates, fats, minerals, vitamins, enzymes—see chapter 3) to use in carrying out their functions, or in building new cells and tissue.

The body's tremendous compensating mechanisms can mask the foolishness of improper diet for years, but not without hidden costs that only later can become apparent. It is much easier to prevent a disease than cure it. The old saying, "you are what you eat," is essentially true.

Symptoms of a Toxic Body

Headaches	Arthritis
Digestive disorders	Fatigue and weakness
Depression	Nausea
Gas and bloating	Chronic and degenerative diseases
Candida albicans	Allergies
Constipation	Skin problems
PMS	

Making Dietary Changes

It is natural to want some general dietary rules to help guide you. Because of individual genetics, and the variable responses to environmental influences, it is very difficult to establish guidelines that will work for everyone. What is nutritious food for one may be harmful to another. For your own choices, check out information on Ayurveda and listen to your body. It will let you know what it needs. Finally, read and research the informative books out there today.

The most important changes are those that you will continue to practice for the rest of your life. Experience shows that, while there are certainly exceptions, gradual changes, changes that can be incorporated into your daily life, are those that will continue to be practiced. Remember that you haven't failed even if you have to revise your plan of action. Adopting one new healthy habit, or dropping a bad one, is a step in the right direction.

Acid/Alkaline Balance

The concept of acid/alkaline balance refers to whether a digested food tends toward raising tissue pH (alkaline), or lowering pH (acid). Although the blood is maintained at a very narrow range of pH, residues of digested foods in body fluids retain a charge that can be positive (alkaline) or negative (acid).

Various sources have long exposed the health benefits associated with the consumption of alkaline-forming foods over acid-forming foods. The waste products of cellular metabolism are acidic. Therefore an acid state is associated with a toxic body. (See acid/alkaline food listing in chapter 3.)

Absorption

Contrary to the opinion you may have formed from the above, eating the right foods will not ensure that the necessary nutrients will be absorbed into your body. The amount of nutrients actually absorbed depends on the health integrity and efficient functioning of all organs of digestion.

To fully understand how easily digestion can be disturbed, it is helpful to understand how the sympathetic and parasympathetic nervous systems influence digestion. These two aspects of your autonomic nervous system have opposing actions, and when one is stimulated, the other is deactivated.

Check into the Ayurvedic medical concept to find out what body type you are. Take the quiz in the Ayurvedic section. What do your natural body instincts tell you? How does your body react to foods ingested, and what herbs can help you?

Digestive Herb

Sources: Better Nutrition *(January 1996);* Dimensions *(January 1996);* Better Nutrition *(February 1996);* Healthy Way *2, no. 1; and* Health News Naturally *(February 1996)*

Herbs have been used for digestive complaints for centuries. Of these herbs, ginger stands out. It is grown in southern Asia, and in the tropics of India, China, Jamaica, and Nigeria.

Ginger (Zingiber officinale) improves digestive complaints: (1) causes a brief increase in passage of gas followed by relaxation of the esophageal sphincter muscle; (2) increases stomach secretions resulting in improved digestion; (3) limits the development of "bad" microorganisms by its antiseptic action; (4) promotes bile flow, facilitating digestion and absorption of nutrients; and (5) relaxes intestinal muscle. The recommended dose for motion sickness is four times 250 milligrams, thirty minutes before departure. Ginger tea is also helpful as a detoxifier in cold prevention. It has recently been used to help lower blood cholesterol.

Body's Metabolic Digestion

Residues of human metabolism exit the body via the lungs, skin, liver, colon, and kidneys. In addition to our normal metabolic waste products, we have the industrial toxic residues such as heavy metals, pesticides, herbicides, food additives, and food preservatives. All this enters our metabolism via our food, water and air. Our scientists call accumulated residues "toxic load."

Author Harvey Diamond, in his book *Fit For Life,* recommends fruits and light foods in the morning until noon to extend that eliminative period. This is especially recommended for people who are toxic and overweight. Ayurveda explains that a poor digestive fire is often the first step in the buildup of toxins. The toxins from incomplete digestion are transported to inherent weak areas in the body, blocking important channels and vessels.

Auras, Chakras, and Essential Oils

The aura is part of our psychic anatomy, and radiates around all living things and us. Always in constant motion, vibrating, and pulsating, our aura is affected by our state of mind, life style, feelings, and attitudes.

The aura has three layers, or subtle bodies. The first is the etheric, composed of energy from beyond the earth. It is our celestial being. This is the force we radiate out to others. Spritzing lotions, massage, and essential oils enhance this field. The sages say that our karmic needs for certain experiences are placed in this layer of energy to guide us into what we came to do.

The second auric layer is the astral body. Astral means connected to the stars. The body helps us see the world and weave our energies through it. Our moods, feelings and the energy we send to others are dictated by the astral body. Our illnesses are filtered down by our state of being in the astral body.

The third layer is our spirit body. It is our soul force that always is and always will be. It projects out from our physical body according to the development of our spiritual nature, and the work we do on Earth. These three layers of the aura are connected to our physical body by the system of energetic vortices or wheels of energy called the chakras. (See chapter 9 for Energy Fields and Chakras.)

Essential oils increase the finest and farthest vibrations and assist all of the subtle bodies. The essential oils stimulate and assist in the process of awakening, healing, opening the chakras, and strengthening the aura. Essential oils are the spirit, the prana, chi or ki force of a plant. This essence of vibration from the plant is the plant kingdom's gift to the human being. The Indian medicine of Ayurveda works with the marma points or energy centers of the body. Marma means secret, hidden, and vital. The Chinese use these meridian points for a system of healing called acupuncture. These points have been known and referred to since ancient times. Marma points are the connection between the physical body and the subtle energetic bodies. See examples below from more than fifty marma points in the body.

Marma points and essential oils from book Ayurveda and Aromatherapy *by Drs. Light and Bryan Miller.*

Abdomen (Nabi) — location two inches below navel; affects balance/creativity/elimination; oils: ginger, clary sage, cypress, cedarwood.
Leg (Oovi) — location front midthigh; affects letting go; oils: trifolia, yarrow, lavender
Back (Vrahti) — location midback; affects heart, lungs; oils: rosemary, eucalyptus, camphor
Head (Sthapui) — location between eyebrows; affects balancing of sixth chakra; oils: lavender, jasmine, basil

Pancreas

Metabolic enzyme potential has to do with the nondigestive enzymes that facilitate chemical reactions in all the cells, including the brain, muscles, nerves, gonads and other tissues. The implication is that one's life span is determined in large part by the rate at which one's enzyme potential is depleted. Thus, eating raw foods and avoiding overeating are two ways to extend one's enzyme potential, health, or perhaps one's life.

Sympathetic Nervous System—controls heart rate, breathing, nerves stimulation and blood flow to skeletal muscles.
Parasympathetic Nervous System—controls secretions of the gastrointestinal tract and peristalsis.

Eating when upset, rushed, or in a stressful mode of thinking will divert blood flow and nerve stimulation away from the digestive organs. This can cause inadequate salivary, gastric, or pancreatic secretions which effect improper digestion, due to lack of or weak enzymes and improper pH.
Results are:
1) inadequate nutrient absorption
2) altered bowel microorganisms with decreased beneficial bacteria, and increased growth of nonbeneficial and potentially pathogenic microorganisms, including yeast
3) depressed immune function
4) absorption of toxins, or buildup of toxic load in the body
5) increased burden on the organs of elimination

Elimination

All cellular processes produce waste products that are toxic to the body. These wastes must be carried out of the body continuously. The colon, liver, kidneys, lungs, and skin are the major organs of elimination. Without these organs' proper functioning, toxins build up in tissues and biochemical imbalances occur, leading to impaired functioning. Chronic maldigestion and malabsorption will prevent the digestive organs and tissue from receiving the nutrients they require for fulfilling their function. This eventually leads to tissue changes, pathology and diagnosable illness. Intentional cleansing practices (colonics) are a recommended part of therapy for chronic disease, disease prevention, and purification.

Fiber

According to Dr. Dennis Burkitt, MD, in his twenty-year study of people who suffer from the same diseases in different countries, it was shown that people of Western dietary habits, and those countries that have adopted these habits, have replaced fresh, high-fiber foods with processed and fast foods. Diseases caused by low fiber intakes include appendicitis, coronary heart disease, diabetes, obesity, gallstones, hemorrhoids, and colorectal cancer.

Fiber helps the body to "detoxify." While there may be many reasons why a person may have insufficient bowel movements, a lack of fiber is a likely one. Because fiber is nondigestible, it travels through the digestive tract and "picks up" harmful substances, such as fat, along the way, then carries them out of the body. When the fat and other debris are cleansed from the digestive tract, nitrogen and sulfur gases are also reduced, allowing for more optimal absorption of the important nutrients, including oxygen which increases the metabolic rate in the body and is important for memory and energy levels.

In the Western countries it takes an average of three days for food to transit the body; in Eastern countries it takes approximately eighteen hours. During food's transit through the body, toxins from fermenting waste products can be reabsorbed in the blood stream, creating problems ranging from fatigue to colon cancer.

Basic Fiber Sources: Whole grain cereals, legumes, vegetables and fruits.

Obvious Symptoms of an Unhealthy Digestive Tract

Poor Digestion	Gas	Poor Skin
Body Odor	Fatigue	Stomach Bloat
Bad Breath	Lower Backache	Poor Elimination

Eight of the Most Common Causes of Toxicity

1) Poor Elimination—The colon is your body's sewage system, from which wastes are often reabsorbed back into the bloodstream, polluting our tissues and cells.

2) Poor Diet—Poor food choices include dead, low fiber, fried, devitalized or clogging foods, which lack proper enzymes to assist in proper digestion and assimilation, and also lack essential vitamins, minerals and other basic nutrients, rather than fresh fruits or vegetables.

3) Over-Consumption—Overeating puts a great amount of stress on our digestive system. The body must produce hydrochloric acid, pancreatic enzymes, bile and other digestive factors to process the food you have eaten. The stomach bloats as the digestive system goes into turmoil, then foods do not break down properly, and tend to lodge in the lower intestines.

4) Lack of Water—Water makes up sixty-five to seventy-five percent of the human body. It is second only to oxygen in its importance to sustaining life. Water cleanses the inside of the body as well as the outside; water flushes out wastes and toxins.

5) Stress—Stress affects every cell and tissue in the human body by breaking down the immune system and all of the major organs. It robs the body of important vitamins and minerals and over time can cause severe acid buildup. Stress hinders proper digestion, absorption and elimination of foods by throwing the digestive system out of balance.

6) Antibiotics - Can have a damaging affect on the intestines. Their purpose is to eliminate unhealthy bacteria in the body. However, antibiotics also eliminate good bacteria; they strip the colon of all intestinal flora and this throws the digestive and eliminative systems out of balance).

7) Lack of Exercise—Exercise strengthens the entire body, stimulates the circulatory and lymphatic systems, builds muscles, nerves, blood, glands, lungs, heart, brain, mind, and mood. Blood is pumped throughout the body by the heart, but lymphatic fluid depends solely on exercise to be circulated, so lack of exercise lowers metabolic efficiency.

8) Eating Late at Night or Too Early in the Morning—The human body uses sleep to repair, rebuild, and restore itself and uses the sleeping hours to cleanse and build. When a person goes to sleep with a full stomach, the body is not at rest, because it is busy digesting and processing. This inhibits the vital cleansing). It is best to have only light fruits or juices before noon.

Understanding Detoxification
by Claire Zieman, NC, IACT, Virginia Beach, VA

The Law of Cure

"All cure starts from within, and from the head down, and in reverse order as the symptoms have appeared" (Christine Hering, homeopath). How important this is to accept and realize. There are no quick fixes, no immediate reversals. Healing takes time, effort, intent, and knowledge. Let's take a look at how we can bring our bodies into balance, and the processes we go through.

Renowned nutritionist Dr. Bernard Jensen defines the process as follows:

Detoxification—Relates to reduction of toxic materials in the body, and to making this toxic material easier to eliminate. Therefore, the first part of his health program involves enabling the body to begin rejecting materials collected in the years before from bad diet and poor health habits.

Reversal Process—Is the retracing of the stages or steps of each disease you have had, reactivating each one and eliminating it. Many people who have suppressed diseases all their lives think of elimination of something like a cold as a sickness instead of a healing process.

Healing Crisis—Follows the reversal process. It is an effort by all organs to become new and strong again. Though it may feel like a disease crisis, it will not last as long, or develop into another disease. Instead, it will bring about renewed health.

Catarrh, Phlegm and Mucus—Are a termination process of toxic materials, acid and debris, which the body does not want. It can be the end result of the body tissues breaking down and has to find a way out of the body. The accumulation of this material can be eliminated through any orifice, skin or any of the eliminative organs.

Disease Crisis—Is when the body has reached its tolerance level with toxins and waste production. The body's defense brings forth an elimination of toxins, in the form of cold, fever, etc. The body is on the defensive and produces a disease crisis.

How Body Detoxifies—The bowels, lungs, kidneys, skin, and lymphatic system are all systems that eliminate. On the average, two pounds of toxins are eliminated from each organ daily.

The Kidney, Skin and Liver all Detoxify—The liver at any given time contains one-fourth of your blood. It is imperative for you to keep it cleansed. Alcohol causes liver damage and will interfere with liver function. Proper liver function is when bile is sent into the colon, stimulating bowel movement.

The Colon—The colon has the poorest nerve supply in the body. One half of all our bowel movement is the body breaking down, not what we eat. That is why juice fasting, juicing, and six to eight glasses of water a day are so important to optimal health. The main elements for proper bowel function include calcium, potassium, and magnesium. Chewing food well injects more saliva into the stomach, making it less acidic. Bowel cleansers, psyllium husks, and colon hydrotherapy will attempt to cleanse the colon.

Colon Hydrotherapy—Is a safe, restorative procedure that gently infuses warm, filtered water into the colon without discomfort to the individual. The entire colon is thereby cleansed stress-free.

A healthy colon is essential to a healthy body. Today's diet is all too often composed of saturated fats and processed, refined, and devitalized foods. This contributes to problems associated with the large intestines: colitis, constipation, diarrhea and toxemia, to name just a few. Eliminating undigested food particles, glandular and cellular debris, excess mucus, gases and parasites is an essential part of the digestive and assimilative processes.

Increases in environmental pollutants—such as pesticides, herbicides, and preservatives as well as antibiotics, chemical and hormonal food additives—heighten the need for these toxins to be removed from the body. Additionally, bacterial toxicity results from waste material that remains in and stagnates in the colon.

Many of these toxins are reabsorbed into the blood stream, lymph, liver, and nervous system, thus straining and eventually weakening the body's defense against viruses and foreign bacteria. The result is a breakdown, which affects the body as a whole.

Cleansing helps provide therapeutic improvement of colon muscle tone, necessary for peristalsis. It also cleanses, and dilutes the toxin load in the colon, resulting in a reduced burden on the liver. In turn, this helps restore internal balances and improves overall health by supporting the eliminative organs and rejuvenating the immune system.

Skin Eliminates Toxins

Our skin, by sweating, body odor, acne, and boils, eliminates toxins. The list goes on. Skin brushing every morning will help stimulate the skin and open the pores, aiding the release of toxins such as uric acid crystals and catarrh. Wearing natural fibers will allow your skin to breathe. You make new skin every twenty-four hours. Our bodies are truly amazing!

Exercise of the Lungs

The lungs are a channel through which the air we breathe passes, so that the blood can collect the oxygen and nitrogen needed to keep us alive. Tobacco is harmful to the lungs, as it destroys and damages the alveoli of the lungs. As stated by Norman Walker, "The condition of the entire breathing apparatus depends on the cleanliness of the colon, as well as the lungs. Fermentation and putrefaction in the colon have their effect on the health of every part of the anatomy."

Exercise helps the lungs to breathe. There are many types of breath work therapy available to assist with this process. The mini-trampoline is particularly beneficial. "Physical fitness is a measure of circulation efficiency. Increase circulation efficiency of the body fluids, the lymphatic and the blood stream that services the cells, and the body is considered physically fit. The muscles are able to continue the same work longer without fatigue" (Albert E. Carter).

When using the mini-trampoline to strengthen every cell in our body, it is important to remember that the feet do not leave the mat. Deep breathing is also necessary. As we begin to clear the body, unprocessed metabolic waste in tissues and undigested food accumulated in the system empty, and the circulating fluid called lymph becomes clear.

Kidney Function
1) Regulates water and electrolyte content.
2) Maintains acid/base equilibrium.
3) Eliminates metabolic waste products.
4) Retains vital substances.

The kidneys are complex and their work is nothing short of amazing! As cells and tissues of the body use food and oxygen, they produce waste. Carbon dioxide is eliminated through the lungs, while the kidneys extract wastes of protein metabolism in the form of urea and uric acid. The kidneys also extract cast-off, used up minerals, other elements, and wastewater from the lymph stream and from the blood.

Water is one of the easiest, most helpful means of caring for the kidneys. Drinking six to eight glasses of water a day does wonders for your system. Especially important is to have a glass as soon as you wake in the morning. This will aid your system and help rid it of urine, which has been there all night. It will also help develop muscle tone.

These are just a few suggestions to help you. Remember, only you can take care of you!

Chelation Therapy
Chelation is a complementary treatment for vascular disease and involves the infusion of the man-made amino acid EDTA, combined with certain nutrients and antioxidants, into a blood vessel of the body. The process takes about three hours to allow the solution to slowly circulate throughout the body's blood vessels, and to nourish the organs and tissues at the cellular level. The EDTA neutralizes heavy metals like lead, cadmium, and mercury by combining with them and allowing excretion through the kidneys. Chelating agents can be used to bind with undesirable calcium from the blood vessels and reduce the serum calcium level by excreting this mineral from the body, also through the kidneys. This also helps to strengthen the bones and to help prevent and arrest osteoporosis.

Chelation therapy treatment has been around for more than forty years, and science is just now catching up on how safe this treatment is for taking heavy metals out of the body, decreasing the production of harmful free radicals, and reversing hardening of the arteries in the entire body. This method also allows reversal of the symptoms of ischemia, which is a lack of adequate blood supply to the heart, the legs, the brain, the reproductive organs and throughout the 60,000-plus miles of blood vessels in the body.

Oral Chelating
Oral chelating agents offer a safe, convenient alternative to patients with serious circulation problems. There are also nutrients available that can aid in detoxifying, chelating, and removing substances from the body. The following chelating agents can be used to help prevent many degenerative illnesses:
1) alfalfa, fiber, rutin, and selenium
2) calcium and magnesium chelate with potassium
3) chromium, kyolic, pectin, and potassium
4) copper chelate, iron, kelp and zinc chelate

Hopefully, your healthcare insurers will add this to the list of therapies that are covered, sometime soon. There are more than 150 doctors in the United States who are certified by the American Board of Chelation Therapy. You can contact one of the following two groups for information on those in your area (referral services only).

The American College of Advancement in Medicine
23121 Verdugo Drive, Suite 204, Laguna Hills, CA 92653, 1-800-532-3688, www.acam.org

The American Board of Chelation Therapy
70 W. Huron Street, Chicago, IL 60610, (312) 787-2228 and 1-800-356-2228

Blood Cleansing for the Liver

One way to help lighten the liver's burden is to use wild plants such as dandelion, wild leek or bear's garlic, young nettles, yarrow, milk thistle, alfalfa, Swedish Bitters, and watercress, which are all ideally suited for this purpose. Obtaining the full value from a blood-cleansing cure requires effective intestinal elimination. It is here that mucilaginous seeds such as psyllium or linseed come into their own. Soaked figs or prunes can also be used.

A cleansing fast helps purify the blood. Drink distilled water, fresh lemon juice, beet juice, carrot juice, dandelion teas and extract. Quality water is important; drink at least eight glasses daily to aid in the cleansing, and to help carry toxins out of the body. Eat raw vegetables for a few weeks, and include "green drinks," since lots of chlorophyll is needed. Alfalfa liquid, wheatgrass, and barley juice are good for the colon, and for the added chlorophyll. Also good is super blue-green algae, a natural plant food.

To purify the blood, avoid white flour and all sugars. Also leave heated fats and oils out of the diet for one month. Herbs are helpful: goldenseal, red clover, dandelion, and barberry. Black radish, dandelion extract, and beet juice are good for the liver and aid in cleansing and healing. Burdock root helps eliminate toxins.

Boosting the Immune System

Echinacea—Helps to stimulate the body's own immune defenses for short-term help in warding off various minor bacterial and viral infections, particularly colds and flu.

Golden Seal—Increases the blood supply to the spleen, works with cells responsible for engulfing and destroying bacteria, viruses, fungi and tumor cells.

Licorice—Helpful in respiratory tract infections such as bronchitis, laryngitis and pneumonia.

St. John's Wort—Has been used for depression, infection, viruses, skin conditions, gastritis, hemorrhoids, bladder troubles, bronchitis, catarrh, consumption, diarrhea, dysentery, jaundice, bronchial asthma, neuralgia, fibrositis, sciatica and rheumatic pain, bruises, menopause-triggered irritability, and more.

Ginkgo—A major aid to circulation and nerves, and a powerful antioxidant. Suggested uses are for memory loss associated with aging, early stages of Alzheimer's disease, poor circulation to the extremities, recovery from a stroke, tinnitus (ringing in the ears), and early stages of macular degeneration.

Food Processing

Modern food processing methods are the primary cause of the nutrient devaluation of foods in developed countries. The less processed your food is, the better. When adding fiber to your diet, do so slowly, and drink plenty of water to help flush your system.

Book Resources

Clean Me Out (herbal program for cleansing, physical and emotional) by Dr. Rich Anderson
Edgar Cayce: Guide to Colon Care by Sandra Duggan, RN, BS

Edgar Cayce Handbook for Health through Drugless Therapy by Harold J. Reilly
Family Guide to Natural Medicine by Reader's Digest
The Complete Home Healer (three hundred treatments of common problems) by Angela Smyth
The Cure for All Cancers and *The Cure for All Diseases* by Dr. Hulda Regehr Clark
Natural Treatments and Remedies for the World's 400 Most Common Ailments by Global Health
New Choices in Natural Healing (eighteen hundred remedies from the world of Alternative Medicine) by Prevention
Prescription for Nutritional Healing by Dr. James Balch and Phyllis Balch, CNC

A wise man ought to realize that Health is the most valuable possession.
Hippocrates

Chapter Nine

Chakras and the Human Energy Fields

Humans Are Energy Beings

Each individual is composed of a system of energy fields or auras, which interact with each other and the environment. Our planet is a living universe: trees, plants, mountains, rocks, animals, rivers, oceans, streams, water—all are energy.

This energy, known as the "aura," or "electromagnetic field," has been depicted as a luminous radiation surrounding the body and our planet. This aura has been shown painted by artists of traditional religions in different cultures, including Chinese, Japanese, Buddhist and Egyptian. In Native American traditions, the aura was in the legend of the white buffalo. Descriptions in the Bible illustrate the transfiguration of the aura of Christ, using colors such as white and gold.

Each of our thoughts, emotions, and actions can be viewed as an energy discharge, radiating from a localized source into the universal field. Our personal energy field or "self," as well as everyone else's personal energy field, resides in and receives "nourishment" from this universal field. That is why, on the inner levels, we are all connected to one another.

If we think three dimensionally (affected by gravity and the Earth plane), we distort reality in thinking of ourselves as separate from everyone and everything else in our universe. A person identifying with only the physical body, conscious mind and physical senses, and believing there is nothing more, will not perceive the universe as it really is, nor will they experience the relationship of interconnectedness, unity, or Oneness.

Scientists are beginning to discover forces that do not fit into the conventional Newtonian science of reality. Various researchers who recognize the vital importance and correlation of these to physical living systems are studying energies of the life force.

The *Newtonian belief* is that the human body is a cellular mechanism.

The *New belief* is that the human body is energy. The body/mind/soul connection has been established, plus humanity's connection to all living organisms upon the planet.

A new breed of physician/healer is evolving to understand the functioning of human beings, of matter as energy. These spiritual scientists are looking to the human body for the inner workings of nature and the secrets of the universe. By realizing that human beings are energy, one can comprehend new ways of looking at health and illness. In conjunction with drug and surgical approaches, vibrational medicine attempts to treat people with pure energy. The infinity of energy is the "beyond," or the quantum outlook for the future of man.

Energy work changes unhealthy conditions in the human energy system, promoting a healthy energy field and producing harmony and balance. In this balanced state, a human becomes more conscious of "self" and the connectedness to the whole, and is able to radiate energy from all of his centers/chakras of power and consciousness.

Central to the work of psychospiritual integration (massage, healing, rolling), is the concept that the physical body is the outward manifestation of thought patterns, many from childhood fears and traumas, that we have allowed to penetrate our energy fields. Within specific locations of our energy systems, sensations, emotions, thoughts, memories, and other nonphysical experiences are what we report to our doctors and therapists. Understanding how our physical symptoms are related to these locations will help us understand the nature of different illnesses that we have attracted to us.

1) Each energy layer appears different and has its own particular function.
2) The layers of the auric field are associated with chakras (wheels of energy).
3) These fields relate back to fears, emotions, teeth, and traumatic experiences. (See charts and diagrams for further information, also the appendixes.)

The Fields of Energy

The Auric Field—Fields of Energy Diagram

The Seven Levels show the physical, emotional, and mental within three groupings: the three physical chakras, the bridge or heart chakra/astral, and the three spiritual chakras.

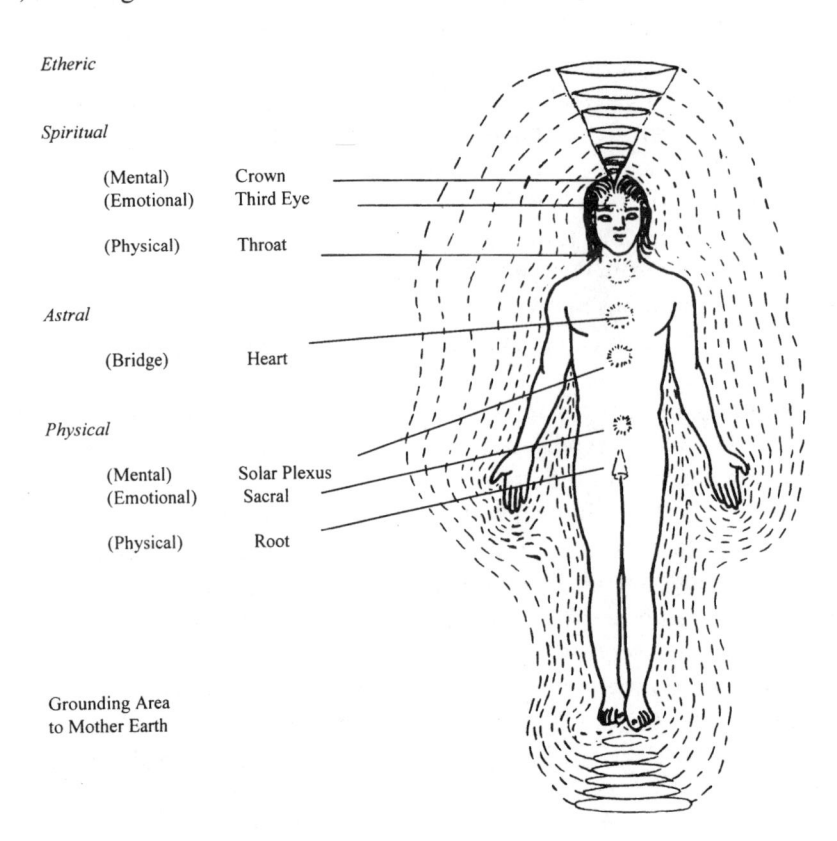

Etheric

Spiritual

    (Mental)   Crown
    (Emotional) Third Eye

    (Physical)   Throat

Astral

    (Bridge)   Heart

Physical

    (Mental)   Solar Plexus
    (Emotional) Sacral

    (Physical)   Root

Grounding Area
to Mother Earth

Physical Plane

Etheric Body (Physical Root Chakra)—The first layer, a state between energy and matter, is composed of tiny energy lines or light beams. The etheric body consists of a definite structure of lines of force or energy matrix, upon which the physical matter of the body tissues is shaped. This weblike structure is in constant motion. The physical tissues exist as such only because of the vital field of energy that is prior to, not a result of, the physical body. This field extends one-quarter to two inches beyond the physical body.

Emotional Body (Emotional Sacral Chakra)—The second layer is associated with feelings. This field roughly follows the outline of the physical body. Its structure is more fluid (clouds of fine substance in continual motion) than etheric, and does not duplicate the physical body. This field extends one to three inches from the body. This field of energy interpenetrates the denser bodies that it surrounds.

Mental Body (Mental Solar Plexus Chakra)—The third layer extends beyond the emotional, and is composed of a still finer substance. Associated with thoughts and mental processes, it extends three to eight inches from the body. The mental body is a structured body. It contains the structure of our ideas. Clear and well-formed ideas produce clear thoughts associated with those ideas. Within this field can be seen thought forms. This is the level at which clairvoyants connect.

Astral Plane—Bridge

Astral Level (Heart or Bridge)—The fourth layer is amorphous, and is composed of clouds of color. The field extends one-half to one foot from the body. Interaction between people takes place at this level. Pleasant or unpleasant, you can feel the difference. People forming relationships grow cords out of their chakras that interconnect them. These cords exist on many levels of the auric field. When relationships end, these cords are torn and can cause pain. Many cords hang by strings if we keep reconnecting with traumatic issues such as divorce, abuse, job-related experiences, personal relationships, traumas, etc.

Spiritual Plane

Etheric Template Body (Physical Throat Chakra)—The fifth layer contains all the forms (like a blueprint or negative of a photograph) that exist on the physical plane. This grid structure is what the physical body is built upon. The field extends out one and one-half to two feet from the body. It is the level at which sound transforms matter. It is at this level that sound is most effective for healing the body.

Celestial Body (Emotional Third Eye or Brow Chakra)—The sixth layer is the emotional level of the spiritual plane. It is the level in which we experience spiritual ecstasy, meditation, initiations, and transformation work, a point of being where we know our connection is with the entire universe. Through it we see light and love in everyone and everything. The field extends two to two and three-quarters feet from the body.

Ketheric Template (Mental Crown Chakra)—The seventh layer is the mental level of the spiritual plane. The field extends two and one-half to three and one-half feet from the body. The outer form is the egg-shaped shell of the aura and contains all the auric bodies associated with the present life an individual is living. It is composed of tiny threads of gold and silver (male and female essence) and holds the aura together. All the chakras and body forms appear to be made of golden light at this level. This is the strongest, most resilient level of the auric field. Its power current pulses up and down the spine, carrying energies through the roots of each chakra, and connecting the energies that are taken in through each chakra. The Ketheric field holds this present life's plan.

Cosmic Plane

The chakras above the seventh have been called the cosmic plane level.

Chakra System

Chakra is a Sanskrit word used by Hindus meaning "wheel of light." Most traditions refer to the seven major chakras as within the body, and those outside the body (eight through twelve) as the cosmic plane.

Visionaries (clairvoyants) perceive chakras as being circular spirals of energy, which differ in size and vibrate at different frequencies. Chakras serve as gateways or portals to collect and take up the flow of assimilated energy into our physical bodies; our material bodies could not exist without them.

Chakras act as pressure valves for the subtle energy system. A blockage in the energy flow of the chakra or an excess of energy can lead to imbalance and disharmony on the physical, mental, and spiritual levels. Our chakras react to every influence coming from outside, which in turn can draw together or open up the chakras accordingly. A blockage is the buildup of energy that, when it reaches a certain saturation density within each of us, causes a crystallization (pain).

Examples: Shoulder pain often occurs when a person is feeling that they are carrying a heavy load of responsibilities. Ankle pain is associated with flexibility in thought and/or action. Lower back stress is often associated with stress over financial worries. Heart pain can mean relationship problems or worry about everyone and everything. Gallbladder problems are associated with anger or hurts.

Channeled 'life force energy' can dissolve, fill or infuse light into the blocked and congested areas, and humans will again experience unconditional joy, which is our birthright. There is spirit or divine source in everything, and it is through this spiritual energy field that the "I Am" makes contact and comes into relationship with everything in the manifest universe.

The seven main chakras correspond to and connect with the major nerve plexus and glandular centers (seven main glands) of the endocrine system. The lower chakras include root, sacral and solar plexus, and correspond to the fundamental emotions and needs; vibrations are at a lower frequency. The upper chakras include throat, third eye or brow, and crown, and correspond to man's higher mental and spiritual directions. The upper chakras' are of a finer energy frequency. The heart chakra is the Bridge through which all energies are processed. One might visualize white light entering the crown chakra (prism) and flowing downward into different colors of the rainbow and entering into Mother Earth for grounding and balance. Each chakra is associated with a different-color ray and is located near the major nerve plexuses of the body.

Chakra Levels Eight through Twelve

The eighth chakra is in the auric field attached to the physical body. Nine through twelve are in the etheric fields, which may evolve as the changes within man change, and as our planet may evolve into another star system. We have the necessary spiritual resources to take our quantum leap when the time comes.

The conjecture that extra chakras, called "energy cysts" or "energy vortexes," appear in the body at different locations is a misunderstanding. This is caused by the "mirror aspect" effect where you see in others what you sense for the self. In other words, you may feel a vortex of energy within your own body, and you seem to see or feel this in others. Thus, you will have drawn to yourself other people needing to resolve the same issues or patterns of thought, not an additional chakra.

Location of Seven Chakras (Wheels of Light)

Location: 21 minor chakra points

2 sole of each foot
2 palm of each hand
2 behind each knee
2 spleen
2 behind each eye
1 solar plexus
1 stomach

2 front of each ear
2 above each breast
2 gonad
1 thymus
1 clavicle area
1 liver

CROWN
BROW OR THIRD EYE AREA
THROAT
HEART
SOLAR PLEXUS
SACRAL
ROOT

Root Chakra

First Level: is related to the quantity of physical energy and the will to live in the physical reality. It is the first location or the first manifestation of the life force in the physical world. It reflects the degree to which we feel connected to the earth and grounded in our present day activities. The ability to link with and function in day-to-day decisions controls basic survival instincts and primal feelings of fear from physical injury. Its influence is living in the present: I am here now and have the presence of power and vitality. Root chakra acts as a generator, a strong will to live.

Not enough energy in this center causes a tendency to react defensively to most situations; can manifest in feelings of paranoia and that life is too much, or suicide. This center is the seat of kundalini. A balanced center—kundalini—is the creative force of manifestation, which assists in the alignment of the chakras, the release of stored stress from the body centers, and the lifting of consciousness into higher spiritual levels.

Egyptian:	Physical Body Womb
	generation of people, humanity, heart of the sycamore, belly of heaven
Linked with:	sacrum, spine, rectum, anus, and urethra
Location:	base of spine, between the legs, sits into sacralcoccyx joint
Glandular:	gonads (testes—men; ovaries—women) - part of the endocrine system
Body:	physical vitality, will to live, supplies energy to spinal column, adrenals, and kidneys
Sense:	smell, basic element in sexual attraction between human beings
Key Words:	grounding, accepting incarnation, self-preservation, instinct of danger, developmental age

Developmental Age

Birth to three to five years of age. Early years are the foundation of life, revolving around the primary needs, such as warmth, food, shelter, and love. Without a variety of experiences and games, the child will not learn the differences between sizes, colors, sorting, counting, matching, putting puzzles together; all of which are the basic skills required for literacy and numeracy. Children of this age like touching different fabrics, hearing music, tasting (but not always liking), smelling, climbing whenever you aren't looking, squeezing (watch those pets), and generally observing their surroundings.

Earth Element

Dense matter, feminine, receptive and yin.

When living in harmony and respect for Mother Earth we also attune ourselves to the nature of Earth itself. By understanding Mother Earth we can understand its rhythms and cycles, and even the planetary threats affecting Earth itself. If Mother Earth dies, we die. The ancient ones remembered the promise of abundance and manifestation that Mother Earth would provide.

Color: Red Ray

Vibratory rate is the heaviest and slowest in the spectrum. This vibration draws out poisons, builds up red corpuscles, and stimulates arteries, sluggish PMS, and the autonomic nervous system. If vitality is lacking, simply wear something red. Chronic diseases nearly always require heating up. Helpful for those suffering from arthritis, rheumatism, lumbago, sciatica, and stiffening of the muscles and joints. For poor blood circulation, sluggishness, or low vitality, drinking carrot, beetroot and red grape juice is helpful.

Manifestation of Disease and/or Stress

Anger, frustration, insecurity, depression, lack of grounding, blood and nerve disorders, apprehension, temper, lack of balance, suppression, and lack of confidence.

Organs Affected: Prostate and cervix

With the first level weakened, you will experience being tired, and may not like physical activity. It can also affect whether you like eating or being touched.

Self-Healing Techniques

- Weed the garden; enjoy the fragrances of nature, walk in nature
- Use perfumed oil that has earthy quality for you; rub on lower back and legs

- Visual meditation—go into cave with the safety of your power animal for your journey
- Work with clay
- Sit with your back against a tree and feel the energy/Earth connection
- Lie in the grass, spine down to allow stresses to flow out of body into Earth
- Cry, scream, and let go of built-up inner tensions and especially any anger
- Participate in a sweat lodge ceremony for deep healing and Earth connection

Crystals to use with Root Chakra
- garnet - grounding, sensuality, sexuality, intimacy, positive thoughts
- ruby - vitality, nourishment, courage, passion, generosity, emotional warmth
- bloodstone - smooth energy flow, alignment, purification, brings abundance

Angelic Guidance: Angel of Patience and Acceptance and Angel of Creative Words
Healing Tone: Do
Day: Saturday
Planetary Influence: Saturn
Red Astrological Influence: Aries and Scorpio
Continent: North America
Level of Existence: All material things
Aromatherapy: Vetiver, Cypress, Angelica, Jatamansi, Musk

Sacral Chakra

Second Level: Related to the quantity of sexual energy of a person. When open, a person feels his sexual power; when blocked, there will not be much sexual drive. The person tends to avoid or disclaim. The nature of one's focus on sensual expression and sexuality can have both positive and negative effects (i.e. overfocusing to the exclusion of any higher spiritual pursuits or creativity). A person centering primarily in this chakra will tend to view relationships for their sexual and sensual aspects, and to view people as sexual objects.

A balance of giving and receiving, experiencing unity rather than separateness, is necessary. The orgasm, bathing the body in life energy, can be a holy experience culminating from the deep primordial evolutionary urges of mating on the physical level, and the deep spiritual yearnings of uniting with Divinity. This can be a wedding of both spiritual and physical aspects of the two human beings.

Egyptian:	KHABIT Shadow/Etheric/Astral: Divine Shadow
Linked with:	reproductive organs, intestines, urinary bladder, appendix, and lumbar vertebrae
Location:	below navel just above pubic bone, sits directly into center of sacrum
Glandular:	lymphatic
Body:	etheric; sensuality and sexuality, supplies immune system and sexual organs with energy
Sense:	taste, relating to color, design, building, fashions, entertainment
Key Words:	security, consciousness of sexuality, creativity, empowerment, sincerity, sense of others

Developmental Age
Age of discovery and individuality, but needing boundaries. Three to eight years of age. Foundation is setup from the root chakra for security within. Routines and repetition help set the patterning and

nurturing framework of security, but with adventure and flexibility rather than repression. It is an essential basis for a healthy individual for future relationships. Unnecessary rebellion against authority or obsessive self-control problems show that early development authority problems have not been dealt with.

Sexuality structure and instinct start at root at the sacral chakra. The consciousness of sexuality and choices starts with manipulation and power plays giving false impressions at this early age. The beauty and level of spiritual sensuality in sex have been greatly overlooked. We have forgotten from this spiritual sex aspect that energy creates a release for being creative in all forms of life (i.e. writing a book, painting a picture, laughter, joyfulness, communication of deep love). Suppressed and guilt-laden sexual attitudes create denial, abuse, degradation, fear, and anxiety. Celibacy by free choice, without guilt feelings, can be enlightening and create with Earth's natural rhythms the needs of the body.

Power is a principle. Empowerment is the process of that principle. Empowered people respect wisdom, authority, and the expertise of another person without feeling unworthy. A true teacher can empower her students and is not into grandeur, applause, or ego. Playing the part of the victim is passive by nature; being co-creative in society is playing an active part in the community. If we see authority figures as being totally to blame for anything and everything, we take power from ourselves. An overly judgmental or demanding environment affects the abilities of children to be sincere, open, and honest. Fully awakening, healing, and activating our sacral chakra heals the schism between matter and spirit, and holds the vitality for life and living. Strongly linked with expression or the throat chakra.

Water Element
Sense of movement, feminine, receptive and yin.

Water is linked to the moon, tides, time and the patterns and cycles for women. Earth and water define each other. Water courses through rock, forging canyons and valleys, and yet earth holds the water and contains it. With water, the earth becomes fertile, alive and reproductive. Water to the sacral chakra relates to the bodily fluids, such as the life force of blood, hydration of the body, and the fluid processes of elimination and cleansing.

Color: Orange Ray
This is an active ray, a mixture of intellectual and reproductive energy. Healing comes through action and the therapeutic release of emotions. Ceremonies with breathing, chanting, drumming and rhythmic movements help release the tension, fear and hostility. The ritual of the sweat lodge, along with herbs and diet, releases poisons and negative emotions. The sweeping of the body with feathers or hand movements moves the energy downward and out, along with breathing out the negatives. Orange ray increases oxygen, helps lungs, encourages interests and activities, releases gas, draws boils, and brings abscesses to a head.

Manifestation of Disease and/or Stress
Repression, mask, smothering, inhibitions, control, holding on to old relationships, lethargy, mental blocks, foreboding, worries, overconcern, lack of fulfillment, lower back pain, colitis, kidney and spleen ailments, chronic fatigue syndrome, dislike of self.

Organs Affected
Muscles (fibromyalgia), lymphatic glandular system.

Self-Healing Techniques
- Take healing baths to soothe or energize
- Use apple cider vinegar and Epsom salts; this also helps clear toxins and cleanses repression
- Drink healing teas: jasmine, hibiscus, chamomile, and orange spice
- Drink water, water, and more water—flush it all out
- Take a walk in the rain
- Connect with earth and water elements
- Fill a goblet with pure water; allow the sun to energize it
- Sit in a warm shower with a towel on your lower back and visualize tensions washing away
- Take time for a personal party, be silly and joyful, and laugh
- Sweat lodge ceremony

Crystals to use with Sacral Chakra
- amber—purification, wisdom, balance, patience, strength, calmness, healing
- jasper—compassion, nurturing, contentment, serenity
- citrine—orange or amber, heals wounded emotions, aids in acceptance of sexuality
- carnelian - appreciation of nature, harmony; acceptance of death and rebirth

Angelic Guidance: Angel of Imagination and Liberation and Angel of Courage and Perseverance
Healing Tone: Re
Day: Tuesday
Planetary Influence: Mars
Orange Astrological Influence: Leo
Continent: Europe
Level of Existence: all biological things
Aromatherapy: Canadian Balsam, Bergamot, Juniper, Clary Sage, Patchouli

Solar Plexus Chakra

Third Level: This is the center and issue of personal power whereby we relate to others in their life, express control over one's life, or are subjected to the whims of others. Issues of dominance and submission are the lesson. The viewpoint is of one's sense of comfort with the universe as a nurturing place, as opposed to seeing the world as bad things waiting to happen. This center supplies energy to the major organs of digestion and purification. Negative programming of the unconscious mind during the early childhood years may manifest imbalances. A person with an open solar plexus chakra will have a deeply fulfilling emotional life that does not overwhelm him.If it is closed he may not be connected to his own uniqueness within the universe and his greater purpose.

This center is very important with regard to human connectedness. If connected, a person is firmly grounded in his place in the universe. He is the center of his own unique aspect of expression of the manifest universe, and from this he derives spiritual wisdom. He has an ego center or ego identity, where the word "I" is used confidently for needs and desires. This is not to be misinterpreted as negative ego, which can manipulate, control, and try to possess.

Egyptian:	KA Emotion/Desire: Image, genesis, character, reverberation
Linked with:	major organs of digestion /purification, stomach, pancreas, liver, gallbladder spleen, adrenal glands, lumbar vertebrae, general digestive system

Location: above the navel, sits directly into the diaphragmatic hinge between T12 and L1
Glandular: Two adrenals (cortex and medulla) linked with abdomen above the kidneys. Medulla is activated by nerve impulses, fight or flight impulse. Cortex is an endocrine gland activated by blood-borne hormones, sent out by the pituitary, and essential to life; an energy generator in charge of energy storage, regulates fire in the body.
Body: astral
Sense: physical sight and creative or intuitive vision; knowing how the wind blows, so to speak
Key Words: assimilation, logic, reason, opinions, intuitiveness, physic energy, rites of passage

Developmental Age

Eight to twelve years of age, an emergence from the cocoon into a butterfly (or independence of being) but with subtle softness, love, and a gentle hold on the reins. Coming into realization of being intelligent, children digest information around them, so keep it rich and stimulating, rather than abusive television programming. A wake-up call to becoming aware of the opposite sex, this is a difficult time to help the child understand their freedom, and at the same time protect them in their choices, which can have long-term implications, bitterness, or even resentment, if they do not feel they have been given choices. A rite of passage is the coming of age that is celebrated in some religions. This can be healthy when children understand the privileges and new responsibilities, and that old patterns are left behind.

Fire Element

Masculine, active and yang.

Consumes, changes things, and enables assimilation, also sets processes in motion. When the solar plexus is underfunctioning, we have been on a one-track notion or treadmill and unable to bring about creative change in our lives. An active well-functioning chakra brings about nourishment, enjoyment and passion, but an overly active chakra makes us irritable, uncomfortable, dry-skinned, and angry. Our body's food can then be burned up too quickly, not properly assimilated, and its nutrients imperfectly absorbed.

Color: Yellow Ray

This is the ray of intelligence or intellect, a mental color. It is possible to heal the mind through imagination. For example, with children, knights fighting dragons; with adults, using the fountain of golden white sunlight flowing. Actual sunlight on the solar plexus can help the metabolism, eyesight, and a physical sense of well-being. The word "solar" links this chakra to the sun and all which is light, fiery, and conscious. Hypnotism works if you get to the root of the problem, rather than just fixing an outside condition, such as smoking. Mesmerism healing can take place at this level, but watch the ego. Christ was said to have charisma without being showy, and he always directed the power from "father in heaven," not from himself. Psychic surgery works if trust is established, and only if the patient wants at some deep level to be healthy. This vibration can help mental illness and reinforce self-confidence and courage. Helps assimilation, stimulates lymphatic system, liver, gallbladder, eyes, and ears. Lemon juice will help loosen congestion and mucus in the digestive system.

Manifestation of Disease and/or Stress

Nervous dysfunction, intestinal disorders, energy blockages, delusion, exaggerated obsessions, abusiveness to others, aggressive anger, inner rage, depression, poor circulation, liver dysfunction, domination.

Organs Affected

At a weak level you will lack mental agility or clarity, and not be interested in academics or intellectual pursuits. These "negative thought forms" correspond to our habitual processes and are difficult to change because they appear to be logical to the person experiencing them.

Self-Healing Techniques
- Go for a walk on a sunny clear day
- Read poetry that is inspirational and soothing
- Go to museums, zoos, and places of pleasant joyful stimulation
- See a funny movie; laugh, loosen up, and breathe
- Make a natural arrangement of flowers, leaves, roots, and stones.
- Meditate, meditate, meditate and sleep
- Do creative art, experiment visually with colors and textures, make interesting designs
- String beads, focusing on each bead; use one color, forget patterns
- Write out goals and achievements on slips, then burn papers
- To release energies, burn during a waning moon
- To attract energies, burn during a waxing moon

Crystals to use with Solar Plexus Chakra
- calcite—deepens intellect, memory, wisdom, channeling, and astral projection
- topaz—happiness, sense of humor, abundance, attracts love
- kyanite—aligns chakras, vivid dreams, clear visualization, brings about tranquillity and calmness

Angelic Guidance: Angel of Discernment and Angel of Order and Harmony
Healing Tone: Mi
Day: Friday
Planetary Influence: Venus
Yellow Astrological Influence: Taurus and Libra
Continent: Asia
Level of Existence: all animals
Aromatherapy: Gold Chamomile, Sandalwood, Lavender, Yarrow, Basil, Fennel, Calamus

Heart Chakra

Fourth Level: Bridge, center for connectedness and nurturing. Related to the ability to express love, including self-love. The highest form of spiritual love is unconditional love towards others. When this chakra is in an open and loving state, you can see the whole individual, the uniqueness, the inner beauty and the light; and not just the negative or undeveloped aspects. In the healing process the current power (energy) moves into the heart chakra before moving out of the hands or eyes of the healer. The heart transmutes the Earth plane energy to spiritual energies, then spiritual energies to Earth energies for the client's use. Heart provides energy to bronchial tubes, lungs, breasts, and the entire circulatory system. It is the meeting and blending place between spiritual energies moving downward and the physical energies moving upward. The throat then becomes the gateway.

Egyptian: AB Heart/Lower Mind: Heart of the Soul, Heart's Desire, intentions, imagination
Linked with: thymus, bronchus, lungs, breasts, entire circulatory system, vagus nerve, upper back
Location: middle/left of chest, sits into T5
Glandular: thymus
Body: feelings, front of chakra related to love, back of chakra related to will
Sense: touch through tenderness and vulnerability, also situations touch or move us
Key Words: compassion, feelings, tenderness, love of spirit, love of others, emotional detachment

Developmental Age

Twelve to fifteen years of age, this age group still needs support and yet freedom to explore; having previously built a trust between child and parent is now helpful. Teenagers are at the stage of tender feelings and vulnerability, passionate about their beliefs, and experiencing the intensities of first love. If a child is to develop into a self-assured mature adult person, the parent of the opposite sex must give permission and recognition from puberty onwards. Adolescence carries a need for rebellion and the focusing of discontentment, but this can be turned into a healthy stage yielding greater consciousness of personal integrity on which to base rules and guidelines, by setting and stating values and why the parent has these beliefs.

At a physical level, trauma connected with this developmental stage can trigger asthmatic and allergic conditions. If in existence from birth onward, the cause can be an overanxious mother, whose own wounded heart affects the child's early response to life. The discipline to see a situation with detachment brings clarity leading to dispassionate appraisal of problems, thereby wisdom. When prepared to be vulnerable and tender, we can then give tenderness, true feelings, and compassion to others. The heart-centered individual brings a feeling of quality to life without being governed or driven by raw emotions. It is possible to have knowledge of and to use feelings without them controlling our lives in an irrational or irresponsible way. Compassion brings nonjudgmental understanding. The Native Americans say, "Judge no one, until you have walked a mile in their moccasins." This reflects the true meaning of compassion.

Air Element for Heart Chakra

Masculine, active and yang.

Airborne qualities give the heart its key word of detachment, and demand a clear discernment between romantic feelings, emotional feelings, and wisdom. Air challenges those ideas about the heart that are symbolically linked to romantic love. Our physical bodies contain air, we exist in air, we are touched by air, air gives us space between things for definition, and without air our physical bodies die.

Color: Green Ray

This ray incorporates wisdom and intuition. Healing through the heart involves the powers of love and nature. If a healer's heart is not really concerned with love of human beings and nature, he will be using the left-brain hemisphere and his own energies may not be balanced. This ray stimulates the pituitary and raises the vibrations, restores balance, builds cells, dissolves blood clots and heals infections. When healing with the green ray, we can use the hands to massage in aromatic oils or use herbal remedies. A healer with no love and a closed heart will be unable to channel the green ray, and it will be almost impossible for him to help anyone with cancer.

Manifestation of Disease and/or Stress

Dissatisfaction, greed, envy, inconsiderateness, covetousness, imposition, coldness, blood pressure disorders, heart palpitations, ulcers, blood clots, itching palm, resentment, gall, bitterness, hostility, and grudging.

Organs Affected

Heart, thymus, lungs, breasts, nerves, circulatory system. Fourth level carries our whole world of relationships, i.e., people, plants, animals, Earth, sun, stars and the universe as a whole. Negative aspects can form mucus conditions in the body, effecting pain, discomfort, feelings of heaviness, exhaustion, and then disease. Fourth level contains all love and joy as well as struggle and pain.

Self-Healing Techniques
- Be in nature—touch or hug a tree, plant some herbs
- Burn sage or thyme, allowing smoke to stream throughout house
- Feel the peacefulness and change within yourself
- Hug something, a pet, a rock, a teddy bear, a child, someone special
- Take a walk on a windy day; allow the wind to sweep you clean
- Use scented oil to anoint your heart area; mint or lavender is good
- Use a feather to cleanse your auric field, sweeping downward and allowing any disqualified energy to flow into Mother Earth for cleansing and being transmuted into light; be in the present moment

Crystals to use with Heart Chakra
- moss agates - emotional balancing, strength, allows one to see beauty
- malachite - stone of transformation, helps clarify emotions, love, friendship and loyalty
- emerald - stone of successful love, enhances memory, brings harmony, instills sensitivity

Angelic Guidance: Angel of Truth and Enlightenment and Angel of Spiritual Strength and Will
Healing Tone: Fa
Day: Sunday
Planetary Influence: Sun (spine) and Neptune (heart/thymus)
Green Astrological Influence: Cancer
Continent: South America
Level of Existence: Man
Aromatherapy: Rose, Eucalyptus, Bergamot, Neroli, Lavender, Orange

Throat Chakra

Fifth Level: Taking responsibility for one's personal needs. The chakra shows what state the person is living in with respect to receiving whatever is coming to him. An open center will attract nourishment. Clearing the misconception of receiving or taking in is then transformed into trust in a benign nourishing universe. Center has influences over the major glands and structures in the neck region, including thyroid and parathyroid glands, mouth, vocal cords, trachea, cervical vertebrae, and parasympathetic nervous system.

This center is communication, transpersonal expression, connection to higher self, and higher creativity of song and music. It is also known as the center of the will and is the way, or how, one communicates. Thyroid affects metabolism, bodily heat control, and some aspects of growth. The parathyroid secretes a hormone that maintains the correct levels of calcium in the blood.

Egyptian: BA Soul/Higher Mind: to shine, be light, give light
Linked with: parathyroid, thyroid, senses:
hearing, tasting, smelling, bronchus, lungs, alimentary canal
Location: throat area, front and back, sits into cervical vertebra C3
Glandular: thyroid and parathyroid
Body: mental, giving and receiving, speaking our truth
Sense: hearing, listening, tasting, smelling, speaking, and being heard—the quality of the voice
Key Words: communication, expression, responsibility, and universal truth

Developmental Age

Fifteen to twenty-one years of age. Expression is twofold: (1) seeks fulfillment through an outlet of talents or abilities, being heard; (2) higher expression is concerned with connection to one's spiritual qualities, being true to self and taking charge of one's life and becoming a responsible adult. Responsibility is about hearing that calling, and responding with conviction to a divine or higher purpose.

Working with the throat chakra can help in the task of listening to our bodies and becoming more attuned to our health patterns. Communication is an expression of ourselves, the exchange of information and ideas. It is a function for creating our futures. The Hindus believe that all is a matter of sound. The universe is a melody of sound that we are not yet attuned to. Is sound the basic pattern upon which the universe came into being? It is a universal truth that the throat chakra is connected to law and order; in the normal functioning of man comes a sense of moral rightness. Individually, we strive for integrity and function best with positive thoughts. It is a universal truth that we are challenged by and concerned with understanding "Divine law." It is the questioning of what peace, justice, wisdom or beauty is.

Ether/Akasha Element

It is the first plane of subtle substance. Etheric body ether or etheric plane—not chemical ether. The Sanskrit word is "akasha," or the imprint of all humankind's individual and collective experience in the etheric, our blueprint. Our thoughts, concepts, and creative imaginings are held here as part of their journey. Sound frequencies are part of the etheric plane. The sacral chakra has a close connection to the throat.

Color: Blue Ray

Through this radiation the atmosphere becomes calmer and creates a protective shell where people feel safe and happy. All healers must acquire a specific amount of this ray. It also deals with sound; Christ healed with his voice, as did many ancient healers, shamans, and medicine men. Singing in the bath is cleansing as water helps to purify the etheric, and the sound will dissolve any negativity that has been washed out and is hanging around in the atmosphere. This ray is good for sleep, fevers, inflections, inflammations, mental depression, irritation, itching and burns.

Manifestation of Disease and/or Stress

Withdrawal, hyperventilation, hysterics, self-concern, possessiveness, control, domination, fevers, respiratory problems, throat infections, laryngitis, coughing, and rheumatism. On the fifth level, divine will is divine intent manifested into pattern and form. We have free will to align ourselves, or not, with the template of the evolutionary plan for humanity and the universe. Negative aspects include being flustered, cluttered, messy, and uncomfortable with your surroundings, a disorderly life, not having inner strength or purpose of life.

Organs Affected
Throat, neck, thyroid, parathyroid, ears, sinuses, nervous system.

Self-Healing Techniques
- Chant, sing, whistle, yell, scream, and laugh
- Express self vocally, in the shower, at the beach, in the mirror, do not hold back
- Lie outside in nature, look at the sky, and breathe with mouth open
- Fill throat with sky energy and blue serenity
- Enjoy some mint, spearmint or orange mint tea
- Write letters to send or not; keep a journal of your feelings, your opinions, and your advice

Crystals to Use with Throat Chakra
- lapis lazuli—inner power, love, sense of wonder and mystery, total awareness, truth
- blue topaz—meditation, psychic powers, spiritual growth, and law of attraction and manifestation
- sapphire—stone of prosperity, stimulates throat, assists in communication, lightness and joy

Angelic Guidance: Angel of Materiality and Temptation and Angel of Illusion and Reality
Healing Tone: Sol
Day: Wednesday
Planetary Influence: Mercury
Blue Astrological Influence: Capricorn
Continent: Antarctica
Level of Existence: Perfected Man
Aromatherapy: Sandalwood, Lime, Hyacinth, Tea Tree, Blue Chamomile

Third Eye or Brow Chakra

Sixth Level: Seat of intuition (clairvoyance) and intuitive prowess, referred to as the third eye. Alchemy is the spiritual marriage of spirit and soul. Spirit is seen as yang, clear, direct, initiator, commander of life and its revolving tasks; it commands action with inspirational insight. Soul is yin, receptive, gestating and sifting through the information to facilitate a response. It is the conscious level of awareness, developed by various types of meditative practices. It also includes the person's concepts of reality and the universe, or how he sees the world.

This higher mental body is a light and subtle substance. It reflects the indigo and amethyst colors, and we wear these colors for communication and meditation with other planes, and for moments of inspiration or mystical experiences. These inspirations give birth to original ideas, before we put them into language. It is the plane of divine principal and arch-angelic beings: Michael, Gabriel, Raphael, and Uriel. The pineal gland is our internal day and night clock and there are nerve pathways between the pineal and the retina. There is some relationship between the pineal and the hormones relating to growth, temperature control, repair of broken tissue and the generation of energy. Hormones regulate basic drives, emotions, sexual urges, identity, anger, fear, violence, joy, sorrow, and sleep.

Egyptian: KHU Spirit Body/Spiritual: heart of light, seed of light
Linked with: pituitary, left eye, lower brain, ears, nose, and nervous system
Location: center of forehead and back of head, tip sits center of head
Glandular: pineal
Body: higher mental
front of chakra—related to conceptual understanding
back of chakra—related to carrying our ideas forth in a step-by-step process to accomplishment
Sense: intuitive, sense of being spiritually inspired, receiving inspiration
Key Words inspiration, insight, spirit, and completeness

Development

Within each of us there is a spark or essence of purity that does not get clouded. Somewhere beyond all the behavior patterns and our daily reactions to life—regardless of our personality, character, or morality—this spark burns on. Sometimes deeply seated, this honor comes forth in battle, or when there is an accident. When the concepts of mass murderers, vicious crimes and con-artists are talked about, we wonder where their spark has gone; yet many of these people feel inspired and have high perception and understanding but on a level of low density. Through spiritual awakening in this area, we can begin work with our spiritual guides. This awakening also brings about a need to enjoy completeness of peace and inner harmony, balance of body, mind and spirit soul.

Color: Indigo Ray

This is a calming, pacifying ray, which affects the right side of the brain. It is the ray of intuition and the key to intuitive levels and is used to treat people suffering from neuroses. Superconsciousness is the ability to master the right brain's intuition and the left brain's logic. Functioning properly, we should be able to transmute anything. Training to develop your intuitive powers helps your awareness about coincidence or the synchronicity of happenings in life. Awakened intuition brings about wisdom and knowledge. When the whole circuit is awakened, we can link with a network of energies that transmit signals at the speed of light often called "flash of intuition." We may more fully develop the powers of smell, sight, or hearing. However, if the information is flowing, it then goes beyond these senses. Information that then comes through is from the whole and to be shared with the whole of consciousness.

This ray promotes the building of inner strength, and through this our security, helping us to do the right thing at the right time. Through this ray we can travel to other dimensions and learn to dance our dance rather than someone else's. On the negative side we can develop ourselves so strongly that we allow intellect, will, or ego to impose itself, rather than to serve the cause. Reach for the inner teacher and bring forth your own intuitive knowledge that lies within. Powers run in seven-year cycles, so be aware of your own cycles. First, relaxation is a must to build your intuitiveness. This will change the brain waves, so that you can gather the necessary power to raise the mind to a higher dimension, to receive information from the collective consciousness.

Manifestation of Disease and/or Stress

Not wanting to see something that is important to their soul growth, egotistical behavior, disorders of the nose, eyes, ears or sinuses, cataracts, arrogance, authoritativeness, obsession, neurosis, headaches, pretension, loftiness, and major endocrine imbalances, because of the association with the pituitary gland.

Organs Affected

Sixth level is experienced as spiritual love, joy, elation and bliss; we reach this level by silencing the noisy mind and listening. This is where we commune with beings of the spiritual worlds of various dimensions, as well as humanity, plants, animals, and Mother Earth. Negative aspect include a lack of spiritual nourishment, and still feeling the "separated from Divine Source" concept.

Self-Healing Techniques
- Meditate, focus on indigo or fuchsia, go into the All-Mind consciousness, and find a sacred place
- Visualize and activate your imagery, see yourself as completing your goals
- Find a quiet place, like sitting by a tree, walking along the ocean, or walking in floral gardens
- Listen to gentle flowing music, listen to the elements or take a luxurious bubble bath with candles and soft music

Crystals to use with Third Eye Chakra
- azurite—stone of heaven, prophecy, psychic dreams, intuition, called "sacred stone"
- amethyst—spiritual awareness, inner peace, relieves tension, positive transformation, mysticism
- halite—enhances good will, provides insight, stimulates meridians, meditative ancient solutions

Angelic Guidance: Angel of Loving Relationship and Angel of Success
Healing Tone: La
Day: Thursday
Planetary Influence: Uranus
Indigo Astrological Influence: Aquarius and Pisces
Continent: Australia
Level of Existence: higher forces
Aromatherapy: Lavender, Patchouli, White Musk, Rose Geranium, Myrrh, Jasmine, Eucalyptus

Crown Chakra

Seventh Level: One of the highest vibrational centers in the subtle body, it is the deep inner searching (spiritual quest) for the meaning of life. Opening of the crown chakra allows one to enter into higher states of consciousness. A conscious activation represents the beginning of awareness of spiritual perfection or ascension. The crown correlates to our reason function. When this level is strong and intact, it forms into a golden egg that surrounds and protects everything within it. It regulates a proper flow of energy out from the entire aura into the space beyond and prevents energy leakage out of the shell. It is the level of the divine mind, and when healthy, it enters the universal divine mind field. It is here that we understand and know that we are part of the great plan of life, and know our perfection within our imperfections.

If you have a strong level you will have creative ideas and clearly understand concepts about existence, the world, and its nature. You will understand how your ideas fit into this plan and how you as a person fit into the plan, and have a strong sense of divine source.

Egyptian: KHABS Divine, to shine through like a star, illumination
Linked with: pineal gland, upper brain, right eye
Location: top of head

Glandular: pituitary
Body: soul, ketheric or causal experience of direct knowing; related to integration of personality with spirituality
Sense: letting go, letting Divine Source take control, total surrender
Key Words: surrender, release, incoming will, and soul

Development

The opportunity of reincarnation enables experience to be gained and balances to be made. The soul governs the pattern of karma, and spurs us into action; the result is the law of cause and effect. When the karmic journey nears its end, the soul becomes a clear chalice in which the spark of spirit can burn. This balance between soul and spirit represents the consummation of the mystical marriage and the birth of knowledge, light, vision, healing, and wisdom.

Release and surrender work together and create a condition of blind obedience. It signifies a trust in the higher self, which enables a relaxed attitude to life, rather than abdicating responsibility and alertness.

The incoming will refers to the purpose of the soul in our present-day incarnation. Surrender and release from the "lower will" to the incoming divine will brings about harmony and is spiritually directed. These accomplishments are not possible except through the crown chakra.

Magnetum Element

Not found in standard list of elements, its symbolic quality is unification, and signifies "being whole." It is experienced when body, mind, and spirit are in harmony. Helps promote the healing of our relationship to Mother Earth and all its life forms.

Color: Violet Ray

This is the ray of creativity. On this ray, it is possible to heal with works of art. Art links mankind to the spiritual levels and reflects his inner longing to go beyond his earthbound realms. This ray is the expression of our innermost aspirations. Helpful choices in healing on this ray are art, fragrance, color, crystals, dance, and music or singing as tools. Better yet, inspire the client in his own creativity of using these tools. This ray is good for headaches, and for some people it can aid in slimming down.

Violet has the highest vibrational rate in the sevenfold spectrum of color. Violet at the crown chakra pertains to balanced and perfected wisdom. It is a good cleansing color; visualization helps cleanse impurities from the energy field.

Manifestations of Disease and/or Stress

Tiredness, weak psychic ability, cerebral dysfunction, psychosis, being overwrought, creative exhaustion, migraines, and nervous tension.

Organs Affected

The pituitary gland regulates the endocrine system. It is largely responsible for the type of bodies we have, and the way in which they function. It opens the physical channels through which the purposes of the higher self can be reflected in bodily and behavioral patterns, by the experience of birth. It regulates substance, which helps kidneys to regulate body fluid, and levels of sodium and potassium.

Self-Healing Techniques
- Dance move, and experience the spirit of music
- Write poetry, journal, etc.
- Vision quest
- Retreat into nature or walk in nature
- Sweat lodge ceremony
- Light a lavender candle, relax, and meditate
- Listen to gentle mood music
- Take a warm luxurious bath with gentle music

Crystals
- white fluorite—helps to clear and energize aura, align chakras, brings accord between spirit/intellect
- white tourmaline—protection and healing, aligns energy centers, balances the female and male energy
- evansite—allows one to see the truth, provides insight, helpful to teachers and lecturers

Angelic Guidance: Angel of Power and Authority and Angel of Unconditional Love and Freedom
Healing Tone: Ti
Day: Monday
Planetary Influence: Moon and Neptune
Violet Astrological Influence: Virgo and Sagittarius
Continent: Africa
Level of Existence: God or Divine Source
Aromatherapy: Violet Absolute, Gardenia, Ylang Ylang, Myrrh, Frankincense, Shamama

Link between Heart and Thymus Gland

The word "thymus" is Greek word meaning life force or vitality. The gland is located in the middle of the chest, behind the upper part of the breastbone. Today we are aware that the thymus gland is the most important organ in the maintenance of our immune system. Researchers are now beginning to discover powerful regulatory hormones, which are produced by this gland, influencing an individual's ability to fight off disease by enhancing the activity of different types of T-lymphocytes.

Various researchers have examined the link between emotions and illnesses, and have found a strong association involving depression and grief, and the suppression of the immune function. Interplay of these blockages with the heart chakra may arise from an inability to express love, or even a lack of self-love. The ability to love oneself is far more important than many psychologists realize. Negative self-images, loss of self-worth, emotions of grief, sadness, loneliness, depression, and an inability to express love cause imbalances to occur with the heart chakra.

Medical researchers do not yet understand that the subtle energy flow of prana (life force) through the heart chakra is an integral factor in the proper functioning of the thymus gland, thus the body's immune capability.

Individuals with strong immunology defenses may be able to remove a virus from their system, or limit its effects to minimal flu-like symptoms. A significant energy factor contributing to a strong immune response is a healthy flow of subtle energy through the heart chakra to support the thymus gland.

A weakened thymus gland can be strengthened within a matter of seconds. A wake-up call to the thymus is to tap lightly with your fingertips ten to twenty times. This will stabilize your system and give you vitality. You can also Reiki your thymus. Strengthen your thymus on a regular daily basis and you will feel stronger. (Rubbing does not activate the thymus.)

Our heart chakra has cords in the auric field connecting us with our parents, much like the umbilical cords. Each parent is a model of how we will continue to create relationships with either the men or the women in our lives. Cords from this level represent loving and the mystery of the balance between loving and willingness in our relationship. These cords are what we refer to as "heart strings." An unhealthy structure starts in childhood, is repeated as that person grows up, and then gets amplified each time the trauma is repeated.

Opening Your Heart Exercise
Start by grounding or anchoring yourself to the Mother Earth crystal, then place your hands in prayer-like position over your heart. Press hands together and visualize letting go of any anger, pain, worry, or grief that might be at the forefront of your mind. Press disqualified energies out of your heart, your being. Then slowly open your hands moving sideways towards shoulders. Turn your hands outward and send this "divine love from the core of your being" out to the universe. Do this early in the morning and on a regular basis.

You will see a difference in your attitude, intuitiveness and soul purpose from this exercise. Help others with this exercise, learning to be centered, opening their heart and drawing energy from the divine source. As you work with opening your heart in groups, you may become aware of a group-purpose consciousness for the planet. We are all here to awaken to our spiritual being; how long it takes us depends upon how close we have stayed to our true purpose, or if we have gotten off track from experiences in other lifetimes. We all came with a contract or purpose; be still and discover yours.

Chakra Imbalances

An understanding of how emotional and spiritual difficulties can create disease in the body is based on a broad working knowledge of how the chakras affect physical and mental illness, and can be the key to understanding and healing emotional blockage occurring in the body.

A healer can do a lot by simply "purifying" the chakras and balancing them, so that the energy flows.

Meditation or relaxation on a daily basis, and visualizing white gold or silver light atoms of energy flowing upward (from the earth) and out the crown chakra assists in maintaining balance. It is important to follow all the way through, so as not to allow the energies to stop and stagnate at any particular chakra. You can also visualize the energies flowing from spirit into the crown chakra and down to Mother Earth; again, be sure to follow through. Saying positive affirmations that relate to distress or problems you are sensing within yourself is helpful. This is energy clearing of your being. It helps to clear the mind of day-to-day concerns of the earthly personality, and allows the higher information to be processed through the individual consciousness.

Mental Blocks
The mental body affects our whole circuit, our "energy field." Mental blocks restrict the circulation of the etheric, which is similar to clots of blood in the physical. If our personal mental world is in upheaval,

and we are perturbed or frightened, this will act upon our heart. These fears then work against our blood circulation, which will alter our energy fields. Disharmonious thinking causes anxiety and disharmony to every cell and every organ in our body, and works on our cycle or circle of life. Every emotion carries a vibration. If we cannot release this through our excretory zones, then we send it through the body, express it through our mouths, and then suffer the effects of our reactions.

Human Auric Field

Our auric field is a quantum step deeper into our personality than our physical body. It is at this level of our being that our psychological thinking processes take place. Our auric field becomes the vehicle for all of our psychosomatic or stressful emotional thoughts. Our auric field is not the source, but only the vehicle through which creative consciousness from the core reaches our physical body. To be healthy we need a balanced auric field.

Our auras are absorbers, soaking up vibrations from everything around, the sun, moon, plants, stones, and people. A large aura is more difficult to control since it could overwhelm someone with a weak aura or influence him or her. The weaker a person's auric field, the more he is susceptible to other people's energies and could take on their projections. The healer's aura should have an inner calm and inner beauty, which is then capable of transmuting negativity.

Chakra Direction

You can use your finger as a pendulum for balancing the chakras. Simply put your finger with rightful intention, to the area of the chakra and the chakra will automatically start spinning in rightful direction. The chakras always spin in a clockwise direction, as you stand and look at the front of someone's body, or when you stand and look at the back of the body,

Cords That Bind Us

Barbara Ann Brennan's book, *Light Emerging,* has in-depth information on cords. The following is a small sample of how cords affect us in our relationships with each other.

There are five major types of cords:
1) Soul Cord—ongoing soul carries from Divine Source connection/spiritual world
2) Past Life Cords—from past life experiences on Earth or elsewhere
3) Genetic Cords—connection to birth parents
4) Relational Cords—growth through relationship with parents
5) Relational Cords—growth through relationship with other human beings

Soul Cords

Connect us to Divine source, home, our guardian angels and guides. When meeting someone, there are times when we feel we have known them from someplace; we just can't seem to put our finger on where we've meet them. We may find ourselves working in the same type of environment and enjoying many of the things we have done before. We have not only incarnated on this Earth plane, but we have incarnated on other planes of existence; this is why so many are now feeling this "star connection," or that they don't belong here. Our consciousness is opening up to remembering.

Genetic Cords

Connect deep into the interior of our heart chakra before conception takes place. Mother connects to egg and child, father connects to sperm and child, mother and father connect to each other. Connections exist between aunts, uncles, cousins, grandparents, and all along the bloodline, thereby creating a genetic tree of life dating back to the beginning. This great network or matrix goes beyond three-dimensional space. Thus, we are connected to everyone and everything that ever existed. It is through these birth cords that we carry our genetic heritage on an auric level.

Relational Cords

- First chakra, represent the stability of the will to live in the physical and on the earth
- Second chakra, represent enjoyment of life's sensual and sexual relationships
- Third chakra, represent clarity and appropriateness taking care of self and others
- Fourth chakra, represent loving and mystery between the loving and willing balance
- Fifth chakra, represent trusting in the higher will of relationship, giving and receiving
- Sixth chakra, represent seeing higher concepts in relationship, spiritual love perspective
- Seventh chakra, represent power to be within divine mind in relationship to other humans

With adoption, the cords between child and original parents remain, plus new cords are established between the child and the new parents. The cords on the left side of chakras connect to female persons; the cords on the right side of chakras connect to male persons. This is important knowledge in understanding the client's problem, and whether the role is parent, child, or peer. These cords change and grow as the relationship grows and changes; the cords attach between chakras only if both people allow them to.

Unhealthy relationships create dark, stagnant, heavy cords. This is where manipulation, codependency, depressed resentment and anger form. The sucking of energy from one person to another also happens when relationships are controlling, needy, and misused. When someone pretends to be your friend, then finds something wrong with what you're doing, he undermines your confidence in your pathway until you begin to identify with him. Thus, he starts sucking your energy.

Our Character Structures

The Celestine Prophecy by James Redfield talks about our character traits, and the simple message of how we use and misuse energy with each other, and our surroundings. Redfield's characters are:

1) Intimidator   2) Interrogator   3) Aloof   4) Poor Me

Hands of Light and *Light Emerging* by Barbara Ann Brennan talk about five major character structures, and have in-depth information on the following. Also check out *Core Energetics,* by Dr. John C. Pierrakos .

1) schizoid   2) oral   3) psychopathic   4) masochistic   5) rigid

Schizoid: This structure is characterized mainly by energy-field imbalances and breaks. Main energy is held deep with in the core and is usually frozen until therapy and healing work are done to free it. These are usually spiritual people with a deep sense of purpose in life, or very creative people with many talents; but they need to integrate their general being and face their inner terror and rage.

Oral: This structure tends to have a depleted field, which is quiet and clam; main energy is in the head. He has probably not done much processing work; character is centered on intellectual and verbal activity and not on physical activity. Defense mechanisms are verbal denial, snide remarks, and the sucking of energy. His Life Task is to learn to trust in the abundance of the universe, and reverse the process of grabbing. Needs to learn to give without restrictions, to acknowledge that he has received, to face fear of being alone, and to not play the role of the victim. This is a natural teacher who has varied interests, intelligence, and spiritual love connection.

Psychopathic: This structure experienced a secretly seductive parent of the opposite sex. The parent wanted something from the child, which caused feelings of being betrayed and led him to try and control others through bullying, overpowering or seduction. Torn between fear of failure and defeat, he fears being controlled and used or being put in position of victim. Main energy is in the upper half of the body. His Life Task is to learn that when higher energies are released, he is very honest, has integrity and intelligence, does well managing complicated projects, and has a heart full of love.

Masochistic: This structure's experience of love given was conditional. Mother was dominating and sacrificing so he was made to feel guilty for any self-assertion or attempt at freedom. Holding in feelings and creativity led to anger and hatred. Driven by a fear of releasing tension and a belief system of being submissive or humiliated, his unconscious tends to remain blocked. Physically he is heavy, carries tensions in the neck, jaw, throat and pelvis. His Life Task is to free himself of humiliation by freeing his aggression, to creatively express himself in intricate design, and to develop his capacity for fun and joyfulness.

Rigid: This structure experienced rejection by the parent of the opposite sex, thereby creating a betrayal of love, sexuality and love being all the same to a child. He therefore controls all feelings such as pain, rage, or even good, by holding them back. Surrender is scary; he will not reach out for his desires, and will try to manipulate. His Life Task is to open his feeling heart center and allow the energy to flow forth into adventure, passion, and love. He is a natural leader, capable of deep relationships and caring for nature.

Hara Vital Center

Key Words: Purpose and Intention

According to the *Donning International Encyclopedic Psychic Dictionary* by June Bletzer; "Hara" is the Japanese word for the vital center around which the whole body is centered.

Hara Level is one step deeper into our nature and one dimension deeper than the aura. It is a laser-like line that runs down the center of our body (it is not a chakra). It is the foundation upon which our auric field is built. It corresponds to our life task or spiritual purpose. The HARA is visualized as a point two inches below the navel, running into the core of the earth, and on upward to approximately three feet above the head. According to Barbara Ann Brennan's book, Light Emerging, this is representative of our first individuation out of the godhead, the reason to incarnate in physical form, the place where we connect to our higher spiritual reality.

In doing healing work, when you center self, it is to go to the core of your being, the HARA, and allow the divine essence to come through, letting go of anything within self for that moment and space. In doing so, the connection is made with the divine, yourself, and the client; the energy flows in a positive constructive communion and the purpose and intent have been made.

Points of the Hara Level

Three points along a laser-like line that is on the centerline of the body, about one-third of inch wide, three and one-half feet above head, down deep into the core of the earth.

First Point—Above head looks likes an inverted funnel, carries the functions of reason, carries the reason to incarnate, and is the place where we connect to our higher spiritual reality.

Second Point—Upper chest, corresponds to our emotions and carries our spiritual longing, the sacred longing that carries us through life, passion to accomplish great things in our life, to do a specific life task. It is what we have come do, and lets us feel why we are here.

Third Point—Tan tien, as it is called in Chinese, center from which all martial artists draw power, appears to be a ball of power, about two and one-half inches in diameter, located about two and one-half inches below the navel. It is your will to live in the physical body, and the one note to hold the physical body in physical manifestation. It is your will, this one note that has created a physical body out of the body of Mother Earth. It is the connection where healers connect to regenerate the body, provided the healer grounds the hara line deep into the core of Earth.

Clear Hara level—actions on the auric and physical levels bring about pleasure and contentment.

Dysfunctional Hara level—illness can be brought about by an unclear, opposing or mixed directional life task, or even a disconnection from one's life task. This disconnection from your deeper life's purpose shows in the hara level and can be healed from this level.

I saw the hara line in a photograph taken during a sacred artistic workshop; the line ran above the head, straight down through the body, and into the earth. The photograph showed the line as blue.

Chakras and the Human Energy Fields ~ 153 ~

Hara Line Diagram   **Kundalini Vertical Power Line**

Connection to Godhead

Soul Seed

Tan tien

Auric Field

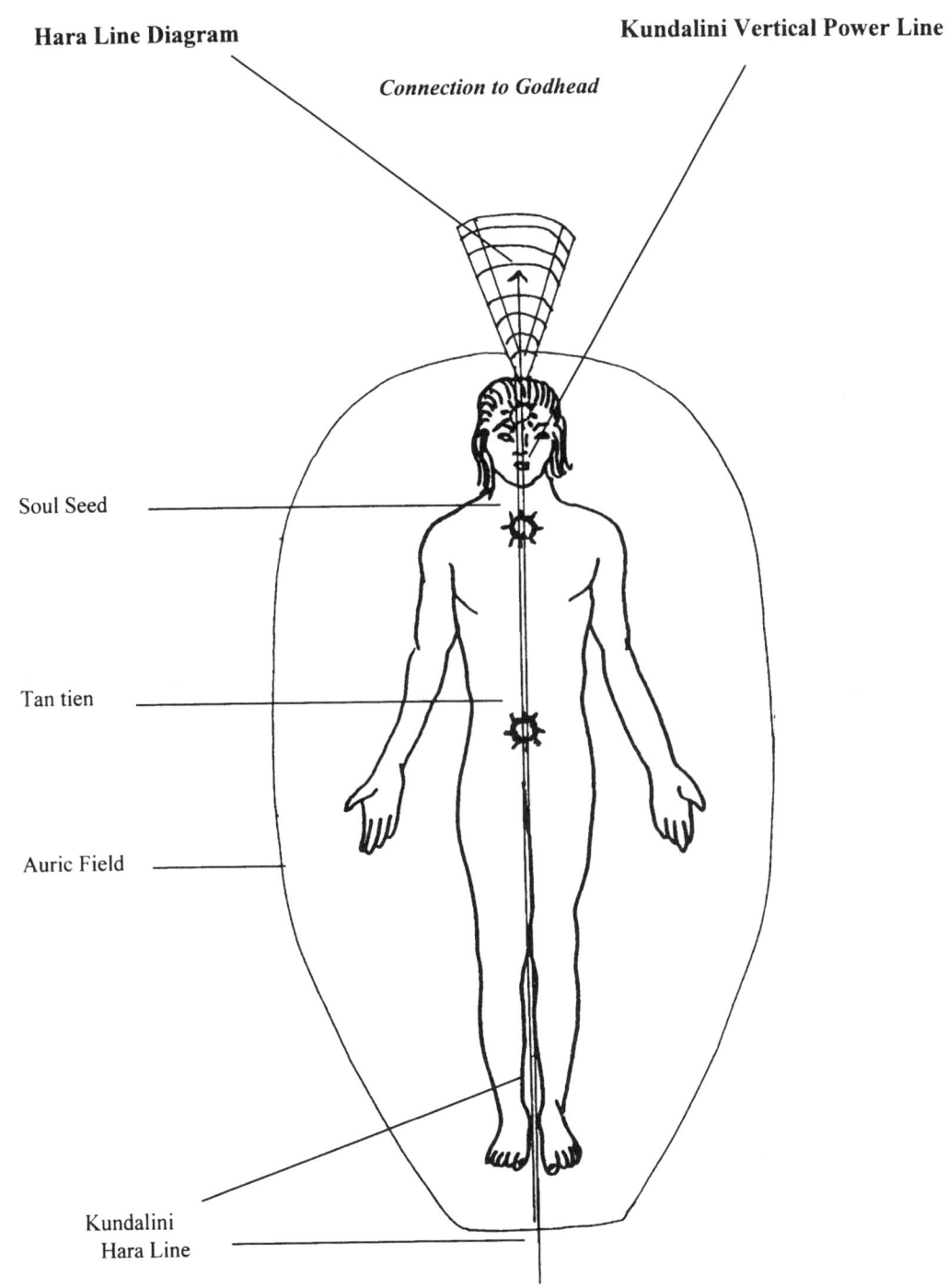

Kundalini
Hara Line

Mother Earth - Connection to Core

Inner Light or Core Star

(Divine Essence)

Location: One-half inch above navel

Theory: All things began as one perfect light, which is synonymous with intelligence. Each star is a part of the infinite. We are the center of the universe. We are one with the creator. We are divine essence.

An inner seeing shows people reflecting this Inner Light as a star, each one different, each one as an individual. This inner divine essence represents trust, faith, hope, encouragement, inner strength, loving, and a deeper goodness. One might say, "they have a pure soul." From within this Inner Light, divine essence is our creative energy.

The core star level is one step deeper into our nature than the hara level, which is one step deeper than the auric field. The concept of natural healing is to use nature to fortify a weakened system so it can fight for itself. We can do our part by becoming aware of who we are, what we eat, and how we think, by believing that we are more than our human body and becoming the spiritual being that we really are. This is the balance and harmony we all seem to be striving towards.

Core star has been within us since the beginning of time; it is beyond limitations of time, space, and belief. We recognize the core star as that which we have always known ourselves to be; the inner essence has not changed with time, no negative experiences have tainted it. Yes, our reactions to negative experiences may have clouded it, but not changed it; it is our basic nature, the deeper goodness within each of us, it is who we really are. When we are truly happy and healthy is when our core essence is most fully expressed.

Disconnection from Core Star

When this happens, the essence is not fully transmitted into the physical world. When you are least happy, in discomfort, or have problems, the core essence is expressed the least. It serves as a signal to us that we have become disconnected from our core essence, the inner divinity, and we have forgotten who we are.

Chakras and the Human Energy Fields ~ 155 ~

Core Star Diagram

Connection to Godhead

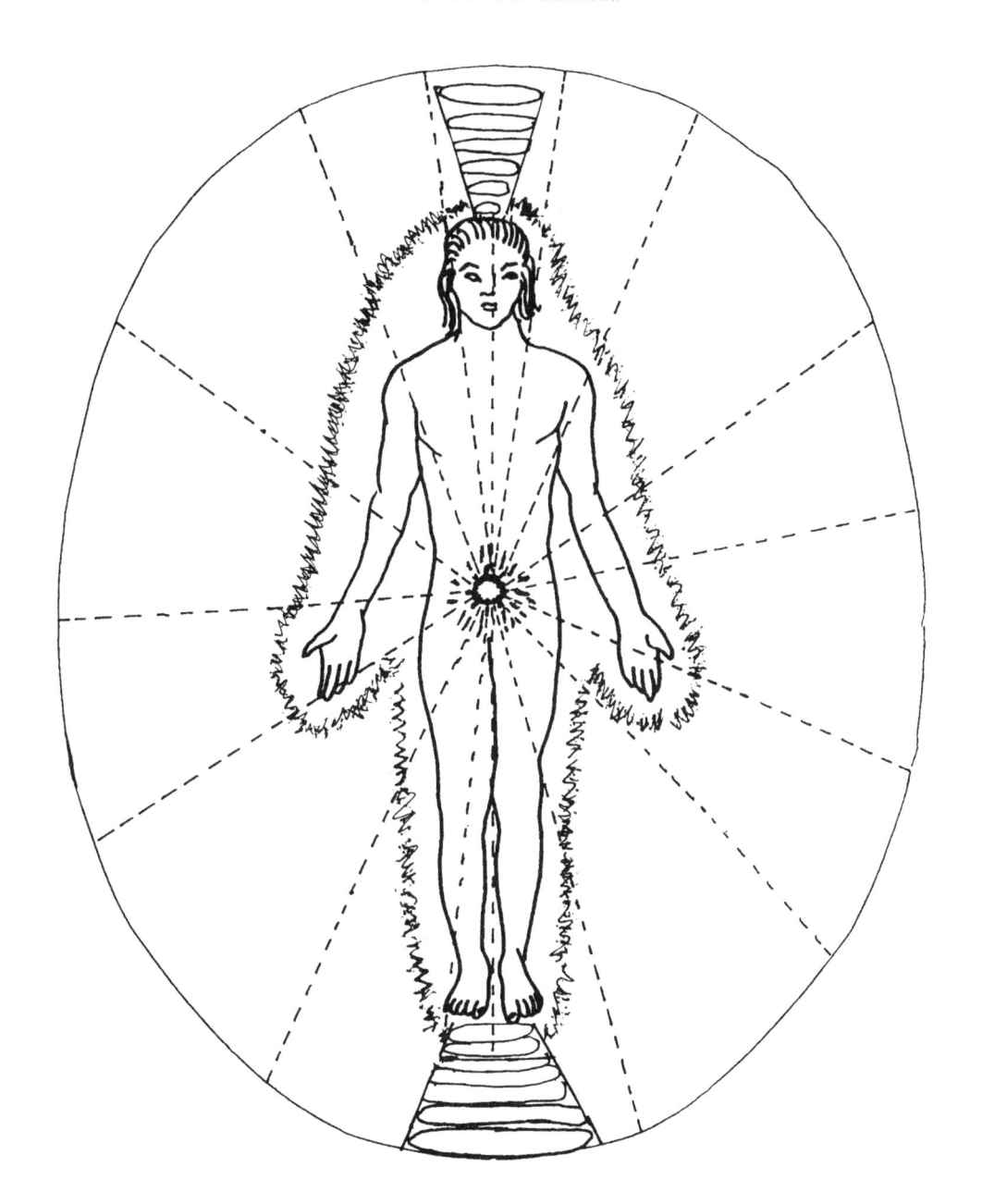

Mother Earth - Connection to Core

Polarity Diagram
Front of Body - feelings
Back of Body - will

Sun - Divine Creator
Upper Body - Positive

Masculine/Intellectual
Right Side

Feminine/Intuitive
Left Side

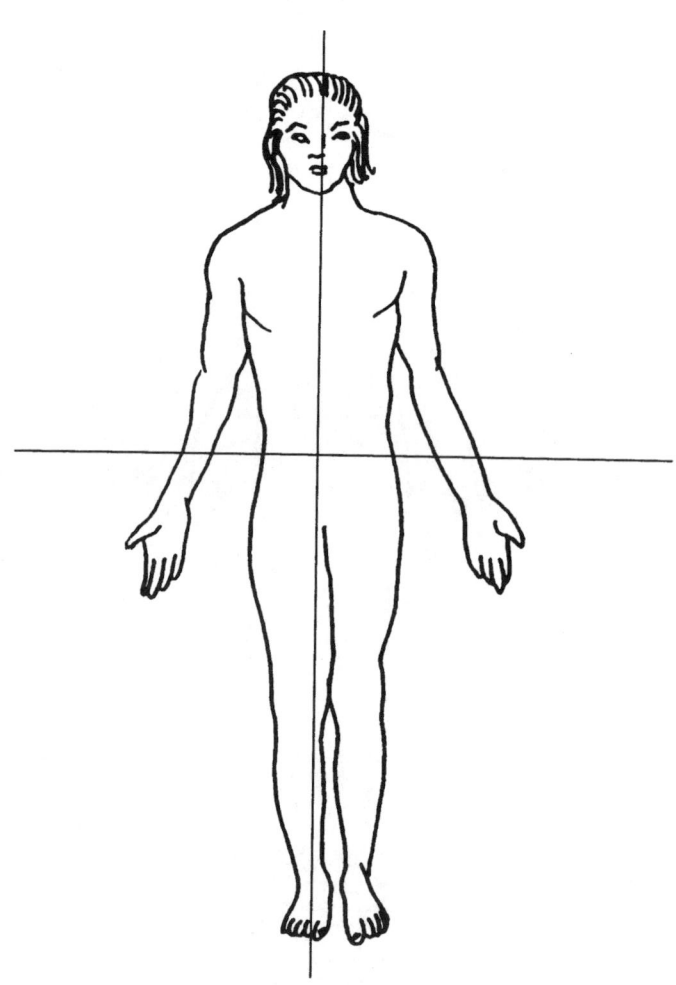

Lower Body - Negative
Mother Earth - Moon

I shall rise above defeat and trouble.
I shall not waste time and energy in useless worry.
I shall look only on the bright side of life.
I shall do my best in all things.

I shall let go
And let Creator be in charge of my life.
I will remember—
I am always and forever connected
To the endless source, Divine, creative love, and wisdom.

by Wind Dancer

When we have children to care for
the world looks different from when we have none;
when we are raising infants, the world seems different
from when we are raising adolescents.
When we are poor,
the world looks different from when we are rich.
We are daily bombarded with new information
as to the nature of reality.

If we are to incorporate this information,
we must continually revise our maps,
and sometimes when enough new information has accumulated,
we must make very major revisions.

The process of making revisions, particularly major revisions,
is painful, sometimes excruciatingly painful.
And herein lies the major source of many of the ills of mankind.

Excerpts From *The Road Less Traveled*

The endeavor to do our part to restore the Plan gives meaning to our Lives.
This we do when we hold the vision of universal brotherhood
And the new era community alive in our consciousness as we take up our daily work
As a global group let us continue to work for a human civilization built upon the cornerstones of co-operation
And sharing that truly promotes peace, social justice and prosperity for man.
Let us contribute to the emergence of a new culture born of love, knowledge and creative striving
That truly bestows greater freedom, joy and beauty on human living.

Excerpts from *Triangles*

Crystal Information and the Body

The receptivity to search for the knowledge about crystals has intensified in today's society. As we cross the threshold of the Golden Age of Knowing, the essence of crystals and stones has developed. Crystals have become tools for healing energy. Crystals are instruments of power to embrace, develop and manifest the light within. It is important that we do not lose sight of the fact that "we are the light," and the crystals are guides or tools, a bond with Mother Earth.

Required when doing a crystal healing:
1) a clear mental focus
2) letting go of any personal emotions, stress, or other problems
3) the art of giving clear, strong intention of healing
4) awareness of the power of the crystals and body's electromagnetic fields

Note: wearing an amethyst can help your focus and intuitiveness

Experience when receiving a crystal healing:
1) more light force and color are brought into auric field
2) opportunity to let go and let God take over is received
3) any mental or emotional blockages may surface to consciousness
4) as auric field becomes infused with light, the vibrations of the field increase
5) losing outdated belief systems can cause a revision of attitude, work with heart and mind centers

Preparation and Prayer for Protection

Center self for work and repeat an affirmation (example below). Imagine the white light coming into the crown chakra and flowing through you continuing down through your feet into Mother Earth, deeply connecting to her. As the Native Americans do, see this light as clearing you, protecting you, grounding you, intensifying you, and radiating out of your heart center for the preparation for the healing to begin.

Crystals are to be cleansed before and after a treatment by putting them outside in direct sunlight or moonlight (full moon phase). If you are aware of a planetary energy grid, place the crystals there for recharging.

I call upon the Divine Source
I call upon the God and Goddess Balancing Energies
I call upon the Light of the Great White Brotherhood
I call upon the Light of the Great Central Sun
I call upon the Great White Buffalo Spirit
I call upon the Divine Light of my own Beingness
I call upon the Endless Source of Light for Strength and Protection

Clearing the room of any misqualified energies or psychic debris is necessary before and after each crystal healing session. An open window, smudging with sage and sweetgrass, or lighting a candle is helpful. Use the Reiki symbols for empowerment and also for a positive frame of mind intention. Music for meditation and the quieting of the mind will also be helpful for releasing and clearing out.

What follows is a guide to crystals used with the different chakras.

Root Chakra
Root or base chakra concern is our connection with Mother Earth, our foundation, the Kundalini center, physical energy and the material reality.

Suggestions:	Red Garnet	Black Obsidian	Black Onyx
	Jasper		Smoky Quartz

Spleen/Sacral Chakra
Deals with emotions, intuition, friendliness, creativity, our self worth, and confidence.

Suggestions:	Tiger's Eye	Topaz	Jasper
	Carnelian	Amber	Citrine

Solar Plexus Chakra
Deals with the center of personal power, natural skills, aptitudes, mental emotion, and our center of intelligence.

Suggestions:	Turquoise	Chrysocholla	Azurite
	Malachite	Clear Quartz

Heart Chakra
The bridge between physical and spiritual; symbolizes the awakening of spirituality, center of our compassion, unconditional love, our most vulnerable wheel of light, connects with our immune system of thymus and Peyers Patches.

Suggestions:	Green Jade	Pink Tourmaline	Rhodonite
	Adventurine	Rose Quartz	Ruby
	Malachite	Emerald

Throat Chakra
Deals with our center of communication, being able to express self, being spiritually open to clairaudience (hearing).

Suggestions:	Lapis	Blue Sapphire	Aquamarine
	Blue Lace Agate	Sodalite	Celestite
	Peridot	Azurite

Third Eye/Brow Chakra
Deals with the center of our intuition and psychic powers, ability to tune into our divine source, astral traveling, past lives, being a visionary, and openness to clairvoyance (psychic seeing).

Suggestions:	Sugalite	Alexandrite	Azurite
	Lapis	Clear Quartz	Gem Silica
	Amethyst	Fluorite (purple, white, blue)

Crown Chakra

When this center is fully opened, spirituality is omnipresent. You live in the light, and the silver cord connects with our pineal and pituitary areas, attaching our etheric body to our physical body and allowing astral traveling without disconnecting from our physical being.

Suggestions: Clear Quartz (double terminator) points towards aura and crown
  Fluorite   Lapis   Amethyst
  Diamond   White Sapphire

Purification Techniques for Personal Healing

(Based on Native American Circle or Wheel of Life concepts)

The value of a purification technique (preventative measure) is to incorporate it into your daily life. Doing this daily helps you to avoid dealing with a health crisis. Spend a small part of each day moving the energy, to either resolve body problems or to keep problems from manifesting.

We are going to use the Four Elements associated with the Four Directions of Spirit.

East—Air   South—Fire   West—Water   North—Earth

This will align our energy with spirit, and remove the effects of being out of balance.

Love represents the organized energy of our universe. The Divine Being, God, created the universe out of his love and this is the universal life energy force and fills the space between the parts of the atoms and molecules.

Old concepts that created blockages: Shutting down, refusing to cry, guilt, worry, and anger, repeating negative relationships, having the same reactions to the same situations, and on and on.

Blockages are caused by our "structured" thinking in this existence, and our resistance or lack of "letting go." This starts the blockage in our auric field from the Divine Source's love energy, which is the energy that literally keeps us alive. Examples: constantly being angry about everything (or it's always your fault), and worry (being in crisis all the time). A ritual will help reprogram the thinking.

Psychologically, there is no difference between feelings of fear and excitement in the body. Whether we shut down to fear or pain, we are shutting down the ability to love to that same degree. Same situations, same reactions. This creates a decrease in a person's life force including the ability to resolve issues. When we react to every situation with frustration or anger (everyone has a bad day), we complicate the process of clearing the energy, and might go further into self-judgement.

The anger we feel is fear and/or pain, and the fastest release of this energy is nonresistance, surrender, or "letting go and letting God." It takes little bravery or intellect to become angry, but it takes great inner strength and trust to continue loving ourselves in the middle of a crisis by holding that neutral place and becoming Heart Centered. It doesn't always happen overnight, this letting go of our ego, because they were a strong pattern in the way we learned to resolve problems. It takes time and patience with oneself.

Purification techniques are some of many processes that remind us of our eternal conscious connection to Spirit. This is a tool for our physical and emotional self to connect with the calmness and peace within. The experience plays an important part in our ability to stay healthy. When we deny ourselves universal love from the divine source, we will not stay alive very long.

Elements Used in Purification

Earth Element
Grounding—Using the natural materials of Mother Earth is very grounding. We respond in a relaxed mood, and have more practical attitudes.
Examples:
1) Foods we eat affect our state of mind coming from Earth.
2) Walking through the woods, gardening or working in the yard.
3) Sitting on the grass for a picnic or even taking a nap outside.
4) Participating in a Native American sweat lodge or drumming.

Air Element
Breath—The breath of life, the bridge between spiritual and physical strengthens our connection to Divine Source.
Examples:
1) Rebirthing, Transformational Breathwork, Tai Chi, and Yoga.
2) Doing exercises in meditation, singing, chanting, laughing, and dancing bring forth the movement of air into your being.

Fire Element
Inspiration—Passion and compassion move energy into our emotional fields, just as fear and pain also move to that area. The conscious use of fire removes energy blockages associated with passion or holding onto.
Examples:
1) Sit in front of a fireplace and visualize the fire burning away the anger in your auric field.
2) You can write your anger and fear on a piece of paper and put them in the fire also, but do this with intention.
3) Take the plunge and participate in a firewalk (letting go of fear).
4) Burn candles with visual meditation of letting go, or take a walk in the bright sunlight, with each step letting go of any built-up emotions.

Water Element
Feelings and Emotions—The physical body is made up of over ninety percent water; it is what keeps us alive.
Examples:
1) Cry. It is a great way to let go. I have heard it said that crying from the core of your being would release years of karmic buildup.
2) Swim and feel the waves wash away any judgment, pain, or guilt.
3) Take a shower or a wonderful soak in the tub with aromatherapy oils.
4) Flotation tanks are very popular, along with meditative music. Bring out the memories of being connected with the womb where it was safe.

Energized Baths

After a day of doing massage and Reiki healing, I have been in the habit of taking a long shower and brushing down my energy fields. As I do this I visualize any disqualified energy leaving my body and running down the drain to be neutralized. If I have more time, I run moderately warm bath water in the tub and add Epsom salts, or natural sea salt with baking soda. You can also add a very small amount of aromatherapy oil, one that will enhance your energy fields. Other bathing remedies are available in your health food stores.

Note: If you have low or high blood pressure, be extra careful if you become dizzy.

Sea Salt—1 pound plus 1 pound baking soda
Epsom Salt—1 cup makes a strong bath
Soak—about twenty minutes
Extras—music or candles are nice

Laundry: Along the line of water, putting natural sea salt or even Epsom salt into your laundry will help transmute the energy on clothing—especially if someone in the house is ill—and also linens from massage or healing work. I have found one large tablespoon or small handful seems adequate.

Blessings

Esoteric Meaning:
A mass of energy psychically produced that is healing, soothing and pleasant to the receiver. Blessing Decree works with the electrical impulses, and is directed to a certain designation, to improve health, to bring about a good experience, to wish well.

Blessing Way:
A special ceremony, in which the whole tribe (Native American, Navaho) participates. It raises the vibrations that can be used to heal and bring abundance to the tribe.

Blessed Water:
Fill a dark blue glass or jar with water; Reiki the water either by sending energy or using the Reiki symbols with the intention of the water being blessed.

I have a friend who does this on a regular basis; her cats enjoy drinking the water daily and are exceptionally healthy. In fact, the cats won't drink any other water but this energized Reiki-blessed water. Intention, and so it is!

Smudging

A Native American practice is to burn a special plant usually sage or sweet grass in an area before any ceremony, such as medicine wheel, sweat lodge, or firewalk. Smudging is used before healing work or other spiritual workshops.

Ritual: Smoke from the sage or sweetgrass is fanned, usually with a feather, throughout the room or area from each of the four directions. The smudging cleanses the atmosphere of any disqualified energy that has gathered from thought forms in that area. Meditative music can also be used while performing this ritual. Smudging yourself before or after healing work is wonderful. It produces a feeling of freshness throughout your own energy system.

Book Resources

13 Original Clan Mothers by Jamie Sams
Animal Speak by Ted Andrews
Chakra Therapy by Keith Sherwood
Core Energetics by John C. Pierrakos
Crystal Healing by Katrina Raphael
Donning Encyclopedic Psychic Dictionary by June G. Bletzer
Earth Medicine by Kenneth Meadows
Hands of Light and *Light Emerging* by Barbara Ann Brennan
Karmic Astrology by Martin Schulman
Keepers of the Earth by Michael J. Caduto and Joseph Bruchac
Love Is in the Earth (a kaleidoscope of crystals) by Melody
Star Signs by Linda Goodman
The Angels within Us by John Randolph Price
The Color Atlas of Human Anatomy by Vanio Vannini
The Electric Nature of the Universe by Walter Russell
The Power is Within You by Louise L. Hay
The Secret Teachings of All Ages by Manly P. Hall
The Way of the Wizard by Deepak Chopra
Vibrational Medicine by Dr. Richard Berber
Wheels of Light by Rosalyn L. Brayere
Working with Your Chakras by Ruth White

Chapter Ten

Fears, Stress, and Worry as Emotional Diseases

Fears—How They Affect Us

Denial

Our mental processes determine the body's health. What we think of life, especially of self, at both the conscious and the unconsciousness levels, affects our physical state.

"Masking the self" is creating a mask of what we think the world might accept, thereby hiding emotional pain. Many times this lies within the subconsciousness of our mind. This mask succeeds in giving us an inner feeling of security or safety, gives us the feeling we are the good guys, makes us critical of others and afraid, puts constant pressure on us to produce, and creates the scenario of not accepting responsibility for our actions. These fears keep on manifesting in ever greater degrees until we learn to deal with them.

Examples of Masking Self

a) A person who has gone through a very traumatic event in their younger years. This event will at times result in a mask for others that everything is always okay or fine, that "I can handle that," which makes them feel they are in control. But underneath they have feelings of guilt, unworthiness, rejection, relationship problems, and control issues. Some people may actually be aggressive or fearful, while others will become the shadow where they do not want to be seen.

b) What we project to others in everyday life. When you have to carry a lot of responsibility, such as raising children by yourself, you will appear to have lots of strength and assertiveness, while underneath you may really want to cry. This is a social issue because of so many women forced into becoming heads of households. However, on the blessing side, this issue is starting to create women in society that are becoming more self-sufficient, and are spiritually growing in strength, thereby gradually confronting the mask they portray to the outside world.

c) A sense of abandonment. An early divorce in the family, being adopted, or the separation of parents can cause many people to have relationship problems. They may have a sense of rejection or unworthiness, be either overweight or anorexic, be aggressive, or display a lack of assertiveness, all portrayed by the masks they have chosen. Choosing the mask comes from our upbringing, and how we view the world, our peers, and those environmental and society issues around us.

d) Codependency. We are in a period of time when the word codependent is used for almost every family. It has helped bring this situation out into the open. Almost every one of us has had some drama we were masking. To what extent we mask depends upon how we want to deal with the everyday world and life in general. Some people use the dramas they have grown up with as excuses for why they act the way they do, rather than changing the way they act. We are a generation wanting someone, anyone, else to be responsible for all of our questionable actions.

Extreme Masks
- being put down—can cause overachievement, aggressiveness or the "poor me"
- seeing family members cheat—gives you an excuse to be dishonest
- work habits or role models—give you an excuse to look the other way, rather than having honesty, integrity
- hearing dad degrade mom—you mask and act out against women, sometimes in violence
- hearing mom gripe about dad—you may decide not to marry or have relationship problems with men
- being raised in an abusive atmosphere—since you were beaten, anger causes you to beat others; this can also be a cause for becoming a controller with those around you.

Denial as a Mask
This is an unconscious defense mechanism used frequently to make our life more manageable on the surface. Denial is diminishing or hiding an unpleasant experience, an alternative to facing hurts and complex situations. Denial of circumstances, and the evasion of a situation, is a way of substituting other things to occupy our time and our minds. Not performing in accordance to one's ability, not handling an underlying current of resentment or jealousy, is putting a denial mask on. Sometimes, as an alternative, people get busy and involved in everyone else's issues. Then they don't have to face their own. This is The Law of Avoidance. These denials can be overcome by recognizing issues, patterns, and set phrases used all the time. Meditation is helpful, as are affirmations, reading a book, and getting a spiritual healing.

Fixed Thought
Fixed thought is a deliberate belief, desire, or idea so intense and persistent that its manifestation is stagnated and solidified to the extent that it will not dissipate by itself. Our thoughts of material objects and the things of Earth are held together by collective fixed thought. For example, when the majority of mankind continues to need war, every time one talks about war, it is visualized as war, and so Earth has wars. When man no longer needs a war, and another object is visualized as a substitute, man will no longer need war. This same example could be something simple like cars, chairs, silverware, or even polluted water, air, chemicals in body products, cleaning products, or our drinking water. The same goes for the masses believing that the human body is susceptible to disease, and therefore maintaining sickness on Earth. The fixed thought desires something to happen with such strong emotions that it possesses one's thinking, causes the atoms to solidify and stop flowing, and one's desire never occurs.

A collective belief manifests as long as it is held collectively by humanity. Thus, a World Peace Day, Earth Day for our environment, Mother's Day, Father's Day, Independence Day, Freedom Day, Harmonic

Convergence for all Earth people. We could, as a whole Earth people, create tremendous changes! Watch for what happens after the Olympics when four million people are focused on working together in a geographical area that holds the Record Keeper crystals from Atlantis.

Our Emotions

Emotions are a highly concentrated form of energy consciousness, which stimulate a pattern of organic responses in the body, and are felt physically and experienced mentally. Emotion is the fundamental manifestation of the universal vital life force. It cannot be seen, or touched, but can be felt in a powerful form. All forms of life possess this vital life force energy in varying degrees. Emotions react in the body from outside stimuli, according to one's entire belief system (i.e. moods, attitudes, or anger).

Emotional Blueprint

The emotions of the body come from the endocrine and gland activity, and manifest as electrical transmitter points along the path of the nervous system, connected to the electrical system in the etheric world. The emotional energy is transmuted to the mental plane in the etheric world, to help make the blueprints of a human's physical body and physical outer environment, by using astral matter for its transmission, linking and influencing astral growth. See endocrine diagram and glossary.

Creating Body Armor

Theory—Our life's experiences write themselves into the muscles, organs, tissues, and cells of the body. These in turn influence bodily reactions, as to one's characteristics and health, and these reactions are solidified when triggered by environmental stimuli. This then creates an energy pattern around and within the body, depicting an aura of body armor. This can be carried through from past life experiences. The client's auric field will show this armor, such as breastplate, chastity belt, or even a full suit of armor; and the experienced spiritual healer will be aware of this when working in the fields of energy.

Disease and Blockages

The typical response humans make to an injury, whether it is physical or emotional, is to block the flow of energy, which ultimately depletes the overall field of energy. At a subconscious level, we believe the less energy that enters a wound, the less pain will be felt. In the moment, this is a good survival technique. However, avoidance of any situation is only a quick fix. This puts a strain on the auric field, where one chakra is overcharged and another undercharged with this imbalance. Complete healing requires a strong, healthy flow of the vital life force. Inner conflicts are the thoughts, and patterns of thought, you have incorporated into ego-self from experiences in everyday life. Examples: pain in shoulder (carrying the world), heart (grieving over loss), and legs (going forward in life).

A release of emotions (laughing, crying, happiness) can occur when healing energy brings about a dissolution of inner conflicts and blockages. Laughing can dissolve a disease in the body. Life is how you play the game and your approach towards healing with your whole heart.

Unresolved experiences from many years ago and unresolved experiences happening now build blockages and crystallizations in the body. These experiences sometimes take over and dictate your life, such as talking about a subject constantly, keeping turmoil inside rather than expressing it, getting caught up in other people's crises, wanting to be involved in knowing everyone else's dramas, and just being overly nosy. These are many of the ways of holding onto blockages, and can form a disease in the physical body. This emotional link can actually weigh you down (make you overweight); it's a mask you are projecting into other people's lives, wanting to always know what's happening. But the mask is that a part of you is not actually wanting to be involved, only wanting to know. The catch is that you have just emotionally linked yourself into their crises or karma.

These crystallizations/blockages usually happen over a long period of time. However, if you are aware, your body is giving you signals. These signals are to help you realize to let go, and let God control your life. Examples of unresolved issues that can cause buildups are: divorce or an abusive mate, legal problems, injustices, abusive work relationships, career dissatisfaction, relationships with children, parents, lovers, companions, friends, and society's pressure of financial difficulties.

Disease, or dis-ease, is the end product of excessive stress, fear, worry, frustration, unchangeable habits, and rigid thinking. These stresses activate the nervous system and the immune system. This cause and effect from the mind to the body sets into motion physical problems, what we would call overload. So the mind starts thinking thoughts, over and over, and our body's cells hear this information over a long period of time, and this manifests into the pain in our physical body.

Block—process in which a person feels he is not accepting a painful emotion that reminds him of a past unpleasant experience (which was not resolved when it happened).
Blocked Pathway — (Huna) ideas, experiences, or thought-forms that are entirely or partially repressed, preventing the conscious mind from going into a higher spiritual level of understanding.
Blocking—to suppress ideas, concepts, memories of past unpleasant experiences, that repeat themselves throughout life. This causes a hold pattern or locked-in area of cells that stagnate and cause abnormal behavior of mind and body systems.
Blocks—these locked-in emotions in the body's cells and subconscious mind prevent one from optimum performance, and grow in mass over the years. Similar experiences will come forth to resolve these issues or this repression gives way to unwanted behavioral patterns, pain, illness, and neurosis.

What's Behind Our Fears
Luke 8:50 "Fear not, believe only and you shall be made whole."

Men of science have discovered that matter is composed of energy and information (quantum physics). The universe, and everything in it, are of thought (God and God in action?) and by observation and attention, we are literally bringing into being particles from this infinite quantum field.

Wherever we put our attention, we draw things into being from this infinite universe of energy and information. Where we put our focus consistently causes conditions, situations, events, and people to come into our lives. Positive attention, love, kindness, peace, balance, and harmony can create the coincidences to inform us of our outstanding question! Negative attention can also be drawn back into our lives.

Being a part of the field of unified energy (oneness) is a way of defining your spiritual reality. Being always and forever connected, and part of the endless divine God infinity, creates the possibilities of abundance, peace, love, truth, beauty, health, etc. The fulfillment of life is all ours and nothing keeps this from us, except attention, belief, judging, uncertainty, frustration, anger, envy, condemning, and impatience (our shadows). We have stepped from the light into darkness, from positive to negative.

Our thoughts draw blessings or burdens from our life situations, but the attention creates chemical messages (neuropeptides) in our bodies. These messages go straight to the heart of each cell with instruction of life, health, sadness, or sickness. The tragedy is that knowing we exist in this unified field of infinite possibilities and unlimited abundance, we still create a hunger, a need, for security and assurances.

Jesus, the master of Christ Consciousness, taught abundance. He insisted that unbelievable power would be ours if we would believe. He demonstrated that all good could be ours by the multiplying of loaves and fishes. Some saw this as lack and madness rather than God's unlimited possibilities.

There is a story of a student going into the forest and talking to his spiritual master, and saying, "I want unlimited wealth, and I want to help heal the world. Please tell me the secret of creating abundance or affluence."

The spiritual master replied, "There are two goddesses. One is the goddess of knowledge and her name is Sarasvati. Pursue her love and give her your full attention. The other goddess is Lakshmi. She is the goddess of wealth, but when you pay more attention to Sarasvati, then Lakshmi will become jealous and pay more attention to you. The more you seek the goddess of knowledge, the more the goddess of wealth will seek you. She will follow you wherever you go, and never leave you, and the wealth you desire will be yours."

We were created to be capable of using focused thought to draw unlimited abundance into our lives. Health, wealth, whatever our goals are, they are within our reach. It is important for us to set goals, to give full attention, and draw to ourselves. Affirmations and prayers about goals and visualizing with clear mental pictures about your goals helps bring them into reality. Focus without desperation or fear.

Pain shows us where the pain is, that something is wrong
Our body is directing our attention to exactly where this difficulty and pain is.
Can space occupy the same place at the same time?
When we direct our full attention, the divine love, to that painful area,
Can the pain and the divine love occupy this same space? I don't think so!

Taking Responsibility—Free Choice

Free choice is when we make a voluntary decision consciously or unconsciously to perform an action, or to think a thought of one's preference. The human is the only organism that does everything of his/her own accord and has complete charge of the body. These voluntary decisions made over many incarnations make our world today, and the decisions we are making today will make the changes for the world tomorrow. So these free choice decisions are what we must live by, or take responsibility for. Free choice is a sacred universal law and no one should be deprived of it. The planet Earth is considered to be the only planet of free choice in our solar system.

Clearing the Patterns

Clearing is to release, flush, and break up complexes in the subconscious mind, so they do not cause problems in one's personality, life style, or physical body. Upon clearing, the conscious mind feels free and begins a new image and method of handling one's daily affairs.

The first step in the process is to identify the fear with the medical problem; this helps open up the energy block in your body to the conscious level. The next step is to pull in as much divine love and energy as possible and to focus it at the exact location of the blockage. Basically, the physical body heals itself. The mind of the physical body takes responsibility, and then the process of the healing can begin. The intelligence in the cells responds to the human being, which is motivated to be a perfect specimen and directs the cells to heal themselves.

Methods to Change Body Chemistry

1) One method of clearing is to go through "rebirthing." The idea is to rid one's self of undesirables in the subconscious mind, for example, our old theories, repressed emotions, guilt, and rejection. Release gives us freedom to function in a clearer consciousness of mind.
2) Spiritual healing along with counseling takes you through step-by-step energy work, where layers and layers of blockages are released. Part of this method has the client taking responsibility for what he has hung onto. Sometimes the client doesn't know, or isn't aware of blockages that could be from past life experiences. Once aware, the client can start working with these issues along with the healer. Learning to love oneself by doing nice things for self is great. Total energetic healing isn't usually done in one session.
3) Other helpful methods are regression, past life therapy, massage therapy, chiropractic alignment, structural integration, acupuncture, dream analysis, primal screaming, flotation tank therapy, meditation with sound and color, and spiral dancing. All help activate the vital life force energy.
4) A desperate method is to go through deprogramming with a forced method of interrogation on a one-time basis, whereby the ultimate goal is to get the blocks out of the victim's head so he can have a clear state of awareness. This has been used in cult programming situations.

Eternal Rhythm

The internal pulsating rhythm of the physical body is in tune with the rhythm of the planet Earth, in a continuation of the rhythm of the universe. Everything in the earth, in varying degrees, beats in time with the earth, the human heartbeat, making all One universal system. Connecting with nature by drumming, chanting, walking, and breathing with Mother Earth, in itself, is very healing. When we are out of sync with this Oneness or universal rhythm, we out of sync with everything. How we treat our peers, family, or each other, is how we are treating our planet Earth, upon which we rely for our very existence.

Reversing Disease and Blockages

Reversal is possible. If the mind created the physical problem, then the mind can undo the physical problem. Healing moves energy throughout the body, helping to change the vibrations, the atoms, and the blockages. Healing helps put the client back into a state of unity and harmony, within himself and with the universe. Aromatherapy, bodywork, various counseling methods, rebirthing, Shamanic techniques, and other techniques that are mentioned in this book, can all be helpful. Art, color, sound, and nature walks can play a role in the individual's integration into wholeness.

Key is Accepting Responsibility

If the client doesn't change any of the thought processes or identify with what caused the problem, the client will continue to create the blockages, and put the problem right back into their fields of energy. The body's cells have memories; it takes twenty-one days or longer in a continuation process for the cells to be reprogrammed. Sometimes the old pattern blockages will reappear in another area of the body, and sometimes in the same area. Therefore, the client's responsibility is to take charge of his thought processes and make changes in his life. Doing this will, in itself, effect a healing by the client.

Deep rooted illnesses (chronic) — Reiki or energy healing treatments will help guide the body through a cleansing process. Sometimes a reaction will happen in the body, even though the body may not actually feel better as it is going through the process. But the healing energy is working. The body has accepted the universal life force energy; the reaction is the adjustment the body will sometimes go through in dealing with deep-seated issues.

Healing through Astral Medicine

Astral medicine involves being taken to the astral planes by one's spiritual or angelic guides during sleep-time. At this time you are shown demonstrations, or taught lessons, to help or aid in changing your attitude in healing the sickness. This only happens to those who truly desire to follow a righteous path. The impressions received in the astral world can aid in changing one's set or unhealthy belief system. This creates healing for the physical body and the emotions of desire. The action to accomplish what is right follows along with the connection of energy from this plane, for the guides to use.

Can Our Minds Heal?

Source: Woman's Day *(April 1996)*

Studies have shown that when people have been diagnosed as having a short time to live, or been given the fear-ridden big "C" for cancer or "A" for AIDS; the mind goes into immediate change, whether it is positive or negative. Fear, anger, hostility are dangerous and toxic emotions to hold on to. We know that positive emotions counteract the harmful effects of negative emotions. The choice is yours.

Case study: A client chose to undergo mastectomy, chemotherapy, and a bone marrow transplant. She was willing to try everything, and was very family oriented. She joined group therapy sessions and started finding the joys in small things, in everyday life. Emotions do have an impact on illness. More and more physicians are realizing that the emotional aspects of disease and well-being need to be acknowledged. The medical scientists draw a clear line between the complex links of mind and body, and the simplistic wishing-the-self-well approach to illness.

Case study: Angry, throwing temper tantrums, acting like a bear, swearing at drivers when behind the wheel, cynical, mistrustful, critical, finding fault with everyone around him, this case was a heart attack waiting to happen. This type of personality is more likely to die early. A choice had to be made and it was. This person joined a group for hostility and anger, and replaced these toxic attitudes with positive ones.

The Bumblebee and Me

by S. Jeanne Gunn

As a child I had an encounter, not with an ET, but with this large black and yellow bumblebee. When you are five years old, they look really, really big! This bumblebee must have decided that I looked juicy, because he started out for me. Upon seeing this action, I reacted. I got into the house behind the screen door before he did. But that did not really satisfy this bumblebee. He kept on trying to get through the screen door to get me.

Wow! This encounter set up fears of being stung by any insect, but especially a fear of bumblebees. Years later, I took my children to a pond where they could swim, and as I sat on the sandy bank, I felt a sharp prick on my little toe. Immediately, I felt a rippling of energy as I saw my foot starting to swell. I actually didn't panic. I stepped into the cool water thinking this would solve the situation. Well, I tried. Soon I realized this wasn't going to help.

I got the children loaded up in the car and home we went. I put my foot in ice cubes and ammonia as soon as we got into the house. I called the doctor and he said, "Well, if you were going to die, it would already be too late, so I'll prescribe something that will help." Much to my dismay, the whole leg swelled up and I spent a week in bed.

About ten years later, after I had just started on my spiritual pathway and had just been introduced to Reiki, I had another encounter with a stinging creature. Walking up to the front door of my home, I heard buzzing. Something was trapped in my hair. Unconsciously, I put my hand up to brush away the insect, only to realize that I had just been stung. It was not a bumblebee, it was a wasp. My first thought was, "I had better get to the hospital." Too late! My son was already pulling out of the driveway.

Well, I calmed myself down and immediately went into the house, got out an ice cube, wrapped my wrist in a towel, sat down quietly, and went into meditation. Soon, I sensed it was time to look at my wrist. There was no swelling. In fact, there was no sign that anything had happened. What a blessing! It gave me encouragement that this spiritual outlook on life and Reiki really worked. The following day, only a red dot was on my wrist, showing me that it had really happened. I had stilled my heart, my fears, my anxiety, and into God's grace I went. It worked! Why not? I believed it would.

Three Fingers and a Door

This story about a lovely spiritual lady named Kay was told to me over dinner one night. On a trip to Mexico with a group of people, when she was getting out of the car, she put her hand up to grasp the support between the front and back windows. Someone slammed the door on three of her fingers. Quietly, but with urgency, she said, "Someone please open the door, now." When they opened the door they found that her three fingers were flattened. Everyone started to get excited, but she said, "Hush." She quietly went into meditation and put her other hand over the fingers, sending them healing energy. After a few minutes, she removed her hand and the fingers were all back to normal, no bruising, no cuts, all okay. By not allowing the other peoples' fears to throw her off center, she had gone into the stillness. She had remembered Jesus the Master saying, "Ask and you shall receive," and she believed it.

Emotional Sources of Disease

Problem	Source	Problem	Source
Accidents	Expressions of anger, rage, frustration	Asthma	Suppressed stifled feelings, inability to take in life, lack of self-worth
Adrenal	Self-criticism, self-worth, depression	Back, Upper	Not feeling supported emotionally by those around you, carrying the world on your shoulders
Allergies	Denial of own power, allowing someone to take your power		
Ankles	Holding onto a limitation, flexibility	Back, Middle	Guilt, stuck in old mental patterns of stuff back there
Anorexia/ Bulimia	Self-hate, rejection, not trusting or feeling good enough, denial of life's nourishment	Back, Lower	Lack of financial support, not having enough, fear about money
Arms	Inability to embrace life	Bladder Problem	Fear of letting go, being pissed off
Arthritis	Feeling unloved, patterns of criticism of self and others, resentment	Burns, Boils	Anger

Fears, Stress, and Worry as Emotional Diseases

Problem	Source	Problem	Source
Cancer	Inner conflict, resentment, deep hurts, entrapment, unresolved grief	Lungs	Ability to take in life or not, denial, emphysema/smoking denial, self-worth issues
Colds	Scattered energy, too much going on at once	Migraines	Resisting flow of life, frustration
Colon/Constipation	Fear of letting go, hanging onto old ideas and beliefs, limited, stinginess	Neck	Flexibility, seeing others' viewpoints
		Pain	Manifesting guilt, seeking punishment
Colon/Diarrhea	Rejection, fear, running away from lack of trusting, not having enough	Pink Eye	Anger
Diabetes	Deep sorrow for what might have been, need to control, sweetness gone in life	Psoriasis/Rash	Irritation, wanting attention, refusing to accept responsibilities for self, anger
Ears	Don't want to hear what's being said, sees no beauty in anything	Snoring	Stubborn, refusal to let go of old patterns, stuck in old thinking
Feet	Not being grounded in life	Sores, Swelling	Anger
Fevers	Anger	Stomach	Assimilation of thoughts and ideas
Gallstones	Hard thoughts, how dare they, bitter and condemning	Stroke	Rejection of joys of life, giving up, soul's way to make transition when time
Heart	Love Center of the Body, giving and receiving, someone to take your power joyfulness	Testicles/Prostate	Represents feelings of masculinity, aging, guilt, mental fears
Heart Problems	Denial of love, feeling rejected, not giving towards others, loss of lover	Throat	Channel of expression and creativity, frustration, fear of change, expressing only one point of view, limited thought
Hips	Balance of the Body, carry us forward in life, making major decisions	Tumors	Holding onto old hurts, false hopes
Jaw	Anger	Ulcers	Not feeling good enough, self-worth
Knees	Ability to bend in life, ego and pride, fear, won't give in, limited thinking	Warts	Feelings of being ugly, expressions of little hates, not a good listener
Legs	Carry us forward in life, movement, willingness or ability to change		

Positive Motivations

Ways to Make Your Days Enjoyable
- Cherish the quietness of early morning
- Be content with what you have
- Stop and take a renewing deep breath several times a day
- Extend courtesies on the road—it is much more pleasant
- Let go and be tolerant with everyone
- Enjoy compliments you receive, as well as those you give to others
- Occasionally relive the past and reminisce with photographs
- Keep a positive attitude, anticipate the good things that are just around the corner
- Take a walk; let the wind blow through your hair
- Fly a kite, roller skate, play volleyball, bowl, or go to a ball game
- Take time out to watch the stars and comets on a clear evening
- Take time to do a good deed, spread some cheer for someone else; this is very healing
- Take flowers to a friend, to the job—this brightens up the room with love
- Take time to journal, meditate, or have a long leisurely bath
- Clean closets, garage, house, just be neat and organized; helps create positive attitudes

Our Operating Beliefs

Source: Article in Avatar *Journal 9 (no. 1), by Henry Palmer*

Objective—To determine if the beliefs we hold are helpful or harmful, deliberately created, or indoctrinated. Look for insights, restructuring of personal reality. Instructions: List three things you believe about yourself, list three things you believe about relationships, and list three things you believe about money. After each belief, note whether you experience the belief as helpful or impeding, and if you created the belief deliberately, or as the result of indoctrination.

Result—To understand where and how you have created your beliefs.

> *Happiness can be defined as pursuing, possessing, protecting nothing!*
> *Happiness means letting go of the limited definitions of what we think we are, own, etc.*
> *Happiness requires that we restore our inner peace. There's no joy without inner peace.*
> *Attachments eat away at our inner peace. Expectations disturb our inner peace.*
> *Seek happiness where you lost it.*
> *Nothing has to happen or not happen to make you happy.*
>
> Henry Palmer

Book Resources

The Arthurian Quest by Amber Wolfe
Earth Medicine by Jamie Sams
Life Patterns, Soul Lessons, and Forgiveness and *The Journey Within* by Henry Leo Bolduc
Men Are from Mars, Women from Venus Series by John Gray, PhD
The Wind Is My Mother by Bear Heart
Women who Run with the Wolves by Clarissa Pinkola Estes, PhD
You Can Heal Your Life and *Heart Thoughts* by Louise Hay

Chapter Eleven

Reiki—A Natural Method of Healing

What Is Reiki?

Rei—Spiritual Wisdom

The Japanese kanji character Rei means spirit, air, and essence of creation. It is a spiritually guided universal life force energy indicating seven levels of meaning, and interpreted as the seven layers of our fields of energy, from the structural foundation to the outer levels. Further esoteric research gives a deeper meaning to the Rei: supernatural knowledge or spiritual consciousness. Rei is the Divine Consciousness of the all knowing, the Core Star, the inner being, the cause and effect, the guidance to heal any situation, and it is wisdom guiding the evolution of all creation, from the unfolding of our universe's galaxies to a more human level. Call upon this energy for guidance in your life. It is Divine Love.

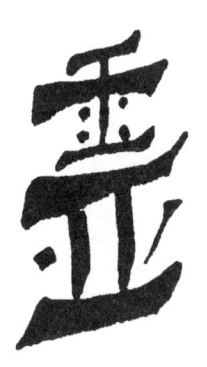

Ki—The Vital Life Force

The Japanese kanji character Ki means power and energy, and has the properties to unlock wisdom and psychic ability. Examples: The Chi in Chinese, first recorded during the Yellow Empire more than four thousand years ago, includes thirty-two different kinds of Chi. In Hawaiian, the corresponding name Aumakau means the connection between the superconscious and the conscious mind. This is pure information brought directly from the Totality of the One through the silver cord to mankind. Ki is the vital life force energy that lives in all things. When a person's Ki is low, they will feel weakness, chronic fatigue, and a lower resistance to illness. When the Ki is high, we feel confident, strong, and ready to face everyday challenges. Our bodies receive Ki through our everyday environment, including sleep, breathing, sunshine, exercise, food, and meditation. Disruptions of Ki—like negative or angry thoughts, fear, worry and stressful situations—will affect our physical organs and tissues.

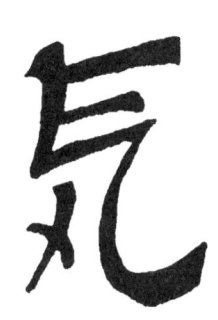

Reiki — A Spiritually Guided Healing Energy

It is the Divine Consciousness, the All Knowing called Rei, that guides the vital life force called the Ki in Reiki healing. Reiki is to be experienced, rather than intellectualized. Reiki is channeled energy from a divine source flowing into the recipient, whose entire system is then charged and revitalized.

Balancing the body's energy fields with Reiki helps us to stop spinning awkwardly off our pathway. Reiki helps us to connect with our center or core star from within, which in turn we extend out to others. The vital force energy guides us back to the reconnection with life's purpose, forgotten during thoughts of separation. In other words, it puts us back on track.

The time frame in which Dr. Usui discovered Reiki was the beginning of a historical time when our planet was ready for these new revelations and insights. The world was ready, especially in the workings of the mind. Many scientists all over the world had new insights about healing and psychology. Freud published the concept of the unconscious and Jung was inspired to carry that work further into the worlds of the past, and researched the meaning of symbols. Rudolf Steiner and Krishnamurti developed their concepts of man's history and meaning.

Reiki — Not a Religion

Reiki itself is not a religion, although forms of this healing practice are known in all cultures throughout the world. Reiki does have a built-in spiritual dimension, where healing takes place at a Divine Conscious soul level. This, we firmly believe, is the reason for the effectiveness of Reiki.

Reiki — Unity Concept

We have spent many generations becoming individuals, while losing the concept of unity. Now accepted globally, Reiki has reintroduced the concept of unity and harmony. Recent discoveries about the background of healing through symbols (Reiki) have shown the unity of cultures throughout the world.

Reiki — Learning About It

Reiki is not dependent upon one's intellectual capacity or ability to learn. It does not take years. It is a personal experience of activation within oneself, and a connectedness to Divine Consciousness. Procedures of Reiki healing use a unique symbolic language. Reiki requires an open mind and a receptive attitude. Reiki does not require a student to change their religious belief system.

Reiki — Harmony with Nature

Through the invention of Kirlian photography, we got our first look at the vital life force energy, and received confirmation of its existence, an existence that many cultures were already aware of, including the Native Americans. These people lived in harmony with nature, not in spite of it, exchanging vibrational information with everything around them. More and more, all Earth people are beginning to recognize the influence of nature around them. Nature hikes, medicine wheel ceremonies, sweat lodges, retreats, spiritual workshops, nutrition and herbal remedies, books, and magazines are all geared towards understanding self and our environment.

Reiki — Today

As soon as Reiki came to the Western world, it was analyzed and became a subject of books and much discussion. The Western mind sees truth in knowledge, fact and documentation. The Eastern mind sees truth in knowing, metaphor, and intuition.

Over the last ten years, Reiki has expanded enormously. Today Reiki masters teach this simple healing art globally, in almost every country of the world. Reiki healing treatments are usually seventy-five minutes long, and give a sense of well-being, trust, and completeness.

Healing means to make whole, accepting and
loving all parts of our self, not just the parts we like.

Origins of Reiki

The Japanese word Reiki (pronounced Raykey) means universal life force energy. Reiki originated in Tibet. This study and philosophy has been handed down from the ancient tradition of the Sanskrit text, the teachings of the Vedas. The Vedas are a compilation of scriptures that were given to the great Rishis (wise men) many thousands of years ago. The oldest known existing text is more than five thousand years old.

Tibetan Buddhism is a mixture of ancient ancestor worship and knowledge of channeling energies. Within this study of energy, a science based on the language of symbols has evolved. Tantra Lotus Sutra, a Tibetan text written in the early first or second century, offers a symbol formula for the technique of Reiki. Reiki is one of the simplest, most direct, and most powerful ways of focusing healing energy. Tibetan monks used various symbols in different ways to deepen their meditation practices, as well as to heal and strengthen the body.

The Polynesian and Hawaiian races of the Huna (meaning secret) religion refer to this universal vital energy force as "Aumakua." It is a symbol of light involving the transformation of the consciousness, coming direct from Totality as pure information without interference from self. Memory stories have been handed down from ancient times through many cultures, including the Egyptian, Greek, North and South Native American, Polynesian, and Hawaiian.

Knowledge of other ancient healing systems sheds light on the Tibetan Buddhist healing technique referred to as the Medicine Buddha. Medicine Buddha involves the laying on of hands and the ability of transmitting this healing through an empowerment from teacher to student. Taught orally from teacher to student, this is similar to the Reiki method of initiation and attunements.

Tibetan Buddhism was the only form of Buddhism that used empowerment in the early stages of its spiritual development. Much emphasis was placed upon healing the physical and spiritual in those early days. Gautama Siddhartha taught the Path to Enlightenment to followers called "Bodhisattvas" or even "The Great Physicians." This Buddhist practice, from its early development, was discouraged as a distraction from the Enlightenment Pathway. Thus, healing was then directed to only the spiritual.

Those thought of as being Bodhisattvas are Jesus (the anointed Christ), Mary (mother of all peoples), Kwan Yin (China), Tar (Tibet), and Native Americans (Earth Mother). These advanced masters came to help awaken and enlighten the future peoples of this planet. They kept alive man's ability to claim love, strength, and hope for a continued future of enlightenment.

The beauty and challenge of the gift of Reiki lie in its simplicity, and its lack of intellectual concepts. The traditional Usui system of Reiki natural healing had no theories, no predisposed thoughts; it was simply transmitted energy, done with trust and pure intention.

Rediscovery of Reiki

The history of the ancient healing method of Reiki and its rediscovery has been told by the appointed Grand Master, Hawayo Takata (1900–1980), and passed on to all Reiki Masters and students in a simplified version and lineage. Further investigation and research into the historical background of Reiki has been done by many of the teaching Reiki masters. The secret attunement symbols are given to each student in Reiki II and Reiki III degrees; reference to these symbols has been given to the general public in the United States and Australia.

Dr. Mikao Usui

Dr. Mikao Usui was born in Japan, and rediscovered Reiki, the hands-on method, during the late 1800s. Usui developed techniques and discovered truths that form the foundation of today's Reiki treatments and teaching throughout the world.

Dr. Usui was a professor in Japan, and taught the philosophies of miraculous healing by Jesus and Buddha. He spoke of the transcendent source of energy when these masters taught and performed healing. Students questioned Dr. Usui about these healing techniques and his theory of this healing energy being accessible. At the students' urging, Dr. Usui started his long search for the ancient truths about this healing information.

For many years, Dr. Usui studied ancient texts from Eastern and Western traditions. He also studied the oldest known texts in Hebrew and Aramaic, as well as the Sanskrit sutras, hoping to find clues for the healing that Jesus and Buddha had performed. Dr. Usui studied Chinese and Sanskrit. Part of his journey took Dr. Usui throughout the countryside of Japan. Then he visited the Buddhist temples and studied their documents. He asked many questions about their healing techniques. In his questioning of the holy men, it was revealed that they were aware of healing techniques for the body, although a great deal of specific information had been lost due to their gradual disuse. The holy men were now concentrating only on the healing of the spiritual self.

Dr. Usui was allowed to study the sacred writings at each of the temples he visited. In the Indian sutras, written in Sanskrit, Usui discovered information for contacting a higher source. The initiation test was a three-week period of meditation. After a long period of reading, study, and discussion with the masters, Usui had an insight that the information he sought would be revealed when he took the test. He prepared for this initiation by fasting and meditating. He then traveled to the holy mountain of Koriyama.

On the mountain, Dr. Usui set aside twenty-one stones, one for each day he would fast and meditate. He waited in total solitude for the healing information to be revealed to him. Before dawn on the twenty-first day, Usui was looking in the direction of the horizon and saw a beam of light coming toward him at great speed. His immediate reaction was awareness that this light had consciousness, and was the healing power he had been waiting for.

As the light became larger, it connected with his third eye area, and Dr. Usui's sight was intuitively opened. He saw hundreds of little bubbles, atoms of light, in all the colors of the rainbow! As Usui lay in an altered state, he saw within this great beam of light the Sanskrit symbols. This is when Usui received his attunement and was initiated into Reiki by this universal life force energy. Thus, the healing method that had been lost for thousands of years had now been reborn.

Dr. Usui set up a practice in the slums of Kyoto, Japan. After many years of working alone with the sick, he realized the people were not bettering themselves. Unfortunately people were looking for help and a free handout. They had not understood or been willing to take responsibility for their actions. At this point, Usui decided to leave the slums, and started his pilgrimage to share the knowledge of Reiki throughout Japan. On his travels he met Dr. Chujiro Hayashi, who studied and received his training to be a Reiki master.

Dr. Usui attuned sixteen teachers; the only one recorded or mentioned was Dr. Hayashi. They worked closely together for five years. Dr. Hayashi was named Dr. Usui's successor to carry on the Reiki work in 1930, when Dr. Usui died. He left behind the heritage of Reiki for all peoples of the world.

Dr. Chujiro Hayashi

Dr. Hayashi accepted the responsibility to preserve Reiki and to carry forward the knowledge and work of Reiki. Hayashi founded the Reiki Clinic in Tokyo and kept records of the treatments given. These detailed records gave Hayashi the information for the standard hand positions we now use. It was Dr. Hayashi who created the system of the Reiki hand positions, the degrees, and the initiation/attunement outline. He trained many people to work in the Reiki clinic, one of whom was his wife.

Dr. Hayashi traveled to Hawaii to help Hawayo Takata establish Reiki in that area. He told her that if he ever summoned her, she needed to come to Japan immediately. He gave Takata her Reiki mastership in 1938. Although Hayashi did not want Reiki to leave Japan, he was aware of a pending war. He knew that most of the men that worked in the clinic would be called to duty. He wanted to preserve Reiki, and made the decision to pass on the teachings and the techniques by naming Hawayo Takata as his successor. This decision would again preserve Reiki for the world. Dr. Hayashi made his transition in 1941, at the age of sixty-three.

Hawayo Takata

Hawayo Takata was born in 1900 in Hawaii. Takata was married, then became a widow with two children while living in Hawaii. Her parents lived in Japan. Takata's traditional family responsibilities directed her back to Japan, but before leaving on the voyage by steamship, she became very ill. Since the death of her husband, the pressures of raising two children had taxed her frail body. Upon arriving in Japan she was hospitalized. The doctors informed Takata that she had gallstones, a tumor, and appendicitis. After resting several weeks in preparation for surgery, she heard a voice saying, "The operation is not necessary." This voice spoke to Takata three times. She then asked her doctor about alternatives, and was told about the Reiki clinic run by Dr. Hayashi. She made the decision to try this method rather than surgery.

Takata received Reiki treatments on a regular basis for approximately four months. She was so impressed with the practitioner's knowledge, and the results of the Reiki treatments, that she made the decision to stay in Japan and learn this technique. Takata took Reiki I in 1936, and worked with Dr. Hayashi for one year as part of her training. In 1937, she took Reiki II and then returned to Hawaii to establish the Reiki healing work there. Dr. Hayashi initiated Takata as a Reiki Master in 1938.

After working with Reiki for many years, Takata realized the need to train others. To pass on this information to the Western world, she devised a value system she believed was necessary to quantify the worth of Reiki. The only way she knew to show the value of the training was to charge a large sum of money, since what is expensive is seen as desirable. This was how the original fee structure of ten thousand dollars was established for a Reiki Mastership.

Takata trained in a traditional way, because that is where the thinking was at the time. Each Reiki master is to carry forth the Reiki Principles, representing integrity in all that is taught. This in itself will serve mankind. All modalities move forward, and Reiki has not stayed totally the same; each master throughout the world will influence their students by sharing their own special knowledge of healing.

Massage therapists today add Reiki energy along with their knowledge of the body and its energies. Some Reiki practitioners are psychotherapists and use Reiki as a form of bodywork. Reiki is enhanced when used along with chakra healing, flower essences, and music. Reiki is completely compatible with all modalities, flowing with every therapeutic concept. Reiki itself does not need to be identified, it just is. Takata became a massage therapist as a way of certifying Reiki almost fifty years ago.

Chronology

The energy of Reiki—the universal life energy force—has been known and used for many thousands of years. Although calling it by different names (Chi, Prana, Ki, Uraes), many cultures did in fact tap into this universal energy. The following is a listing of some of the times and places this vital force energy first became known.

Prehistory	Various Shamans tapped into the universal vital force energy all over the world.

Middle East

8000 B.C.E.	Egypt conceptualized the energy as the Uraes, and developed a system based on the Seven Hearts of the being. This system not only dealt with the physical; it strove to integrate all the parts of the being (physical, emotional, mental, and spiritual).
1500 B.C.E.	China began formulating the concept of Chi, based on Egyptian teaching, and their own Shamanic traditions.
1500 B.C.E.	Eastern Indian concept of prana was also formulated at this time.
1800–500 B.C.E.	Explosion of concepts in many lands and peoples, including Celtic, Aborigine, Native American (North and South), Japanese, Polynesian, African, Greek, European, Hebrew. This explosion of concept and technique was brought about by communication amongst the various peoples.
620 B.C.E.	Birth of Gautama Siddhartha and Sakyamuni Buddha, India—Nepal border.
500 B.C.E.–100 C.E.	The fusion of Greek, Egyptian, Hebrew, and Buddhist concepts in the Middle East led to many codifications of the concepts of the universal energy. Not only were the healing concepts written down, but neo-Platonism, Pathogranism, Qabala, and Freemasonry (plus others) came out of this time.
7 B.C.E.	Historical birth of Jesus.
5 B.C.E.	Three Wise Men came from the East, seeking the reincarnation of an Enlightened One. They went with Jesus and family to Egypt and India.
27–33 C.E.	Jesus returned to Jerusalem for his work, the crucifixion, and his ascension.
46–49 C.E.	Records of Jesus returning to India.
110 C.E.	Death of Jesus in Srinagar, India. Legends say he lived to 120 years of age.

Japan

1880s	Dr. Mikao Usui's search and vision quest for the universal energy he called Reiki.

1925	Dr. Chujiro Hayashi received his Reiki Mastership, worked under Dr. Mikao Usui.
1930	Death of Dr. Usui; he initiated more than sixteen Reiki masters.
1941	Death of Dr. Hayashi. He initiated more than fourteen Reiki masters, including his wife, Chie, and Takata. Aware of impending war, Hayashi chose transition, rather than fighting.

Hawaii

1900	Birth of Hawayo Kawamuru (Takata)
1935	Takata's return to Japan, for healing at hospital in Akasaka, then at Reiki clinic in Tokyo, where she was healed in four months.
1936–37	Takata received her Reiki I and II from Dr. Hayashi.
1937	Takata opened first healing clinic in Kapaa.
1938	Takata received mastership from Dr. Hayashi on February 22, and was named his successor.
1980	Death of Hawayo Takata. She initiated twenty-two Reiki masters in the ten years before her death. Her granddaughter carried on the legend of Reiki and became the Grand Master. From this point on Reiki blossomed throughout the world.

Masters

Before Takata's transition she initiated twenty-two Reiki Masters, between the years 1970 and 1980. These original teachers have taught others, and there are now approximately ten thousand Reiki Masters, with as many as five hundred thousand people practicing Reiki throughout the world.

George Araki	Harry Kubol
Dorothy Baba (deceased)	Ethel Lombardi
Ursula Baylow	Barbara McCullough
Rick Bockner	Mary McFadyen
Barbara Brown	Paul Mitchell
Fran Brown	Bethel Phaigh (deceased)
Patricia Ewing	Barbara Weber Ray
Phyllis Lei Furumoto (Grand Master)	Virginia Samdahl
Beth Gray	Shinobu Saito
John Gray	Takata's sister
Iris Ishikura (deceased)	Wanja Twan

The Reiki Alliance

Source: Henry Crow Dog Raindrops *by Lumis Two Hawks*

As I work with Reiki in my life on a daily basis, I have discovered I use this method more and more. I am often reminded of something I read from a dialogue of Henry Crow Dog in 1974.

He made the statement in reference to the Ghost Dance and its revival. Its true meaning was one of peace and unity for all people, regardless of their color; all Earth people living in harmony. He spoke of bringing back a love for Mother Earth. He spoke of Mother Earth as a living spirit, with energies like raindrops making a tiny brook. These many raindrops each were making a stream, these streams making mighty rivers, bursting forth across the lands. We are the first raindrops.

This is very profound to me. With Reiki, I, too, feel we are like the first raindrops. As more and more of us begin to use Reiki on a day-to-day basis, we become the mighty river, flowing over all boundaries and limitations, to heal and nurture and create a loving harmony in all that we touch.

The above list was the beginning. Twenty-two raindrops started the flow.
Now Reiki is storming the world.

Organizing Reiki would be like organizing these raindrops—impossible. Still, those that commit their lives to Reiki want to come together, to share their stories, to learn from each other, and to simply enjoy each other's company. One way is through the cottage meetings that I call Reiki open house or Reiki clinics; the other is The Reiki Alliance. The Alliance is supportive with information, and is available to any Reiki master, from any country. Once a year there is an organized global conference, with attendance from all over the globe.

Only a few of mankind continue to make an effort,
to explore this mystery of reality
refining and redefining their understanding of this world
searching for what is true and what is illusion,
remember it is how we play this game of life that is honor and truth!

Planetary Need for Spiritual Reiki
by S. Jeanne Gunn

Spirituality and awareness of life has increased and become more apparent in the last few years. Words that were taboo and hush-hush twenty years ago are now household words. There is a sense of urgency felt by many peoples on the planet to clean house, to become aware of our actions and those reactions that are affecting our global environment. The Reiki healing technique has been one way many aware individuals are spreading and escalating healing for changing behavior patterns.

The well-being of our planet is at stake, and it is the only place we humans have to live in. It is us, the Earth people, that this book has been written for. It is taking a step forward, not only in our personal development, but also in our personal actions. These actions need to be for the good of the All. This will create a better you and a better world.

One of the basics of Reiki is learning who you are, learning about the environment around you. Some of the other basics are the universal laws. These laws are about our actions in relationship to each other, and how our inaction against injustices moves the energy towards negative results. We are awakening to the realization that the messes we create in our life are up to us to uncreate. This learning process and how we react to it is what our spiritual pathway awakening is all about—how we exist together on this planet.

The basic concept of the Native Americans' Great White Spirit was with them, in their thoughts, actions, and deeds. Honor was their word. Their actions were of utmost importance to them. The circles of life exist everywhere, and are viewed in many concepts today. Wedding rings, the tree rings showing the years' life of a tree, the circle of Earth, sun, moon, crop circles, the body's cycles, planetary cycles, and the medicine wheel all show the everlasting evolving cycles of man. This is Spirit's way of showing us that we are an ever-evolving species with opportunities to flow with life, rather than against the natural flow of life. It is our free will, our choice!

We are looking to assist you in your awareness and development to create a better world. We want to help people change the way they interact with each other and with other living things. Through Reiki, you are making a unified connection throughout the world. Like Henry Crow Dog's raindrops, we are all connected and linked up on a vibratory level to help heal the body, the mind, the spirit, and our planet.

We, at the Reiki and Beyond Spiritual Center, want Reiki to be available to everyone. It was not a coincidence that Reiki was rediscovered. Dr. Usui was guided by inner instincts, as each of us now is being guided. The time is right, it is our inheritance, just as it was our inheritance when Jesus taught his disciples, and this information was to be handed down to the people. Through suppression by the early Christian church, which reflects the disciple Paul's writings more than the teachings of Buddhist-influenced Jesus, Reiki was lost for many hundreds of years.

Knowing about our interconnectedness to all life and acting accordingly,
Being responsible for our thoughts and actions
is the first step in becoming an Earth person.
Helping Mother Earth and ourselves in the process of evolving into
One planet ♥ One people!

Working with Reiki

Outline

1) Reiki allows the light particles (the Oneness) to enlighten and heal the part of you that is diseased, is feeling bad, hurts, is traumatized, or has developed crystallization, all of which lead to the cause of disease or dis-ease.
2) Reiki is channeled energy. This energy flows through you but is directed by Divine Source. You do not use your own energy, so yours is never depleted. It is necessary to be centered and grounded.
3) The practitioner (you) receives a healing as the channeled Reiki vital force energy flows through you to the client.
4) Reiki is self-guided by Divine Source and works where the client needs it most. Reiki flows throughout the body on chakra pathways and fields, or levels, of energy. (Fields of energy and chakras are discussed in another section of this book.) The Reiki vital force energy nourishes your cells, organs, molecules, atoms, and electrons, and the very essence of all that you are.
5) Remember to say thank you for the blessing of the healing. This is an acknowledgment to Divine Source and the guides, and helps keep the flow going. Then be patient. When one has taken years to develop an illness, this illness may need several treatments for the client to let go of the stuff he has hung onto. I realize we are a quick-fix society, but change in the body doesn't always happen overnight!
6) Reiki works on all levels, the emotional, the mental, the physical, and the spiritual. You can start using Reiki after you have received your first attunement. The set intention of giving Reiki starts the flow of energy, wherever you are. You do not have to be in a meditative state to use Reiki. It is important to be centered and grounded. Do not allow the ego to dictate to you that it is you alone doing all the work.
7) It is important that you do not force yourself upon a person who does not want Reiki and is not open to any healing work. In this case, you can allow yourself to send energy out for the best

interest and highest good of that person, knowing that your intention is for the good of mankind. Insisting you heal is probably ego. It is not our responsibility or directive to force a change on someone who does not want, or is not open to, a change in their illness. By doing so, you have stepped into a universal law called cause and effect, which in this case would be judgmental and interfering.

8) Reiki is the Divine Source that puts our disqualified (negative) energies into right action. Remember that when doing healing work, intention is most important. Misguided intention (ego) is interfering, butting in, and judgmental. Who are we to decide who needs help, and who needs to make a change in their life or their illness?

9) The more you work with Reiki energy, the more you can use it in your everyday life. Reiki is not just hands-on. Reiki works when driving down the street and seeing an accident or an injured bird. Reiki works when you are around someone who is very angry and upset. Reiki works in hospitals, out fishing, when checking out yard sales, or at the supermarket. Reiki works anywhere and at any time.

Reiki is a way of life—it is life.

Addictions

Reiki helps people who have unwanted habits or conditions, for example, smoking, alcoholism, and overeating. These habits, if excessive, are like poisons to our body. Reiki II is where you are taught the symbols that reach the subconscious and work on that level of awareness within our body.

Reiki Guidance

Reiki triggers the knowledge and memory that dwell within the soul, the impression of the individual consciousness. Your intuition plays an important part in giving Reiki, sensing, feeling, and seeing. By getting in tune with the consciousness of Reiki, you enter a state of mind that connects and works with you and your individual spiritual guides.

You may feel intense heat or cold, tingling sensations, or holes in the energy fields. Ask your spiritual (Reiki) guides to direct the energy for the best interest and highest good of the client. The client will give you feedback on where the energy is flowing. Trust the experience. Allow yourself to believe you have been guided to work where the client needed it most. You will soon learn a physical hurt isn't always where the energy field requires the Reiki.

For example: Legs represent going forward in life, and your legs could be affected by a first or second chakra imbalance. The imbalance could be from childhood and at a subconsciousness level, suppressed anger. Always work from a state of intention for the greater good and effectiveness of the client.

Reiki No-Fault

Reiki is Divine Consciousness, the universal life force energy. Reiki will not harm anyone or anything, it is always helpful. You can never give too much or even too little Reiki. If time is limited, short treatments can be beneficial.

Some of the ailments Reiki can help are headaches, toothaches, earaches, stings, cuts, and bruises.

Reiki also works on house plants, gardens, trees, dogs, cats, birds, fish, automobiles, computers, or whatever area you send healing energies to. Reiki can go out into the universe, to work with governments, countries, health problems, emergencies, disasters, storms, unborn babies, global situations, and our universe. By using this energy, we are aware and helping create a better universe, a better environment, a better commitment to ourselves. We are becoming the mass consciousness that can cancel destructive forces. We can do anything, we can create anything, and all it takes is the remembering and the intention of good.

Reiki is Universal Love, Compassion, and Intention.

Spiritual or Reiki Guides

Appearances in spirit form of angels, or messengers, have been reported since the beginning of time, and throughout every nation. Man hears voices, receives messages, sees spirit forms, has prophetic dreams, and has been privileged to encounter many miracles. All you have to do is ask, and a Reiki guide will work with you in a way you will be comfortable with. Upon receiving your Reiki I attunement, you will have Reiki guides working with you whether you are aware of them or not. The more you do, the more aware you become. Intuitively, this is your Reiki guide working with you.

The great master Buddha teaches that
"you are what you think, having become what you thought,"
in essence saying that for every cause there is an effect.

Reiki Hugs

As you give or receive a Reiki hug, you feel, sense, and are aware of that person's energy. This exchange of energy is whole and pure, and is so much more enjoyable than having someone slapping you on the back. The person receiving the hug, if not familiar with Reiki, may simply feel a sense of warmth or well-being or peacefulness. For that space and time you have shared energy, replenishing, building and extending your own as well as that of the other person. It is like a mini-healing.

Begin noticing the way you hug. You will notice the difference and look forward to a shared hug rather than a pat on your back, which is disruptive and jarring. You will take pleasure in the greeting, knowing you made a beautiful connection with another human being.

Important Steps Towards Healing

Sources: On Death and Dying *by Dr. Elisabeth Kübler-Ross and* Light Emerging *by Barbara Ann Brennan*

1) Denial serves to keep us from seeing what we don't feel prepared to see. When we express a pretense of handling a problem with a glib remark, it temporarily gives us time to mentally process what is happening, sometimes ignoring messages that our body is trying to tell us.
2) Anger brings up the question, why me? This anger is then usually projected into our home, work, environment, and especially our body; and then directed towards Divine Source.
3) If anger didn't bring what you wanted, bargaining with Divine Creator is the next step, and then facing guilt over what could have been or should have been done. Those should-haves can then lead to depression, trying to heal through avoidance and rejection of self, rather than truthful seeking of a solution.
4) Depression is a feeling of lost hope in getting what we wanted, the pretense that we don't care when we really do. This creates a depression in our energy fields, starting with denial from bargaining. Depression is a form of self-rejection, self-judgment, and withdrawal from reality.

5) Acceptance is when we've had enough, when we can focus on the previous four steps, when we have mourned our losses. It is time to get to know ourselves. Acceptance is the process of making necessary changes in our life, a time of deep surrender and of letting go of those feelings of powerlessness to always be in control.

6) Rebirth is a time to see ourselves in a new light. It is necessary to have some personal quiet time, the coming forth or emerging, as a butterfly from a cocoon into the light, seeing the beauty around us. An opportunity to reshape your journey and relationships, be humble, learn to trust the inner self, and remember that all is provided for from our Divine Creator.

7) Creating a new life is learning to live honestly with yourself, being more accepting of self, having a broader sense of faith, love, truth, and internal humility. Inner healing brings forth external changes, whether it is in your job, your relationships, or even your environment. Allowing the fear in step one to be dealt with was the beginning of creating a new life and being healed.

Live your daily life as if everything you do will eventually be known!

Harmony of Nature
by S. Jeanne Gunn

I was newly embarked on what you would call a spiritual pathway when I took the Reiki I course. I definitely needed healing after my marriage of twenty-five years ended in divorce. What better way was there to heal, than by taking a course on healing?

Taking Reiki helped me to understand some simple basics. There was information available that I had not received because I had been spiritually asleep: information about universal laws, giving and receiving, cause and effect, intention, reincarnation, limitation, strength, spiritual guides, chakras, energy, and much more. It enabled me to reclaim my sense of worth, gave me hope, a new beginning, a light at the end of the tunnel. Many thanks to my Reiki Master teacher, Helen Borth.

Two years later, I was intent upon taking care of the four acres on which I lived. I enjoyed yard work and had always done most of the raking, but hardly ever any mowing. And the moles, what do you do about moles, except swear at them?

The moles loved my beautiful geraniums! I had planted deep red geraniums along the rustic fence by the driveway. They made a beautiful backdrop until the moles discovered how tasty the roots were. Imagine my surprise, as I stood admiring my flowers, only to watch them slowly getting smaller and disappearing! Then I took a closer look, and saw that moles (the rascals) had eaten the roots off the whole row. The plants were just sort of leaning there! Now I had to plant two more flats of geraniums, and if I did, would the same thing happen?

I asked the advice of a spiritual friend who said that I should talk to the "King of the Moles" and ask for the moles to stop eating my geraniums. I believed. I had the new faith of a child. So I asked the King of the Moles, "Please enjoy another part of the yard," and stated I would not bother them if they moved. I also made it clear that if they insisted upon eating my flowers, I would take action. They moved!

Well, that was the geranium story, and now about my strawberries! I was fairly new at gardening, but had just read about the Findhorn Gardens. This is where they grew crops in very rocky soil, and worked with energy beings. I figured, if it worked for them, it should work for me. But the large strawberries kept disappearing. My son wasn't eating them, I wasn't eating them, and the birds weren't eating them. One day as I was reaching down to pick a juicy strawberry, a baby bunny snatched it, right before my eyes! It scared both of us. I knew if I wanted to enjoy my garden, I would need to strike a bargain with the rabbits. I told them they could have all the strawberries, but the rest of the garden was to be mine. I asked the "Head Rabbit" if this was an okay deal. And so it was. Then there were the gypsy moths, but we'll save that story for another day!

I have now come to understand that there is mutual respect and balance in our environment. I honored the animals with their rights. It is important to work together for what is best for man and beast. After all, we are One, we are all Divine Sources, and we are all living on Mother Earth, one large planetary community.

I am certainly grateful to loving spiritual guides and angelic beings that guided me to understand the harmony and balance of nature—the living planet we call Mother Earth.

Mass Consciousness vs. the Hurricane
by S. Jeanne Gunn

We all like a good story about the weather. But this is a story woven together from different peoples, working together as a whole, thus becoming the mass consciousness.

Last year in a channeling session, a friend and I picked up that the Angels wanted us to be aware of the eastern coastline. We visualized the Angels putting beautiful healing crystals (violet ray transmuting) into the waters and to send healing to the coastline area.

Another friend was traveling north along the coastline road, and we asked her to send healing energies along the route. Then another friend called. She had received channeled information about problems along the eastern coastline. Then another friend called and said, "My guides are telling me we need to go down to the ocean and play, have fun, because the water and the sea animals all need healing." Several telephone calls later, we gathered at the beach for a healing ceremony. We called upon the archangels of the four directions, the elements, our guides, and the healing energy of Divine Source to be with us. We had brought along candles, blankets, and sage. We danced, acted silly, and sang. We had a joyful time.

All of this happened a month before a hurricane...

We all continued sending out positive thoughts, and learned later that others were doing the same. Soon we heard a storm was coming. The TV news talked and talked about doom and gloom. Everyone seemed to be dashing around in a panic to get his or her supplies. I finally told my friend, "If you would spend as much time praying for the situation as you have being hysterical, there wouldn't be a storm. It is your attitude and panic that will build the storm into destruction." This fell upon deaf ears.

The storm is coming! The storm is coming!

Well, I decided to go to the beach and pray. The winds were gathering intensity and clouds blackened the sky. When I arrived, I beheld a miracle. Hundreds and hundreds of people had gathered, riding bikes, playing, and flying kites, surfing on the larger than normal waves, sitting on blankets and picnicking. Everyone came out to wait for the arrival of and greet the hurricane. This was really something. No invitations had been sent, except by the angels! We all waited in anticipation. The sky seemed to be getting darker and darker. Television crews had staked out and claimed their space and run their cables, and were doing interviews.

Soon, the winds died down. The storm had decided not to attend our party.

The hurricane, according to the weather report, had taken a sharp right-angle turn and moved out to sea. The sky turned lighter and lighter, into the most beautiful colors I had ever seen—a new peach coral and what I called an electric blue. The clouds were magnificent.

This was mass consciousness vs. the hurricane, and the people had won.

I wonder how many people in Virginia Beach, Virginia know they lent a helping hand! I wonder if others, in other parts of our world, joined with us.

What, then, could we do about the even more damaging problems we face upon our lands, problems of famine, disease, our polluted environment, and education? Would you be willing to help? *We live in a time frame when no matter what we have or own, power and money seem to be our first priority, a time when many children sense no future, and -do not believe in honor, trust, caring, or helping anyone or anything.*

Secret Reiki

by Linda Schiller-Hanna

My friend and I were driving together along the expressway from Florida, back to Virginia, when we came upon an automobile accident. We pulled over, both thinking at once that maybe they needed Reiki. There was no ambulance on the scene, just one policeman and a bystander who had stopped to help. The victims of the accident, a mother and her toddler, stood by the side of their overturned pickup truck.

Apparently a tire had blown and the truck had skidded off the road and flipped. Miraculously, no one was hurt. With my background in first aid and certification as a nurse's aide, I instinctively reached for the blanket that I carry in my car. My friend and I approached the young mother and wrapped her and the child with the blanket, holding it around them as she stood talking to the police officer. All the important details of clearing up the accident proceeded easily, and the driver drove the ambulance away empty, due to the fact that the mother and child "felt okay."

My friend and I left the scene satisfied that using Reiki was a positive response in this situation. We had independently decided to help, and mused joyfully as we drove up the highway about how these people had no idea that we had really come to their assistance.

By the way, I took the blown tire as a warning to have one of my bad tires replaced. This I did at the next exit. There was a gift in this for all concerned.

Fish Story!

We all have fish stories in our lives, but this is really a fish story.

One day, while friend "C" was cleaning out her children's fish tank, three goldfish fell into the kitchen sink. Have you ever felt fish? Do you think they feel slimy and slippery? Would you be afraid to touch them? She kept them wet by pouring water on them so they wouldn't die. But she just couldn't pick them up.

Panic time. Pouring water on the fish went on for what seemed an eternity, but the goldfish were gradually drying up. Finally I just happened by. I immediately put the goldfish back into their tank. At first, the goldfish weren't doing very well, and then C remembered her Reiki training. Proceeding to use the skills she had just learned, she visualized a beautiful light surrounding the fish tank. She placed her hands on the fish tank and sent Reiki energy into the goldfish and the water. Soon they were swimming around and acting normal.

Normal isn't the state they are currently in. After a year they grew so big, they were moved into a large aquarium tank. They are beautiful and still receiving Reiki energy!

Humankind has not woven the web of life.
We are but one thread within it.
Whatever we do to the web, we do to ourselves.
All things are bound together. All things connect.

Chief Seattle

Waiting for Proof
by Jennifer A. Link, RN, BA, CEN, SANE, RP

I have a bachelor's degree in biology with a minor in physical science, and work in an inner city emergency room as a nurse. I tend to be a concrete thinker, methodology being the means. I am also a Christian. When I was initially introduced to Reiki, I had to analyze its implications, mentally dissect stories of its success, and decide if it went against my religious beliefs in any way.

I was still skeptical when I attended my first session. The idea of putting into use a greater portion of my brain, using scientifically proven electromagnetic energies, was appealing; plus, Reiki is not a religion.

After the attunements by Reiki Master Jeanne Gunn, better known to me as Mom, I started "seeing" and "sensing" different colors during the practice healing sessions. I prayed in the name of Jesus to be certain these things were of God. I kept quiet about all this until several of the more open-minded students began to discuss these same colors. I was totally astounded that I had seen the same colors they had.

If I had not physically attended the class, I would never have believed. Reiki is a marvelous tool for me at work. I have already used it to calm drug-dependent violent patients, to comfort family members, and to soothe frightened children. It has had an amazing effect on my professional practice and my life as a Christian.

How I Apply Reiki
by Lucinda Fury

After taking Reiki First Degree, I wondered about its application in my everyday life. Wow, now that I have this wonderful tool, how do I use it?

In fact, I soon learned that I use Reiki every day. I chant to myself "Reiki, Reiki, Reiki," and the vibration cancels out my headaches. I use it when my children have fallen or are ill, or when they come home from school and need my special Reiki Hug. When my contractor husband comes home with bruises and cuts from the job—again I use Reiki. I also send distant Reiki healing when I am doing counseling work on the telephone.

I am an artist, and create Native American ceremonial art, teach classes on making your own Dream Catchers, give lectures for the school system, and hold medicine wheel ceremonies on our property. The energy and love I put into all aspects of my work is sensed when people pick up one of my pieces of artwork, and just can't put it down. This is a special joy to me, because I know I am connecting with many people around the world, my own little Reiki international community.

We can either destroy the planet or we can heal it.
It is up to us as individuals to take a few moments each day
And send some loving and healing energy to the planet.
Treat Mother Earth as you would your other possessions, with respect!
Use your heart and mind as a newly born Earth person.

Wind Dancer

Reiki Feedback
by Danny Cunningham

Most healing I had taken part in as a Reiki I practitioner was with other healers in a team effort. I felt they were skilled and had psychic abilities, and I, in comparison, was "just there," channeling the spiritual healing. I was assured I was doing my job well. Those receiving a treatment could feel the energy coming through me, or see my auric field change, but I had little tangible feedback myself.

A friend and I teamed up to do a Reiki treatment on another friend. Both were psychic and one was a visionary who saw way beyond ordinary eyes. Both friends told me that my energy was powerful and helpful. The client, afflicted with Lupus, told me how much our treatment helped relieve the tension and pain she was accustomed to living with. She had been able to relax and fall into a normal sleep, rather than run on nervous energy and collapse into unconsciousness. That was some feedback!

However, at the next session with this client, I alone treated her. We had only fifteen minutes, and so I treated only the upper chakra areas and her hand, which was the most disabled body part. The veins on the back of her hands and arms stood out noticeably. After I had worked on her arm and hand for a few minutes, she told me that the pain had lessened noticeably, and she pointed out that the veins had gone down. I could see the difference. By the time I finished the treatment, the veins on her hands and forearm were barely noticeable, and the limbs looked more normal.

It was not the aesthetic effect that mattered to me, but the undeniable, visible evidence that something had changed since I started the treatment. A great feedback for me!

I had taken part in other healings, and had witnessed the healing of people who had burned their feet at a firewalk, and the healing of emotional traumas. But this was a simple solo healing. This was the confirmation I needed to know that the Reiki healing power of the universe flowed through me, since I was attuned to Reiki. And, as the psychic Edgar Cayce has said, "Use that at hand and more will be given."

Reiki as the Wind Dancer
Dancing, dancing, brilliant colors and dragonflies
Winds of air brushing by, aliken to seagulls in the sky.
Whirling, spinning atoms, doing their dances of light
Is this what the Reiki life force energy is like?

Standing still, going within my center, my trance
Reiki healing energies swirling around created the dance.
Where earth, sky, fire and water, the elements we need,
on Mother Earth, where brotherhood should be heeded.
Are we like the wind dancer, in our dance of life
Are we listening to our personal pathway, or staying in strife?

Wind Dancer

Reiki and Ancient Native American Cultures
by Lucinda Fury

The history of Reiki, as we know it, tells us that it originated in Tibet thousands of years ago. Like anything in history, we usually date learning from recorded pictures or written material. Reiki, in practiced form, existed long before any scriptures made note of it. It was practiced long before the term "Reiki" was connected to it.

Ancient primitive cultures in all areas of the world were intimately connected to the Universal Life Force, which would become the Reiki we know and use today. It is still used in more primitive (by our standards) forms, which have been handed down for many generations. Some of these methods have indeed been termed "secret" in their practice and are only performed by designated individuals in their purest form. As it can be stated that Reiki is not a religion, we can state that our Native American counterparts' attunement to spirituality was not in the past, and is not now, a religion. In their case, it is a way of life.

A connection to universal life force energy, to be utilized every day, to enforce and keep all things in balance, was their spiritual way of life. Native Americans of long ago were aware of their universal connection to all things on the earth as well as in the heavens. They relied heavily on the planetary influences for their very survival. They paid close attention to the "life force" of the earth, waters, and sky. They never questioned that all life was connected, all energy of life force flowed from one to the other, from a source they knew in every being as "Spiritual."

Appointed medicine men, and in some cases whole medicine societies, had the duty to conduct rituals and ceremonies of healing. Regardless of who directed the energy of healing, all people in the community worked together to create a spiritually balanced flow of life force among all that they were connected with. Though we may find the use of feathers (to sweep clean energy fields around the body), rattles, and drums (to balance and enhance resonance of rhythm within and outside the body) unusual, it is nonetheless another way to use the vital life force, called Reiki.

The medicine man who diligently danced, chanted, and used his tools of the trade over the ailing member of his community was indeed performing a Reiki technique in its purest form. Early Native Americans knew that all life was connected to the Creator, and that the Creator's loving, life-giving, life-sustaining energy was available to them as their birthright.

It would seem that Reiki has not evolved to its present state; it in itself has remained ever constant. It is we as its users who are evolving spiritually, to a higher understanding of Reiki's inclusion in our lives.

We are finally remembering our own connection to the life force energy, which is a never-ending supply from Creator. The vital life force will heal us, our planet Earth and all our relations, called Earth people.

Reiki energy swirling 'round, healing gentle and profound
Joining hands and hearts with Love
To bring the lifeforce from Above
Helping us to heal each other,
Transfers the healing to the Earth Mother.

Lumis Two Hawks

Reiki and Role Playing

by Linda Schiller-Hanna

I heard about Reiki back in the mid-1980s when I lived in Los Angeles and hosted a TV cable show, *The Natural Psychic*. One of my guests had studied Reiki and shared some of her experiences with me. I remember thinking they were amazing—healing of severe burns, distant healing, and so forth—and put learning about Reiki on my list of things to do.

Not until I moved to Virginia Beach, and was guided by my inner voice to study Reiki, did I follow through and take the Reiki training.

I have experienced Reiki with some wonderful people, and at one point in my life, two friends practically forced me to lie on their table to receive the blessings of Reiki. I was so overwrought that the energy they gave me felt like the recharging of my batteries. What a joy!

My friend told me about a client she had been working with using Reiki where doctors could not diagnose the problem. The client had been in and out of the hospital, was losing weight, and seemed potentially close to death if the trend continued. He was depressed and seemed to have lost his will to live. She asked if I might go with her to the hospital, where he was on a heart monitor. His doctor was curious about the Reiki she had been giving him, and wanted to see how Reiki would react on the monitor. Would I help?

I was very intrigued by the possibility of a controlled test in a hospital setting under a doctor's sanction. Unfortunately, things did not work out exactly as planned. The machines were not working properly. The nursing staff had not been given written orders to allow our activities, and there was a lot of curiosity and suspicion on their part, as they watched us with our hands on his chest. After about a half-hour of rigmarole from the staff, who were trying out different monitors, using various adjustments, and coming and going repeatedly, I realized our uncontrolled "test" was doomed.

Nevertheless, I felt it important to follow through and do a good healing, regardless of the scientific proof we were seeking. As my friend and I put our hands on the man, I began to talk with him quietly, as he had a semiprivate room. I did not want to lose the attitude of protection he'd need for deeper emotional work.

I asked him how long he had been sick. He said several months. I asked him if anything unusual had happened just before he became ill. "Yes," he said. I asked him, using a gentle tone of voice, if he would like to talk about it.

"No, but I will." He began to tell the story of a woman he had loved very much, who, just before he became ill, had broken off the relationship. I felt this was the "red flag" of cause that I was seeking. After getting him to tell a little more about their relationship, I was given the guidance to use my psychic role-playing technique with him. This technique is a hybridization of certain psychodrama techniques, psychic reading skills, emotional release, and visualization. My spiritual guides trained me in its development, and it has been extremely useful in helping many of my clients.

Once clear on the direction I needed to go with this, I got to work. I told him I'd like to do some role-playing and that it was quite easy. I just needed him to answer normally how he felt in response to what I would say. Meanwhile, my friend and I proceeded to give Reiki. We felt this was soothing for him, while I led the emotional release work.

I started the role of the estranged woman, but speaking from higher-self attitude, loving, responsive, enlightened. (Every person has a higher self.) I acknowledged the man's hurt, anger, and justification for feeling this angry and disappointed. I gave space to all the held-in emotions I sensed he was carrying in his body.

This gentleman visibly began to release tension and finally tears as we continued to speak to one another. I encouraged him to say back to me in his own words how he felt as a result of being treated badly by her. I stated I would not further antagonize or reject him, but really cared and was willing to understand his point of view. The man seemed amazed at this, but I held my ground, and repeated that his feelings were important and deserved to be validated. After we worked this angle for awhile, I sensed it was time to switch roles.

I suggested that he now play the woman part in his imagination, think and act like her. I would play the part of him. He seemed dubious, but I told him I'd start, and he was able to get into the swing of it. I became a strong advocate for the man, now verbally expressing deep hurt and rage, which I psychically felt he was still emotionally carrying. I believed this emotion was toxifying his body. He visibly responded by a change of facial expressions, body relaxation movements, and more natural breathing as a result of his surrogate "I" expressing his hidden hurt and anger. It was as if an emotion lawyer had suddenly come to his defense and was winning his case! Perry Mason comes to the rescue on a white horse! The emotional energy in the room changed dramatically as we cleared more and more of the man's anger.

I did round three by taking back the role of the rejecting woman, and again took the point of view of higher self, responsive, sensitive and understanding. I expressed to this man, who was again playing himself, how I heard his anger, respected it, and expressed that he was justified in feeling it. Relief became more and more evident in the man's demeanor. Within twenty or thirty minutes of this type of exchange, the blocked emotions surfaced, no longer toxifying this man's energy system. I cannot prove that is what happened, but that is how it appeared to us.

Within forty-eight hours, he was released from the hospital, and began to immediately improve. Six months later, he is still doing fine. In fact, he has been out seeking a new relationship.

> *All of us have a gift, a calling of our own whose exercise is high delight,*
> *even if we must sweat and suffer to meet its demands.*
> *That calling reaches out to find a real and useful place in the world,*
> *a task that is not wasted on pretense.*
> *If only that lifegiving impulse might be liberated and made the whole energy*
> *of our work, if only we were given the chance to be 'in' our work,*
> *with the full force of our personality, mind, body, heart and soul . . .*
> *What a power would be released into the world!*
> *A force more richly transformative than all the might of industrial technology.*
> Theodore Roszak

> *Fear comes from not trusting the process of life to be there for you.*
> *The next time you are frightened, say:*
> *"I trust in the process of life to take care of me."*
> Louise Hay from her book, *Heart Thoughts*

Preparation for Giving a Reiki Treatment

Your Role and Function as Healer

Your function as the healer is to allow yourself to be a channel for the creative universal life energy flowing through you. You accomplish this partly by placing yourself in an unconditional caring mode, a non-judgmental mode, an "I am here to serve" mode.

Your role as a healer is not to get involved in the curing process, but to be the liaison between the client and the creative force. Counseling may become necessary, as well as giving information about vitamins and health care, alerting them to their body language, encouraging thoughts and visualization, etc. These are all a part of the person who is facilitating the healing process. You may also encounter helping someone through a past life trauma that comes to the conscious surface during the healing. You may sense that some action in the client's life is taking a stressful toll on their body.

Tips for Healing

Thought forms that become crystallized in the physical body are the diseases that need healing. Counseling may be needed to connect to the source of thought forms that have produced the ailments. Being a practitioner of the healing arts, it is important to keep in mind at all times that it is the client's focus that has created this. The following may help facilitate the client's awareness:

1) The client must want to let go of the condition on the conscious level. The client may reject healing if they are not ready to let go on a subconscious level.
2) The practitioner can help the client recognize how the ailment or disease has served them, and why they may have manifested the ailment. Now that they have become aware of how they have held on to discomfort and allowed it to manifest in their body, they can let go of the limiting thoughts and actions.
3) Clients need to identify and become aware of the limiting thought patterns they are holding on to, accepting that this is an experience or lesson learned for their soul growth. Clients need to learn to take responsibility but not feel guilty over their patterns of thought. Healers need to accept that they are not physically or even emotionally responsible for another person's healing. Clients sometimes think they are responsible for another person's direction or life; there could be a karma bond between these people.
4) Crystallizations can be formed in relationships between child and parent, between male and female, and between friends. Limiting factors such as greed, dishonesty, manipulation, and control also can form stagnation in the physical body.
5) Counsel clients that all things are possible for those who believe. Know that hope and miracles are within each person's grasp.

Protection of Self

In spiritual healing, intent is of utmost importance. A prayer of protection or affirmation is used along with knowledge of the symbols. Visualize the Light of Christ within and outside of yourself, like being in a bubble of divine light. Use the power symbol on the front of body over the chakra areas.

Ground your feet into Mother Earth; she is the nurturing aspect of the universe. You can feel the energy moving from Mother Earth, upward through your body and out the crown chakra, then back to the heart center, and out the arms and hands for the healing channeling work. Having your feet rooted or grounded keeps your self in balance during the work. Always remember to see this energy flow within yourself, either from roots to crown or from crown to roots, so you don't block the flow within you.

Self-preservation is the first cosmic law. We are all spiritual beings, but we are still in the physical body, and bound by the physical laws of the universe. A prayer, symbols, and an affirmation enforce protection in your own fields of energy. This helps to prevent the empathic from taking the diseased condition onto self. It is not our right to interfere and take on another person's ailments. It is essential to go within self, and ask for the Light of Divine Creator to surround us and seal us in a protective shield, while working on someone else's energy field.

Spiritual Healing in Our Society

When you are doing any spiritual work in your community, caution needs to be exercised when doing hands-on bodywork.

1) Clarification is needed as to whether a client is under a doctor's care.

2) Part of the healing process is to involve the family as a unit (especially in extreme cases, such as cancer, AIDS, strokes, etc.).
3) It is valuable to have information available about local organizations where the client may benefit from group counseling, funding, local herbalists, naturopathic doctors, and health food stores. Books are helpful when doing counseling work, even having a list of stores, activities, etc.

Diseasement lives in our unforgiveness.

*Forgiving self and releasing the resentment will help dissolve crystallizations
we have built up in our body.
If internal changes are not made, the disease will either come back,
or we will create another diseasement.*

*Changing the "cell programming" in our bodies takes more than
an occasional prayer. It takes determined changes in our attitudes.
It is also necessary to understand the body/mind/soul connection,
For what we think and what we eat work together in our bodily forms.*

Scanning Client or Self

Once you have received initiation and attunement into Reiki, and you are starting a treatment for a client, you will find the attunement process has activated and increased your intuition and psychic energy.

After protecting yourself, take your hands (about three to four inches above body) and, starting at the top of the head, work slowly down the body and over the chakra centers. Any distortions of energy, hot or cold spots, tingling, warm fuzzies, or having your eyes guide you to the spot where the energy field is moving irregularly, can show you where Reiki energy is needed.

The more you use the Reiki energy, the quicker you will respond to any distortions in the client's fields of energy. Do the treatment. The Reiki will heal the auric fields of energy and the physical body connected to the chakras.

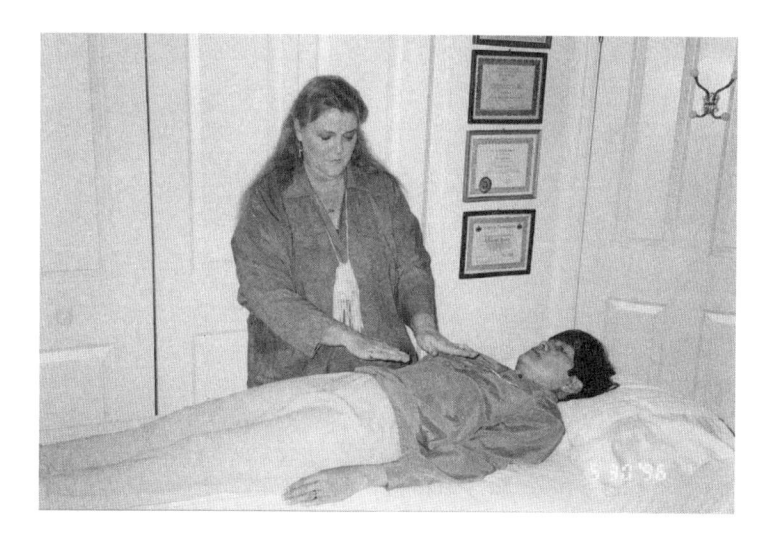

Note: Scanning is the same for you. Tuning in to your own body brings you into an awareness, or consciousness, of your body talking to you. Be as non-judgmental with yourself as you are with your client. Allow your self to love you.

Changes

An individual power hand was chosen at the time of traditional attunements. During these past years, many nontraditional masters have chosen to empower both hands at the time of attunement.

Radiating or Beaming Energy

To beam or to radiate energy before and after a treatment helps set the mode for the healing. What is radiating or beaming?

First protect yourself, then get centered. Focus your consciousness.
Hold your hands up and allow the universal life force energy to flow through you.
Allow the molecules, atoms, and electrons of light to flow forth.
Project and visualize in a laser stream from your channeled being to the client.

Keep your mind on the flow of Reiki vital force energy. Stay centered and focused. If your mind strays, bring the mind back to that altered state, which allows the pathways of Reiki to flow. Having your spiritual Reiki guides work with you, as you channel, strengthens the flow of energy.

We have used beaming and radiating in rooms of the house, on rice, my art studio, automobiles, an animal that has died alongside the road, my flower and vegetable garden, the medicine wheel, sending distance healing from my prayer list, sending traveling mercies, my computer, even when mailing packages. The opportunities for using Reiki are endless; it depends upon how creative you are!

See illustration, below.

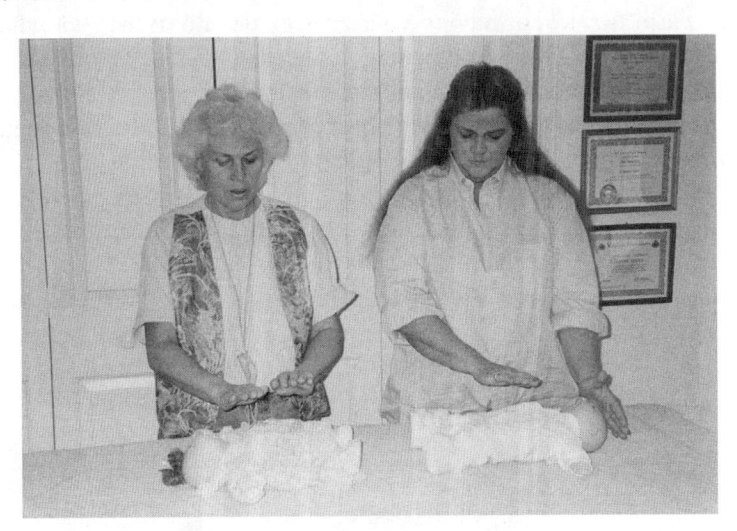

Three-Point Treatment

If there is a small amount of time and space in which to work or help someone in need, e.g., on a hospital visit, the three-point treatment can be beneficial. Remember to ground yourself, protect yourself, and set your intention. This can all be done in a matter of moments.

1) Place one hand on top of head (crown chakra area) where miracles work, the mind center
2) Place the other hand on the navel area (solar plexus/sacral area), the power or personal issue center
3) When finished, ground by touching their feet and, holding them briefly, sense your connection has been made
4) Close up

This technique can be used with the client lying either on his back or his stomach, or even sitting in a chair. You can either physically touch the body or hold your hands two to four inches from it. Have the client visualize peace, and move the energy (the atoms) throughout the body, from the head to the feet, and out. Have the client address the area in his body that is feeling distressed, which will activate the healing in a shorter amount of time.

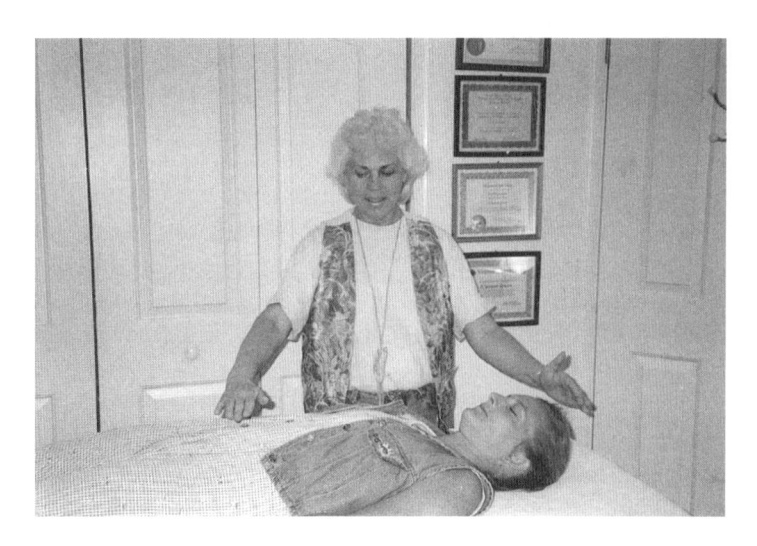

Group Healing

Any group of like-minded individuals can do Reiki healing, as long as the intention is focused by the group. Examples: Goddess or new moon groups, healing groups, medicine wheel ceremonies, healing and prayer groups, Reiki open house groups, and so forth.

The following are some methods commonly used:

Intention is always set, for the best interest and highest good of the person receiving.

1) One at the head/crown for sending the energy, one at feet for grounding, one or two working the middle section of body then moving energy down the legs for grounding. We use this method for our Reiki open house meetings in a mini-treatment agenda.
2) Form a circle of people and beam the Reiki energy into the circle. Each one can send in names of those that need healing at that moment, or in a future event.
3) The inside/middle/center of the circle is the vortex or spiral point; you could also put slips of paper in the middle of the circle with your name and request. We then burn these papers to send the vapors of thought into the universe; a fireplace will do, intention is the key. The new moon is a time for a new beginning.
4) Remember, when two or more are gathered together, there is an endless source of divine energy.

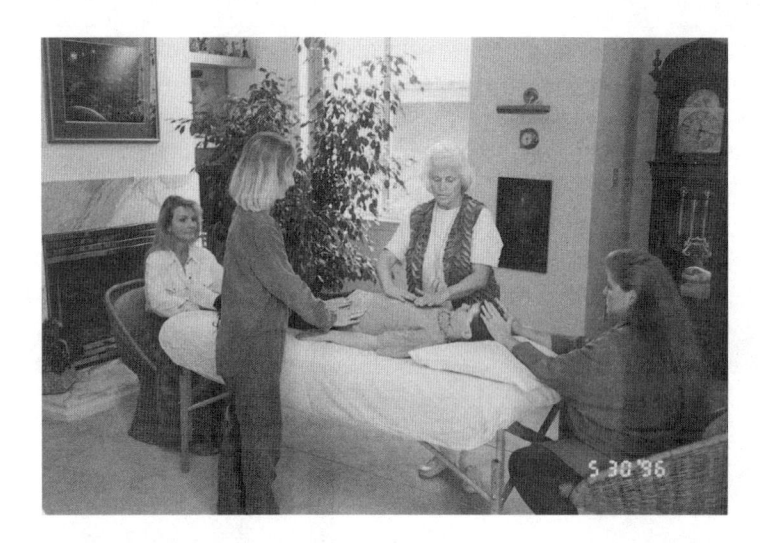

Reiki Team Facilitated Treatment
by Reiki Team

Reiki today is coming to a new age of use. There is no wrong way to use Reiki when the intention is for the best interest and highest good of the client. Setting your intention is the key.

Reiki helps unite people in a cause for greater consciousness and well-being. Reiki is not just for the chronically ill client, though it does work if given enough time. However, we are a society that wants immediate results. Reiki is also for maintenance of well-being. Healing is a daily process, as ongoing as cellular replenishment.

We have been devoting time for the past several years to what we call "team" or "group" work, referred to as "Reiki open house" or "Reiki clinics." We have enjoyed working on each other for maintenance, but we also have given mini-treatments for those that are new to Reiki, or in need of a Reiki healing. Several of us get together with one objective in mind, that of making another individual feel better. It is a time of laughter, sharing, and caring.

When we have three people, we use the three-point treatment:

One person is at the head (crown), one at the navel area (solar plexus/sacral), and one at the feet. We have learned to speak nonverbally and have learned when to move on in the work. When there are only two people, one starts at the crown area, and one at the navel area/midsection; both gradually work down the body.

Our teamwork has evolved in different aspects. Some individuals may have a strong leaning towards working with crystals. The Native American belief system uses feathers, crystals, herbs, rattles, etc. Others may be in tune with the angelic kingdom, or the healing pulses (vibrational), or toning (sound). Ascended masters channel either messages or feelings. All healing with divine intention is using the universal life force energy.

Our Reiki work goes along with some of the ancient rituals and customs that seem to have incorporated aspects of Reiki into their ceremonies. When Native American medicine men performed a healing, they were working for the good of the whole, as well as that of the individual. The medicine man may not have been using the exact methods that are used in Reiki today, but the format and results were the same. Some healing has been done with several people participating, lending their thoughts and visions to the healing work, with the central conductor being the medicine man. The helpers would often wear masks, had feathers for smudging, and used other tools for specific healing purposes. The medicine man would often perform his healing with a rattle (vibrational) or feather (ruffling) or both. The group focused on healing the individual in need. They were indeed working for One Planet ♥ One People. Church healing groups, often called prayer circles, also focused their intention for the best interest of the person needing help.

We have even changed our attitude about traditional handshakes. Moving into a new dimension, we sense the touching of spirit and not just a social greeting like a handshake. Thus, hugs are given to new unknown people. The traditional handshake seems to be confined to strictly business.

Our special Reiki hug is in another section of this manual: a way of giving a hug without interrupting another person's energy field. No slaphappy hugs for us!

Procedures for Treatments

Reiki I and using the Reiki II Symbols

1) Room preparation—before starting the treatment, either place the Power Symbol to the four directions with your hand, or visualize it filling all areas of the treatment room. Burning incense or sage helps neutralize the energies. Say a prayer, asking your spiritual guides, angels, and the healing forces of the universe to work with you and with the client, for their best interest and highest good, and to set your intention.

2) Practitioner—Be sure your hands are washed up to the elbows, before and after treatment, as a neutralizer. Prepare yourself by placing the Power Symbol over the front of your body and the chakra areas and in the palm of each hand.

3) Talk to the client and have them fill out an information form, or verbally ask them about their physical symptoms. I am used to this procedure because I am also a certified massage therapist. This gives you a basis from which to start. A good connection between the practitioner and the client brings about a better focus for the energy to work.

4) You can help direct the client's healing process intention. Have them picture for themselves what their problem looks like and smells like, its shape, and what its texture is. Saying a prayer of thankfulness together helps open the client's field of energy for the Reiki to flow.

5) Before scanning the body, visualize the Power and Emotional/Mental Symbols over the client's body. Then gently scan down the body. You will usually sense, or feel (sometimes heat or cold), areas where there is a need for healing. During treatment you will then remove any stagnant or yucky areas of energy, and then fill up these voids immediately with light energy, or else you will be leaving holes in the auric field.

6) Do the treatment. (If you need clarification for some point of reference, see following pages.)

7) Beaming Reiki energy from a distance at the end of a treatment helps facilitate a finalization. It also allows the client's consciousness to realize the treatment is over.

8) After the treatment, always close the body's rhythm and vibrational frequencies, the fields of energy. Use closing procedure of ruffling, smoothing, and infinity symbols. Starting above the head, work from the side and down the body and past the feet. Shake your hands, letting go of the energy you may have collected while working. Think a conscious thought of disconnecting from their energy field.

9) After the client has left, visualize the Power Symbol again on the walls and in the center of the room. This is done with the intention of clearing energies from that area. Burning incense or sage, or spraying crystallized water, will reactivate and reenergize the room.

10) Thank any spiritual guidance or angelic ones for helping with the healing process.

Body Treatment Guidelines

Source: Hawayo Takata's lineage to all Reiki masters.
1) Always begin the treatment with a complete basic treatment, working each area until the need is met. (This means using all hand positions.)
2) Then go to the affected part that is outside the basic treatment area.
3) See the following for specified problems.

Specific Treatments for the Head

Sinuses, Postnasal Drip:
Basic treatment. Then work on the head.

High Blood Pressure:
Basic treatment. Then treat the hard and brittle glands on the side of the neck, which also helps the heart.

Voice:
Basic treatment. Then treat the larynx, using the whole hand.

Mouth:
Toothaches (cavity) — First treat the cheek and jaw. If client is a child, treatment gives relief. Adult treatment relieves pain temporarily.

Earache, Draining, Hearing:
Basic treatment. Then work on the head.

Canker Sores, Coated Tongue, Cancer of the Mouth:
Basic treatment. Then treat the bottom of the feet.

Headache:
Basic treatment. Then treat ovary/uterus or prostate area.
Headache from cold: treat head, throat and bronchi.

Migraine:
Basic treatment. Then especially areas of ovaries/uterus or prostate.
Then treat the head, thyroid, liver, and endocrine system.

Goiter:
Basic treatment. Then throat, ovaries or prostate, if this is not acute.
Palpitations may be a symptom of endocrine imbalance.

Specific Treatments for the Front of the Body

Colds, Fever, Heart:
Basic treatment. Then treat above the diaphragm to the heart area.

Diabetes:
Basic treatment. Then treat pancreas.
Client must adhere to diet, have blood tests, and take only the needed amount of insulin.
When client's insulin need declines to three units, check with doctor. Continue treatments until stabilized.

Ulcers, Stomach Acid, Cancer:
Basic treatment. Then make stomach alkaline. No fried, greasy or harsh foods.
See chapter 3 for acid/alkaline food listing.

Gallbladder, Nausea, Balance:
Basic treatment. Treat above and behind the ears. Gallstones can be removed by constant treatment.
From reaction to climax may be four to six consecutive treatments weekly, then taper off to three times a week.

Heart Condition:
Basic treatment to front only. Then the heart area.
Note: Do not turn client with heart problems on their stomach.

Pleurisy:
Basic treatment. Then you can turn the client back over to treat the front lung area.

Pneumonia:
Treat front only. Treat entire lung area by putting hands under the back until crisis is over, and temperature breaks. If client sweats, give as much warm lemonade or ascorbic acid as possible. Gently towel toward the heart to remove sweat. Do not put client with pneumonia on stomach.

Childbirth:
Frequent basic treatments all during pregnancy (three times a week) helps prepare for a painless childbirth.
Treat abdominal area for mounting delivery pain. Treat coccyx and rectal area for birth preparation.

Cancer:
Complete basic treatment. Then work especially with the lymphatic glands on the side of the body.
Then again back to affected area, daily for at least a month.

Breast Lumps:
Complete basic treatment. Work with female organs, ovaries, uterus, thyroid, lump, affected area, and then breast area. Results in toxins cleansed, organs revitalized, and lump beginning to dissolve.

Specific Treatments for the Back and Feet

Arthritis:
Basic treatment. Then work with abdomen. When organs are balanced and vitalized, change begins in the kidney area. Also a change of diet is needed.

Epilepsy (An electrical storm in the brain):
Give complete basic treatment.
Then treat head, front and back *daily* for one month. With improvement, taper off gradually to one treatment per week until well. Healing will take six months to a year.

Mental and Emotional Stress:
Basic treatment. Then treat head first, then move to the first position, front and left side of back.

Stomach Acid, Gallbladder, Liver:
Basic treatment. Then treat second position, and right side of back.

Backaches:
Basic treatment. Then on back, down the spine, and kidney area.

Lower Back Pain:
Basic treatment. Then lower spine, prostate, and rectum.

Hemorrhoids:
Basic treatment. Then lower back, prostate, and rectum.

Babies:
Treat the bottom of the feet. A sharp cry means stomach pain. Treat twenty to forty minutes.

Leukemia:
Complete basic treatment. Then work with spleen and organs of the body.

Sties:
Complete basic treatment. Work with liver and kidneys to release built-up toxins.

*The body, like everything else in life,
is a mirror of your inner thoughts and beliefs.
Every cell responds to every single thought
you think and every word you speak.*
— Louise Hay from her book, *Heart Thoughts*

Reiki—Hand Positions

Front of Body/Emotional

When working with the front of the body, be aware that this is the emotional part of the physical body. A highly concentrated form of energy consciousness, which stimulates a pattern of organic responses in the body, can be felt physically and experienced mentally. Emotion is the fundamental manifestation of the vital life force. It cannot be seen or touched, but is felt in a powerful form.

Back of Body/Physical

When working with the back of the body, this is the physical will. This is the mind-governing principle that activates the atoms into manifestations of all degrees in the universe. The essential attribute of the mind acts as a lever on matter, and the consciousness makes the action occur. This in turn affects the aspects of the body's energy fields and chakra system. Again, the differences in these energy wheels depend upon the client's thoughts and will interact with the connecting organs of the body.

Directions

Wash hands up to your elbows, before you begin doing healing work and after you finish the healing work. Release all negativity, disqualified energies, and/or turmoil within. Sense your connection to Divine Source and your spiritual guides. Remember that you are the channel. The Reiki vital force energy will be directed to where it is needed. Ground yourself and trust.

Example

The body's organs supplied by the chakra (energy wheel) will not get what is needed or can get too much focused energy, depending upon what the mind is focused on. If a lack or stress continues over a long period of time, this will start interacting with the other chakras and their body organs and functions. Ultimately, this will start the disease and breakdown of the immune systems.

Below: Basic Method and Alternate Method of Hand Positions for giving treatment.

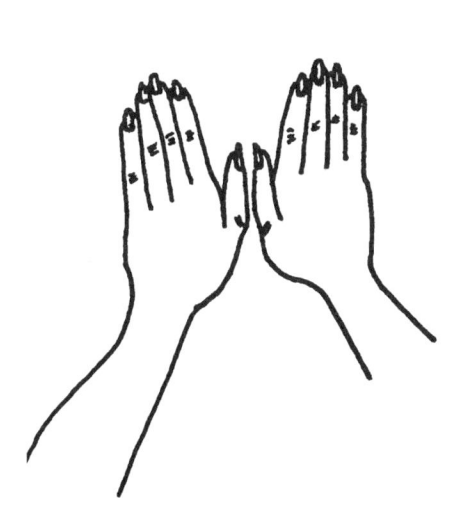

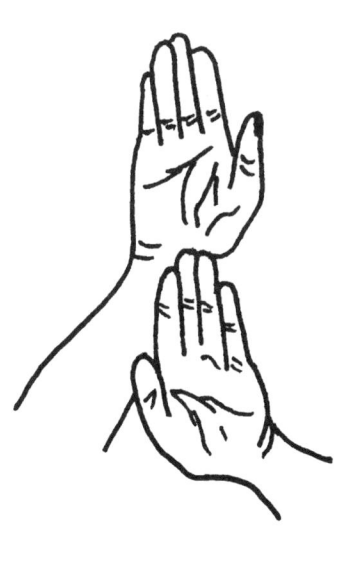

Reiki Hand Positions—Front of Body

With the client lying on his back:

Position 1
Head—with the base of your hands together, place them on the crown chakra (top of head) with your fingers facing toward the feet.

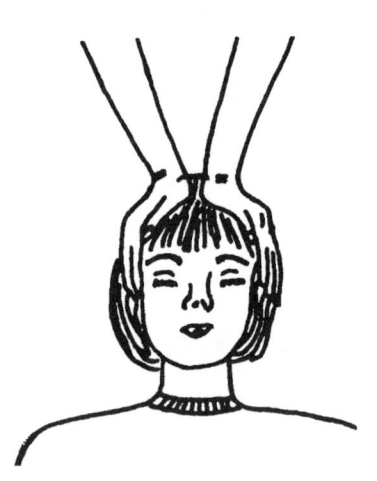

Position 2
Eyes—hands cupped together, thumbs touching, gently place your hands over the eyes with the fingertips resting on the cheeks, fingers pointing toward the feet.

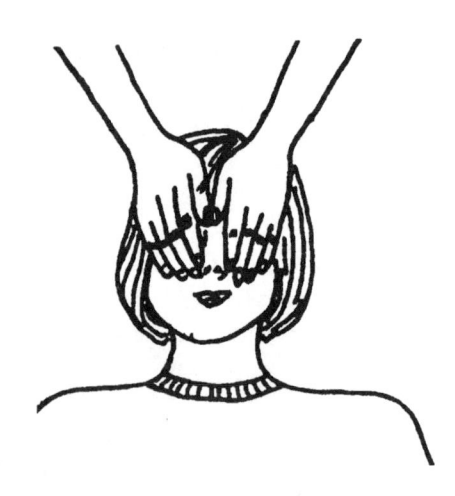

Position 3
Ears—hands cupped, place individually over ears with fingertips pointing toward the feet.

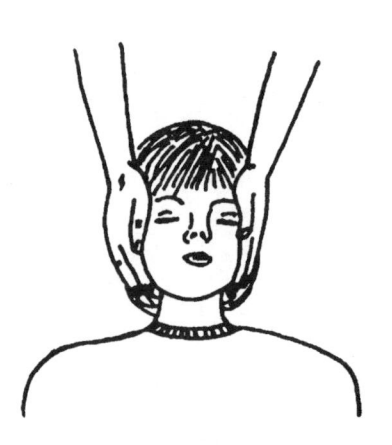

Position 4
Base of Skull—slowing turn head to side and place one hand under base of skull, then gently roll head to side to place other hand under base of skull, both hands touching, pointing towards the feet.

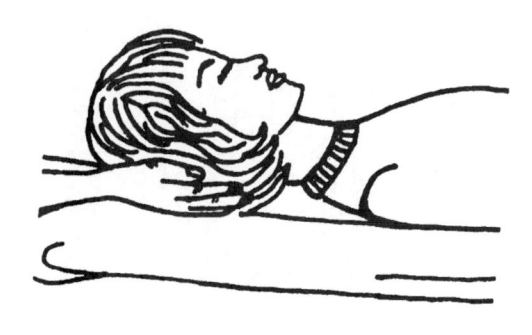

Position 5
Shoulders—place hands on top of the shoulders, with the fingertips over clavicle and pointing towards the feet.

Position 6
Throat / Thymus area—left hand under neck, right hand on throat/thymus area.

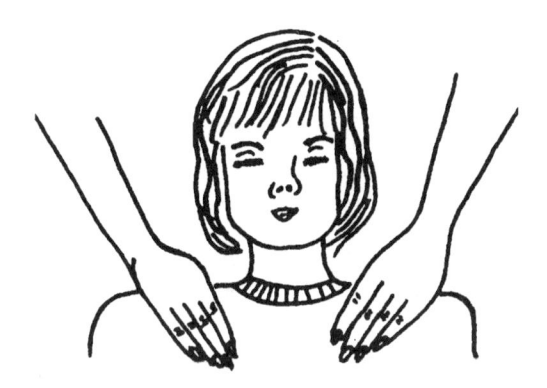

Position 7
Heart—T-position, or hands side by side, over heart area.
(T-position recommended when working on the female body.)

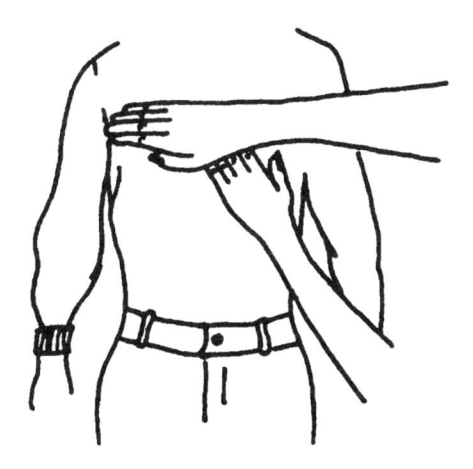

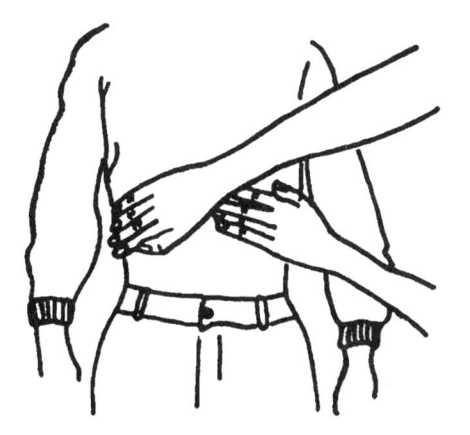

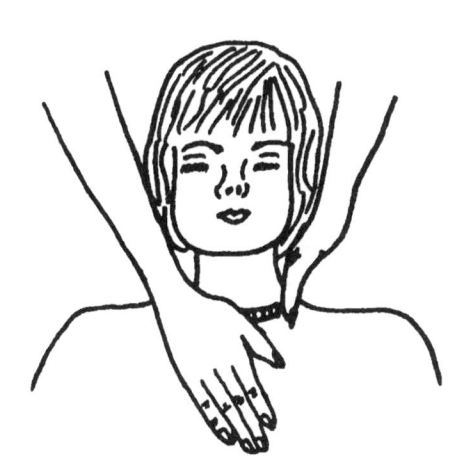

Position 8a
Abdomen—(8a, 8b, 8c) place hands side by side moving across midsection of the body, starting below the breasts and moving to the hip area.
(Major emotions are held in this area.)

Position 8b

Position 8c

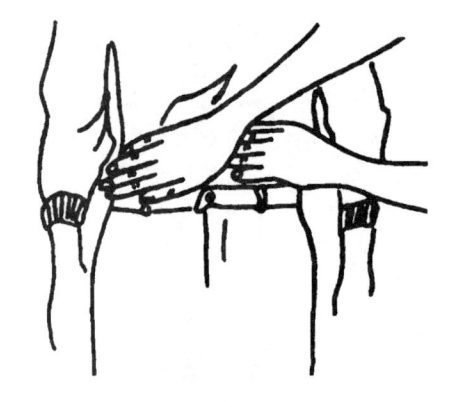

Position 9
Knees—do one knee at a time, one hand on top, one hand underneath. (Legs are going forward in life; this area holds past life energy and may need lots of clearing.) If energy field feels blocked, ruffle from the hip area down and out the feet to clear.

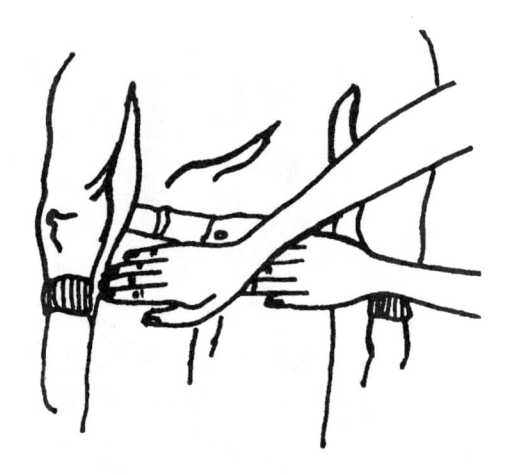

Position 10
Feet /Ankle area—place hands on ankles, then feet.
Ground the client and yourself, put energy field back together. This is the closure procedure.

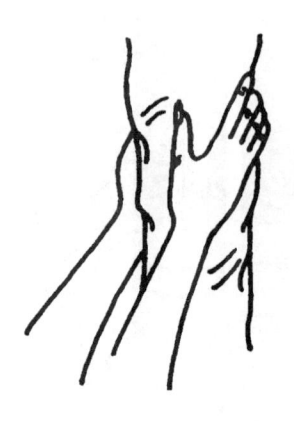

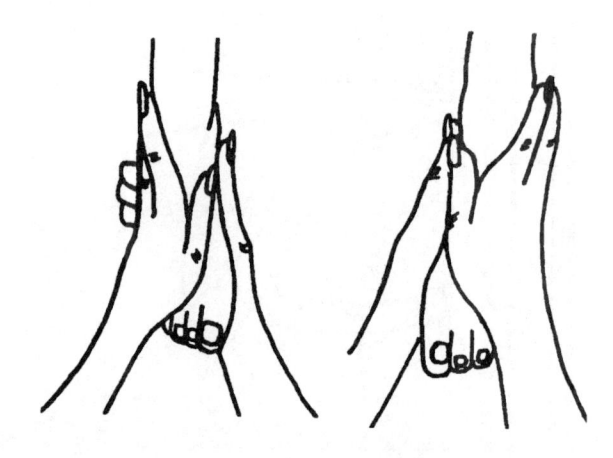

Reiki Hand Positions—Back of Body

With client lying on his stomach:

Position 11
Top of Shoulders—while standing looking towards feet, place hands on top of shoulders, fingertips toward feet.

Position 12
Back: Upper/Middle/Lower—position hands side by side (or alternate style) moving across the body, from upper back area to hip area.

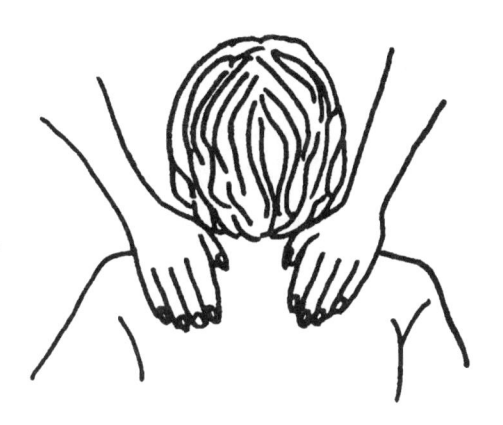

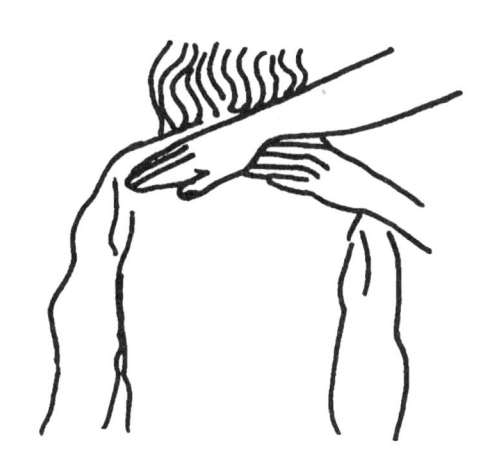

Position 12b

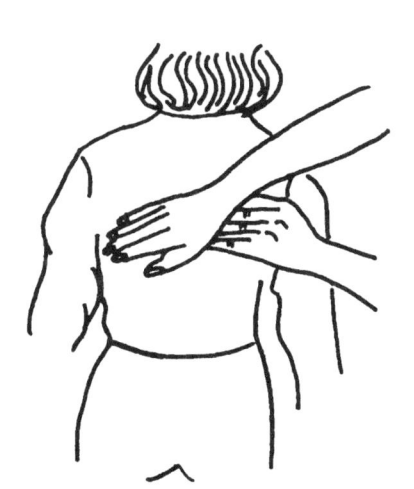

Position 12c

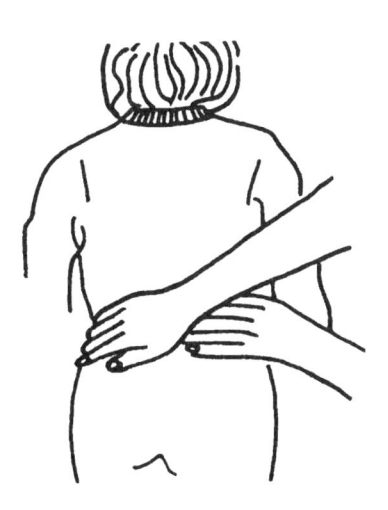

Position 13
Leg Areas—place hands on back of knees, pulling the energy down and off the end of foot. Position the hands on one knee at a time, one hand on top and one hand underneath. Legs are going forward in life, this area holds energy from past lifetimes and will sometimes need a lot of clearing.

Position 14
Feet—place hands on feet. When finished energizing that area, ground the client. Remember to ground yourself at the same time, so you do not hold their energy in your energy fields.

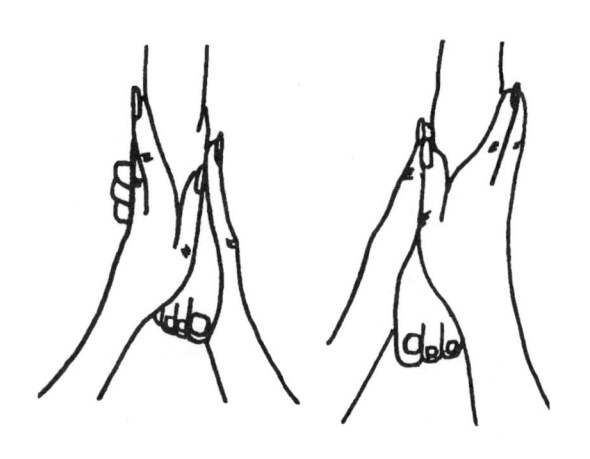

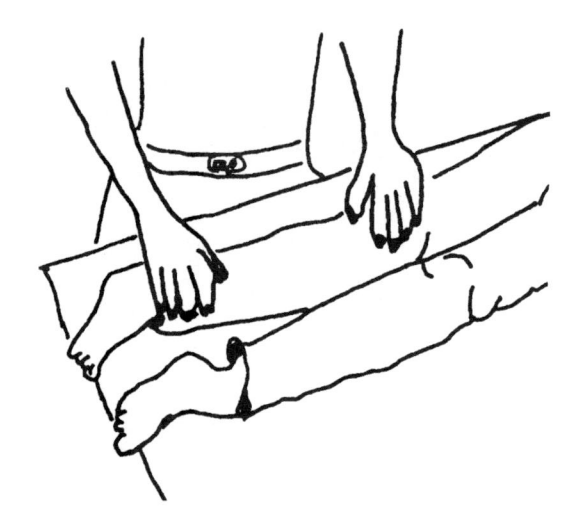

Balancing—hold one hand on knee and one on ankle on each leg, for clearing and balancing.

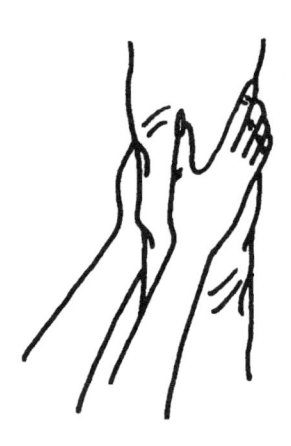

Closure:
Gently ruffle energy down the body from head to feet, three times, then use infinity symbol (like a figure 8) over chakras, or alternate method, woven over entire body. See diagram, next page.

Self-Attunement: one hand over top of head (crown chakra) and the other hand moving downward over the other chakras (wheels of energy). See diagram of energy systems.

Self-Polarity Balance: one hand on top of head (crown chakra) and the other hand on lower back, then reverse positions.

Center in Divine Source and ground yourself. Your personal emotional feelings and/or moods can affect the outcome of the healing.

Closure Method for Energy Field

Gently ruffle with your hands in a movement down the whole body; this pulls the energy back into the client's energy field. Starting at head and working towards feet, close with infinity symbols across the body, or infinity symbol over whole body.

I do this, not only on the front of the body, but on the back of the body, when I am doing healing work or massage work. This is helpful for anyone that works with energy.

Closure

We have found the following to be extremely beneficial:

a) Gently smooth the energy field from above the top of head down to the feet with a ruffling effect.

b) Starting at the top of the head and working down to the feet, make large circular motions. Bring the energy in towards the spine. Work slowly and finish at the feet in two or three circular motions, shaking your hands when finished as a cut off. Do this three times.

c) Using the figure 8 (infinity, yin/yang, male/female) and starting above the head, work sideways across the body's chakras, down to below the feet. Visualize the weaving of a silver and gold thread as you do this, weaving the body's auric field back together. At the end of treatment, it is useful to use the distance healing symbol, which makes a conscious disconnection from working with someone else's energy field.

d) Be sure to wash your hands from elbows down when finished to pull off any clinging energy. Washing helps to neutralize the energy you have been working with.

Reiki Closure Technique

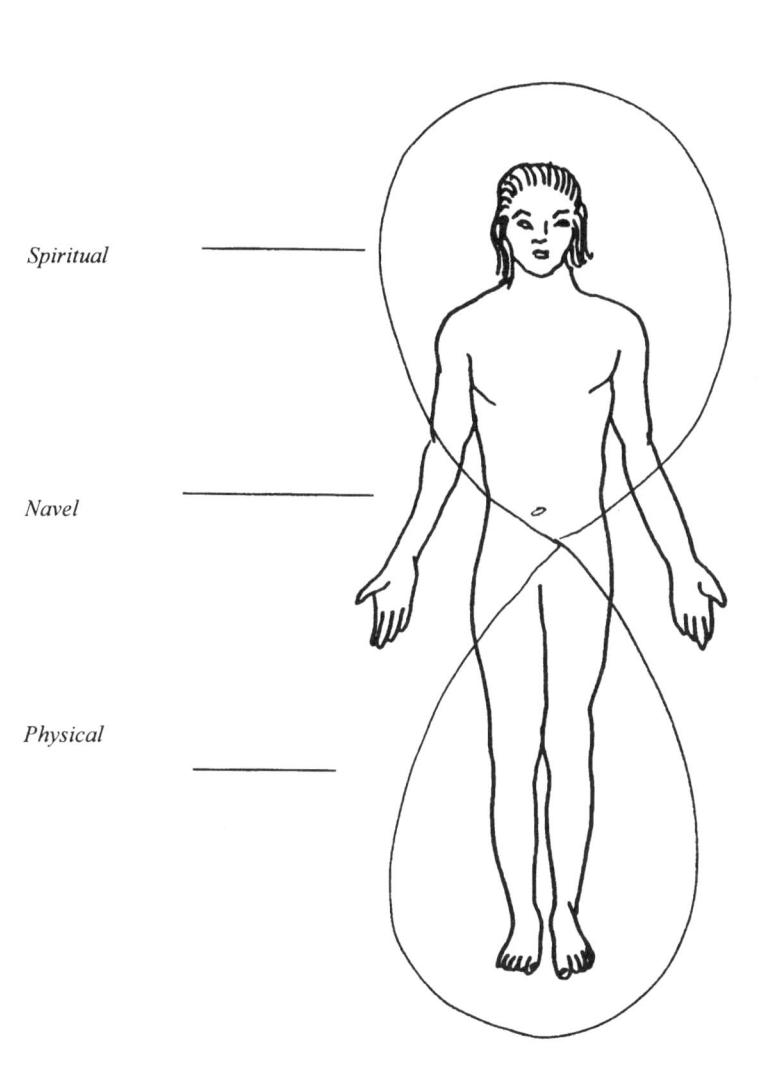

Spiritual

Navel

Physical

Initiation into the Power of Reiki

Symbols

Symbols influence your body's energy and physical being on mental, emotional, physical and spiritual levels. The symbols given through Reiki are the very essence (the key or ki) of, and a reminder of, the divine power within each person that becomes activated upon receipt of an attunement. Three symbols are taught in the Reiki II class: the power symbol (ChoKuRei), the mental/emotional symbol (SeiHeKi), and the distant healing symbol (HonShaZeShoNen).

The symbols can be used in many different aspects of your life. Examples include: sending healing, empowering yourself, your career/home surroundings, meditation, plants, animals, children, peacefulness, protection, harmony, balance, people who are ill and living a distance away, and almost anything else you can think of. Symbols directed with proper intention can be used for anything, whether it is to focus healing energy on your foods, medicines, vitamins, drinking water, pets, garden, home, automobile, or more.

When working with the Reiki energy and the symbols as taught in Reiki II, remember it is the intention and integrity, plus Reiki guidance working with you to provide for any shortcomings you may feel. Reiki is healing. The more you work with this energy, the more you become aware of Reiki guidance. These guides will help you make the transition from feeling insecure to feeling joy and wonder at the results. All you need to do is have intention of what is best for the client or the situation, not what is best for you.

Misusing Reiki

Symbols are to be used with integrity and intention or you will put into motion a cause and effect sequence. Any misuse of Reiki (such as in anger or vengeance against another person) can cause the energy flow to stop. I once heard about someone who was very angry with another person and subsequently lost her healing energy. She actually thought the teacher had taken Reiki away from her. But she had not looked into her own heart to see the intention. This little story shows that Reiki cannot be misused, as the spiritual guides will not allow it and it goes against the universal laws.

Reiki universal life force energy from the One, our Divine Creator, cannot be misused. It is energy of light, to enhance our lives and all of our surroundings. The rediscovery of Reiki influence has come at this time to help our Earth people return to a spiritual nature. The Reiki energy is available for every living being. You could say that it is our first step in the evolving sequences coming to Mother Earth. The simplicity of Reiki is there, to help development and evolution for the Earth changes coming upon us.

Symbols and Permission to Help Others

The symbols were given to mankind to be of benefit to everyone. It is also important to have the right intention, and to realize that healing is given only with permission. When working with a Reiki group of people, if someone gets on the table for their Reiki turn, then they have given you permission to work on them. If a distant family member or friend requires healing, you can ask them on an astral level about sending healing. This is done with the idea that they are ready or open to receive. If they are not open to receive, you request that the healing energy be directed towards the healing of Mother Earth, or someone else who needs it, which is what we call recycled Reiki energy. Now, that is a great environmental plus!

When sending healing energy I usually say, "for their best interest and highest good," not knowing what that may be for the individual person. This is done when healing has been requested. Do not take it upon yourself to just do Reiki on someone, because you think they need it. That is going against their free will. You really do not want to violate someone else's free will—that goes against the ethics of healing. If driving down the highway and you see someone who needs healing energy, give them healing for the best interest and highest good of the situation. Since you do not know if they are open to receiving, always ask that the energy be given to someone that needs it if they do not want it.

Attunement or Initiation

The process of receiving an attunement is through the scientific language of symbols, and comes from ancient Tibet, India, Egypt, and Assyria. Initiation was considered designated to a special few, those with characters worthy of this knowledge. Determined by their akashic records, the rite of passage was set up in steps, to help the person eliminate present beliefs from past karma and lifetimes.

Reiki Initiation

A sacred ceremony that symbolizes the beginning of a spiritual life, a Reiki initiation is without interference by anyone else's personal religion. The Reiki attunement for an individual is powerful. The attunements open gateways to wholeness and the sense of totality. The attunement process is guided by the divine consciousness (Rei), and is directed according to each student's needs. It is the rising up of energy and going beyond the limits of man's thought. The attunement process opens the chakras, moving the kundalini up the spine to create that special link between the one receiving and the universal life force energy. The attunement is handed down from the Reiki Master to the student in a lineage process.

Experiences by students include warm fuzzy feelings of being wrapped in a blanket of energy, feeling very connected to divine consciousness, tears of wholeness, and a sense of belonging. They also experience the opening of the third eye, healing, acute intuitive awareness, personal messages, past life experiences, a sense of being part of the whole, one's purpose and life's work coming into consciousness, and, for some, the opening of their visionary senses. Creator has given this spiritual attunement process to mankind as a lifetime gift.

The attunement cannot be taken away from you. However, you do have a commitment to follow the universal/spiritual laws of the One. The process of receiving an attunement is based on truth and mysticism. How much the attunement benefits you is partly based upon your being open to receive. Doubt, fear, or your limitations could affect the sacred ceremony for you. Believe in yourself, believe you are worthwhile enough to receive, and know that truth is Oneness, but the paths are many. By being open to the belief system of Reiki, a connection to divine consciousness will be made, regardless of whether you can put a label on the event!

Reiki Ceremony

I really like a sacred space for the students receiving their initiation. I usually set up candles, crystals, sage, or incense. I have found that in larger classes, if I give directions first, doing the attunements doesn't take that much time. For example, I tell them to remove any jewelry or watches and how to hold their hands during the ceremony, and I have each student prepared to come into the room as soon as one leaves. In Reiki I, the chakras are opening and connecting to the Hara line. This starts a physical cleansing. Many students have mystical experiences, and because of this, I have never liked giving attunements in a "row of chairs" style. The traditional method for Reiki I is four attunements. I have discovered that with each new attunement the student opens up more, expanding the kundalini and the Hara Line. Many non-traditional teachers place symbols in both hands for all three degrees.

In Reiki II, the attunements continue to expand the fields of energy, opening the mystical and divine empowerment to Creator. This attunement power continues, sometimes for several weeks, touching in with the mental and emotional bodies. Some students go through a physical detoxification, and a processing of emotional/mental levels after the attunement. In Reiki III, there will be more spiritual manifesting than physical. The absolute empowerment of the attunement touches into and works directly with the body's spiritual essence, and bestows awakening and awareness at new levels. Attunements can be given to anyone dying, seriously ill, or undergoing surgery, and also to family, infants, and pets. Attunement acts as a major healing, and, if necessary, distant healing can be done in the astral plane.

Power Symbol (ChoKuRei)

The spiral motion of the power symbol represents the seven chakras, and charges and assists the flow of Reiki energy. This spiral also represents the goddess energy or feminine energy coming into balance with mankind during this time on our planet. The feminine energy, previously lacking or out of balance on Mother Earth, is now in a more balanced atmosphere with all the Reiki training existing throughout the world.

This symbol is used to focus and increase the energy around the client while giving a treatment. It is also used to clear rooms before any spiritual seminars or bodywork. Using this symbol enhances and helps create a sacred energized space to work. Using the power symbol can also boost the energy around newly planted trees, protect your mode of transportation, pets, home, etc. You can direct energy into the divine consciousness, or use it for specified areas of healing, on such things as rain forests, famine, weather disasters, war, troubled parts of the globe, etc.

This symbol is used as a protector on the levels of physical and verbal protection, as well as emotional and spiritual protection. Some other uses include blessing your food, cleansing your water before drinking, and blessing your clients before a treatment. You can also send this power symbol forward in time. For example, you can beam focused energy for distant healing, future appointments, and even past events. You can protect your property, your belongings, your meditation area, your garden, or yourself driving down the highway. You can send this powerful energy symbol towards any accidents along the road, traffic jams, etc. Do this with a blessing of unconditional love and intention of good will.

The power symbol represents focused energy or the Pathway of Light; it is a decree of unconditional love towards all Earth people.

The spiral form of this symbol has been used down through the ages by many peoples. The spiral is a form of a circle which has no beginning and no end, always continuing, ever flowing. Circles are seen in our everyday life. For instance, Stonehenge, the Crop Circles in England, Easter Island, Peruvian sacred sites, the traditional churches using a circle for prayer, the Wiccans, and our Native American ancestors' Medicine Wheel. Circles are a part of many celebrated sacred ceremonies.

Direction of Symbol

Since the initiation of the original twenty-two masters, explanations have been brought forward that these Reiki masters received different symbols. Were the symbols given differently, or was it the perception of the receiver? I would like to add these thoughts. As in all things, changes come about because man likes to intellectualize. The key is intention.

So you have some choices to make regarding the direction of the spiral.
1)   In speaking with one of my masters, initiated by Phyllis Furumoto, I discovered that the power symbol was taught to her in a counterclockwise direction (traditional way). She teaches that the symbol needs no directed direction, it just is. It is the intention that gives direction, not the trying to "think it through."
2)   Wiccan thoughts on this symbol for the Northern Hampshire are: Counterclockwise represents decreasing and dispersing energy and Clockwise represents increasing and/or invoking energy.

One last thought on this. These symbols worked when used by the ancients, they worked when rediscovered by Dr. Usui, and they work now. Remember Reiki in all intent and purpose was an opportunity for mankind to bring about healing. Reiki is very simple, and does not need to get complicated as man seems to do with most information.

Mental and Emotional Symbol (SeiHeKi)

This symbol is used to repattern the brain, to balance the right and left sides of the brain. It awakens and purifies, activates the kundalini, the source within. It is God/Creator and Man/Woman coming together in harmony and peace, healing the mind/body connection and the subconscious mind. It is used in emotional or mental situations. Examples include: Psychic counseling, minister's work, fear, anger, depression, sadness, relationships, and suicides. This symbol works out of the areas of the Heart/emotional chakra, and the Solar Plexus/mental chakra, jointly working together for the harmony and balance of the client.

This symbol is helpful in locating a misplaced item, working with the subconscious mind to bring to the surface what is needed, for meditating and doing affirmations, and when working in a difficult career situation. This symbol will help balance out the energies in these situations.

Using this Symbol

The symbol can also be used for addictions such as smoking, eating disorders, drinking, or drugs. Use to clear any areas, body's blockage, house, auric field, hospital room, or questionable foods. For changing long-term goals such as smoking or weight loss, write down the unwanted habit, your name, along with a healthy result, and then add the symbol onto the paper. Keep this in a place where you can send energy on a daily basis for twenty-one days. You can put it under a crystal or in your medicine bag. After the twenty-one days burn the paper, and send the energy out to the universe for total healing and release. The best release time would be three days before a New Moon cycle; you can check your calendar for dates.

Disease of Emotions

Disease of the body and painful emotions work hand in hand. Either a present emotional state, or a past emotional state or trauma can cause the disease. The disease itself brings to the forefront the mindset, or patterning of the emotional mind, which is why this symbol is called the mental and emotional symbol. When pain remains within the self with no release, it manifests into a physical illness. The level or the effect of our emotions greatly depends upon our physical constitution. In other words, what may cause harm to one person may not bother another. This is because of our family upbringing, our tolerance in situations, our ability to ground ourselves and to release our emotions at some level, our spiritual understanding, and so on.

Being sensitive, I have discovered I don't have a tolerance for watching television. I have empathy for abused victims or the injustices in our governmental system. When we understand our body/mind/soul connection better, we can make the necessary adjustments in how this effects our life.

Animals and Emotions

Animals feel and experience emotions the same as humans do. They manifest disease as a way of handling emotions they cannot otherwise release. They do not have the same level of understanding and control as we do. You may notice a dog, cat or other pet that is particularly bonded to their human person. Pets may actually manifest their owner's disease or emotion, thereby they end up sacrificing themselves in the process. Our pets have taken upon themselves the job of clearing "their human people," and "clearing a house" from disturbing energy. I know this to be true. One case was where a man coughed all the time. Soon only the cat was ill, and the man's coughing stopped. Unfortunately, the cat died. Another case was where a dog was jumpy and nervous, with signs of parasites and fungus. The owner worked in a hospital and was unaware of the bacteria and fungus that was carried into the house. A good habit is to take your shoes off at the entry door. Bacteria get on our shoes from wherever we have walked.

You are in a state of grace when using this symbol
Recovering and regaining your sense of pure spirit.

The Spiritual Warrior

Distant Healing Symbol (HonShaZeShoNen)

This symbol is representative of The Magic Wand, The Blessing.

This symbol is best known for absentee healing, part of which is the healing of past karmic problems, life's set patterns, and repeating relationship issues. Absentee healing is the sending out of Reiki universal life force energy to those at a distance. This symbol is a blessing and represents the Power of the Universe, Bestowing the Truth, and transcends time and space. It is an entrance into the Akashic records, and therefore important in healing karmic issues, goals, debts, contracts and life's purpose. The symbol connects you in finding your true Oneness, the essence, and illuminating the light and wisdom within. This symbol works with the subconscious mind.

The distant symbol means bridging time and space. You can send this energy forward in time, into the future with the proper intention. When using HonShaZeShoNen in a healing, present life traumas, life's patterns, past, present and future can all be changed. Use it when working with childhood traumas or incest. This symbol's energy can go to a time frame before an event, or to change the "thought of the event." Then add the SeiHeKi, which will work with the client's emotional mind. During the process you will work with the client's inner child self. The conscious mind of the client can tell or ask the inner child what it needs to feel better, and can then make the necessary mental adjustment. This sounds simple, but in doing healing work you will find that almost everyone has some pattern from the past, that needs to feel safe, secure, not guilty, that it wasn't their fault, that they were the victim, etc. This will help heal the mental pattern, and therefore release the emotional damage, though nothing can erase the action itself. The important thing is to release or to change the pattern, so it doesn't need to become a karmic pattern that repeats and repeats itself.

This symbol can be used to prepare a room for meditation, healing treatments, massage, counseling or any psychic work. Use along with the power and mental/emotional symbols when beaming energy, doing your prayer list, traveling, aiding hospital patients, friends, or relatives that live away from you, etc.

Send this energy ahead if you are going in for hospital testing, or have a court hearing, important business meetings, dentist or doctor appointments, etc.

Healing with the Symbols

Ground yourself first. Ask permission either from the patient or from the astral plane if the patient isn't able to give permission (as in coma victim). If you receive permission in meditative request, you can proceed, if not, withdraw with love and peace and end the session. Remember that it is for the best interest and highest good of the client, and any recycled Reiki energy can be directed towards the healing of Mother Earth. Set the intention of sending healing energy. I start by sending light, with no color determination (that is limiting). I just allow whatever color is needed for the client to come through. I let the colors fill the client's auric field, then I send the Reiki symbols as a visualization of being whole, not in segments. You may see the symbols encircling or lengthwise as they come through space and time to the client. In distant healing you will always use HonShaZeShoNen, the power symbol ChoKuRei, to empower and increase the healing energy, and the SeiHeKi to treat the emotional aspects of the disease or problem. You may get a message from your Reiki guides, or the client receiving the energy may be given directions, that something more needs to be done. A guided message will always be positive in nature, or life-affirming; refuse anything else. For example, if someone has a broken arm, visualize them using this arm, or if someone has a broken leg, see them running. When someone needs a house sold, visualize a sold sign.

You may work on balancing or clearing chakras in this meditative state. If sensing heavy energy, pull the '"yucky" stuff out, and always remember to fill this area with light whenever you have removed energy from the body. Then you can put the Reiki symbols into that area, whether chakra or other.

Group Distant Healing

Any group of like-minded individuals can send distant healing, as long as the whole group focuses the intention. Examples include: Goddess meetings, spiritual groups, medicine wheel ceremonies, healing and prayer groups, Reiki open house groups, etc.

The methods commonly used are:
1) form a circle of people and send the Reiki energy into the circle
2) the inside/middle/center of the circle is the vortex or spiral point
3) using the power symbol, the mental/emotional symbol, and the distant symbol, focus the energy into the center of the circle
4) pictures/photographs can be placed within the circle for healing
5) names can be called out for healing energy, including your own
6) energy can be sent out for global or universal conditions
7) all energy is sent out into the universe for anyone in need
8) you can sing, chant, or drum
9) intention is for the best interest and highest good of those receiving
10) remember, where two or more are gathered together in His name, there is an endless source of intensified divine energy, especially when set with intention

Empowering Your Goals

If you have a pet project, or a global environmental goal you are working with, you can use the Reiki healing symbols. In the last fifty years since Reiki has been reintroduced, the world has become aware of the potential of what Reiki offers. The use of Reiki symbols gives you the opportunity of reaching out, of directing the healing energies, of becoming a part of the recreation. How exciting to know you are part of the adventure and myth. Take the challenge!

Reiki works for all Earth people—in the creation of One Planet ♥ One People.

For personal goals, or goals that may be blocked:
1) write your name on a piece of paper
2) write your goals on this paper
3) draw the symbols on the paper
4) work daily with these goals by energizing them with Reiki for twenty-one days
5) try connecting with the earth in a new and deeper way
6) surround yourself with unconditional love and harmony, this will strengthen your energy flow, dissolving the emotional conflict at the subconscious level
7) at the end of twenty-one days, burn the paper and release out to the universe; a good release time is approximately three days before a new moon

Master Symbols

In Tibet, a Buddhist master or teacher is honored for being part of a line of adepts, whose lineage refers back to Gautama Siddhartha, the Buddha. The gurus in India also take this responsibility seriously, with no ego and with a teacher/student trust. Today, a Reiki master also has a lineage, and a conscientious commitment for excellence, dating back to Dr. Mikao Usui, Chujiro Hayashi, Hawayo Takata, Jesus, and the Sakyamuni Buddha, and before this to Shiva and beyond. The privilege of receiving the sacred attunements is akin to receiving Christian sacraments, or the rite of passage ritual. This is an empowerment of sacred power that enters the body, your connection to the Creator, a new level of awareness. The awareness will always be with you, on a day-to-day basis, healing obstructions and working with your consciousness.

Traditional and Tibetan Master Symbols (DaiKoMyo)

I have always felt the traditional master symbol seemed geared more towards a masculine energy and that the Tibetan DaiKoMyo seemed more flowing and feminine. Since we are trying to rebalance the male and female energies here on Mother Earth, I use the Tibetan DaiKoMyo. The traditional DaiKoMyo is placed in the hands only with Reiki III, and placed into the Crown chakra during all attunements. Nontraditional teachers are putting this symbol into the hands during attunements of all three levels.

This symbol heals at the soul level, or the Oneness of life, spiraling in and out of the Void, working with the heart chakra. This symbol relates back to the philosophy of the Bodhisattva Pathway (enlightened and heroic being). This philosophy involves the giving of the One-Heart, enlightenment for others, and will not accept the bliss of Nirvana as long as anyone remains behind in pain and delusion. Enlightenment requires the perfect balance, or union of wisdom and compassion. The Bodhisattva resolves to dedicate their soul to endless incarnations doing good service, and helping remind others of their responsibility in the world, waiting for the day when all will enter the Bliss. The Tibetan DaiKoMyo is spiral shaped, and reminds me of the spiral dance I teach to help rejuvenate the energy fields which feels great after doing healing work.

Tibetan Energy Symbol: Raku

Raku is the absolute, the Ninth Consciousness, ether, spirit, the Void or Oneness. It creates movement of energy along the spine (lightning), and grounding at the end of the attunement process. A point of Enlightenment itself, it involves the learning of completion, or of letting go of the lower existence, opening our eyes to the illusion of the material world, and freedom from selfish cravings. With the completeness of Enlightenment, our beliefs and conditioning give way to Nirvana/Void or Oneness. Object and mind are one, and these seeds are imprints upon our consciousness. Raku represents the Vajra (diamond) of Vajrayana (vehicle) Buddhism, meaning shining, clear, unbreakable, and invincible.

In the attunement process, this symbol is drawn from head to feet or from the universe into the body. It grounds the conscious level of enlightened energy into the body. The five symbols used for Reiki III, bring about the light of knowledge, information and Ki, the life force of the Raku and Reiki healing. In Buddhism, this symbol is used in the opposite direction, from foot to Crown. This takes the person out of body and into the Universal Void or Oneness. Reiki is the worldly use for the five symbols and the five steps on the pathway to enlightenment. The Buddhist belief from hundreds of years ago, and still today, makes healing the physical body irrelevant. It is the spiritual healing, or the healing of Enlightenment itself, that is most important. This symbol is the center of Buddhism, and also the center of the Reiki healing system. Many Reiki teachers have not been taught this symbol.

Reiki Master Symbols

ChoKuRei—
Power

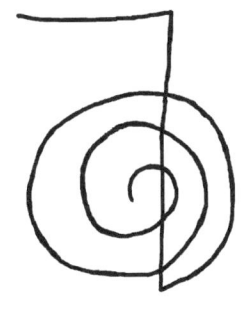

SeiHeKi—
Emotional/Mental

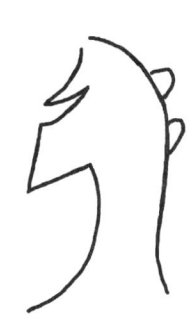

HonShaZeShoNen—
Distant Healing

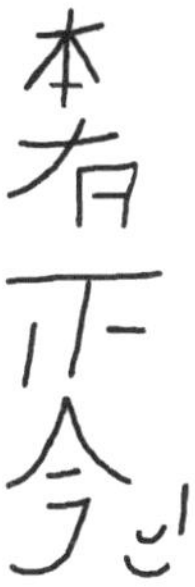

DaiKoMyo—Traditional
Master

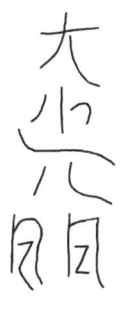

DaiKoMyo—Modern
Master

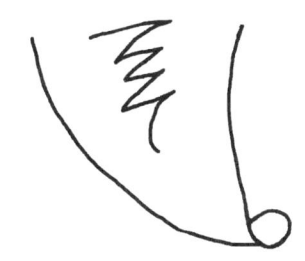

Raku or Dragon/Serpent
Tibetan Energy Symbol

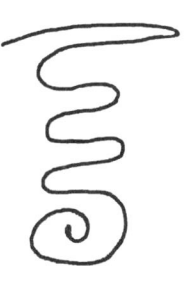

My Initiation into Reiki

by Ruth Hutton, RN

My knees felt weak as I descended the stairs from the initiation room upstairs to the living room, where our class was being held. The other members waited with anticipation for their turn. As I settled onto the sofa, relieved to sit and catch my breath, someone asked, "How was it?"

"Profound," I responded.

Profound, was the only word that came to mind at that moment. It is the only word that can describe what was an intensely personal and spiritual experience. I was affected physically, emotionally and psychologically at the moment of initiation. Things moved. I felt a spectrum of emotions from joy to despair, to relief, pain, and disappointment, all in a single moment. It was cleansing.

I felt the movement of Kundalini so intense that it caused me to jump in my seat. There was breath, which hit me in my solar plexus, so hard that it left me gasping. It was movement. Then there was the feeling of uncompromising love, so encompassing that it made me giddy and left me trembling. It was enlightenment.

What followed for days after was as important as the initial experience. The initiation into Reiki does not end when one walks out of the initiation. I began viewing the world and those around me differently. My psychic abilities were highly tuned up. I was extremely tuned into events, thoughts, and the people around me. It left me feeling as though I was finally emerging out of a dark tunnel into the light of day, after a long period of confinement.

My dreams became very intense and vivid. I had tangible dreams about "unfinished business." These dreams were usually about people and events that had less than positive memories for me. They brought closure and peace to many "issues" which I had been shoving to the back of my consciousness. I would wake up remembering my dreams, which is unusual for me.

People around me noticed a change. I was different. Overnight, I had become a more patient and positive person. My enthusiasm at the workplace was noticeable. I was less likely to complain and criticize, and more willing to go the extra mile, and was more productive. That has continued and cannot be explained by my supervisor.

I have since learned that each person, after experiencing the power and love which is Reiki, experiences an adjustment period after their initiation. My experiences are unique to me. My connection to God, as well as my search, brought me to seek the knowledge of how it is to use Reiki. No person will ever experience exactly the same thing during initiation.

Opening myself up to the healing power that is Reiki has empowered me, given me strength and foresight, and changed my life in many subtle, wonderful ways. I look forward to the road on which I travel, and the experiences that I will encounter on my journey to enlightenment.

The endeavor to do our part to restore
The Plan for Earth gives meaning to our lives.
This we do, when we hold the vision of universal brotherhood
and the new global community alive in our consciousness;
as we take up our daily work of speaking, thinking and acting.

Beginning Visions
by Brenda Stone

When it was suggested to me to take the Reiki healing classes, my thoughts were, "What in the world is that?" I had been to various other classes in my search along the spiritual pathway; my pathway is really new! So I thought, "What would Reiki do for me?"

While sitting in the Reiki class, I seemed to be following what was happening, but I did not quite make the connection. When I attended the second day, my awareness had sharpened and something seemed to click in me. Lights went off in my head. What was all that? I was in a daze, not sure what feelings were going through my mind. A few days later my awareness came like a flash! My opinion is that Reiki is different for everyone. The process, attunement, and initiation are all a special part of you, and Divine Source, and the experience is yours, and yours alone. For me the healing experience was very warming and intense, a far cry from the personal belief that I would ever be interested in any healing work.

The understanding I have received with Reiki has since developed into finding inner peace and strength within myself. My awareness was heightened, I felt unconditional love, and visions became clear and more prominent on a daily basis.

Two Years Later

During our Reiki clinics or Reiki open house groups, I have realized I can be helpful with these visions. I thought everyone saw what I saw. It was really exciting for me to share the visions, about the body's grid make-up, body parts, colors and the energy proceeding throughout the body for healing.

I have started tuning into past life experiences for people, in association with doing Reiki. I also started channeling, and have been connecting with galactic energies. I see their energies bathed in light and feel comfortable with their presence. This has helped me identify with my own past experiences, and has given me encouragement to forge ahead during some difficult times.

I am grateful for the encouragement of my friends who talked me into these classes, and for now knowing. I have found my place in the scheme of life. I am looking forward to helping others, guiding them in their understanding of what their bodies say to them, and how the energy moves through them. The healing of their bodies and minds is one. Life is sweet.

Our union with a Being whose activity is worldwide
and who dwells in the heart of humanity cannot be a passive one
In order to be united with Him we have
to divest our work of selfishness and become
Visvakarma, "the worldworker."
We must work for All.
In order to be One with this Mahatma, "the Great Soul,"
one must cultivate the greatness of soul
which identifies itself with the soul of all peoples
and not merely with that of one's own.

Rabindranath Tagore

Beyond Mind Power

by Suban Potijinda (White Lotus)

My spiritual awareness has been with me ever since I can remember. My visualizations allow me to see beyond our third dimensional realities.

After a routine surgical operation for tumor removal, the doctors diagnosed me with cancer, at an evolved stage; however, my conscious knowingness said to me, "So what, I am not afraid." My belief system was telling me that there is a method far beyond out there, to overcome this situation.

So, after I was released from the hospital, I started intensified meditations and visualizations for healing my illness. Six months later, the doctor diagnosed me as being free of cancer. This experience led me to understanding that meditation, with a quiet mind, was important for all of us.

This pathway had guided me towards interest in spiritual and natural healing. I soon found myself being led into setting up a Meditation Park. This park would have pathways for quiet moments, a sacred sphere for meditation and a center for Reiki healing, all housed on thirty-five acres in North Carolina, only twelve miles from the ocean. I see the land as being protected and sacred. My guides have shown me and I have followed the vision, for all future peoples seeking alternative well-being.

The next step was to add official certification in natural healing to my background, along with my thirty-five years of nursing. I then made the decision to take Reiki universal life force energy. Since receiving my certification, I have been using this knowledge to work on clients. I also send distant healing on a regular basis to family, and friends and upon request. In using Reiki, I have also found myself to be more energized.

Recently, I had a mystical experience during one of my meditations. I could actually see my own aura expanding around me and out from around me—wonderful colors with lots of violet and white. Then, I looked at my hands and saw the energy flowing forth. I decided not to waste this wonderful stuff and proceeded to bathe myself with this energy. I was really excited and overwhelmed at seeing this vision. I have been blessed with many visions lately, like seeing a house that was going to be purchased by a friend. I also saw property in the mountains of North Carolina, where my Reiki teacher is going to move her center. I am strengthened by this guidance, and inner peace stays with me moment by moment.

I am looking forward to many more adventures or just to seeing what's next.

The possibility of stepping into a higher plane is quite real for everyone.
It requires no force or effort or sacrifice.
It involves little more than changing our ideas of what is normal.

Deepak Chopra, MD

All work becomes spiritual when rightly motivated,
when discrimination is employed and soul power is added
to the knowledge gained in the free world.

Alice Bailey

When you cease to make a contribution you begin to die.

Eleanor Roosevelt

Reiki On a Larger Scale—Your Planet
by Lucinda Fury

Reiki to heal a planet. Ridiculous, I thought. How in the world (pun intended) can we save a planet, our earth, by a simple Reiki healing technique? Well, that's a good question, and one that needs to be asked.

In order to answer it, I need first to say there are a growing number of people who believe that we have to heal ourselves first. Then changes will occur that will in fact heal the planet. We need to change our patterns of thought. We need to unite in prayer and action. If you have action and intent, you get reaction. I'm not talking about a bunch of people getting together and praying that the earth heals. You can't think pollution away; or move mountains of trash through meditation. You can, however, generate positive ideas through both.

With positive nurturing ideas comes action. If action is for the good and betterment of our environment, the reaction is Earth healing. If you think you will plant a tree, that's a good idea, a positive thought. It starts there. When you plant the tree, you've taken action, positive action. When the tree grows, it is a reaction to your action of planting it. It becomes manifest. It is!

The reaction doesn't stop there. That single tree has its effect on the environment, which in turn also reacts. All of this started with an idea. If you get enough people planting trees, you'll soon have a forest.

Through Reiki, we aren't planting trees in the literal sense. The seeds being planted are healing our minds, bodies, and spirits. They are putting us in contact with each other on a very intimate level of truly caring about another person and knowing we can cause a reaction through action. We may not even know the person, or about their life, what they do, or even their name. They are important to us, and the intimacy is on a much higher level, a spiritual level. We don't have to know you to care that you are.

Through Reiki, we seem to start caring on a different, more expansive level. Becoming in tune with this "life force" and recognizing this in people leads to "seeing" it in all things. The Native Americans knew and reacted with the "life force." Their respect for the environment and knowledge that certain procedures would lead to regrowth after their collection and harvest showed a spiritual connection to all life. This was their way of acting and receiving a reaction.

Spirit breathes the alikeness into every flower and tree.
And fosters our connections to life's Sacred Mystery.
The net that binds us together is the spirit we hold in kind.
This abundant, unlimited expression is the Creator's breath divine.
Humankind is always looking for ways to measure the soul,
Never really seeing the Spirit that makes Creation a whole.
Fragments rest in every part of the natural world we know,
But when we forget the Oneness, we failed to honor Creation's flow.
Sprit flows in unity through the Source from which all came,
Visible to every seeker who has found the Eternal Flame.
That fiery connection to all life rests in the love that lies within,
A Oneness that gives us no resource but to see the spirit in all our kin.
Jamie Sams from her book, *Earth Medicine*

I Count Myself as a...Rainbow Warrior

by S. Jeanne Gunn

I was going to write about a time when I was very young and very small (three or four years old) and I believed in angels. Then I thought, well, I will write about when I was eight to twelve years old, when life seemed too much for me and I would go out into the woods and soothe away my cares, by becoming Snow White. It worked. I would sit very quiet and very still and the squirrels, chipmunks and one red fox would go on about their daily routine. I would softly cry my tears and gain my strength back. When I knew it was time to go home, I would leave this haven for another day.

I had no one to tell me that Mother Earth's strength was there, or about meditation. Maybe we were not thinking those things back in the old days! Only a handful of enlightened people scattered around the world would understand the crying out of a small child. Thank goodness for them. But then something happened. What was it?

Well, communications on Earth became so advanced, we finally woke up to realize this planet is not really that big. We have started to wake up to the fact that the people that live across the oceans are probably scared of war just like we are, probably want to have freedom of religion, and probably have the same thoughts that we do. Isn't that amazing, they probably aren't the enemy! What will the movies do when there isn't "a bad guy?"

Well, to stay on the subject. I was married and we raised three children. They were honest, had integrity, and concern, and were polite. We were very fortunate. We all worked together, helping each other, and were good neighbors, supporting our community and government. I think—no, I know—we thought this was the American Dream. We enjoyed working in the yard and around the house to make it beautiful. We went without vacations and fancy clothes, but we worked together. We went to church. Still, there was something missing. We got partially caught up in the American myth—that life on this planet was about getting ahead, getting rich, and having cars in the driveway and material things.

The new myth is the Rainbow Legend—the very personal soul development, the understanding of self, the knowing that life on our planet is really about waking up to Divine Source, our Creator. It is about waking up to treat where we live, how we live, and our neighbors with respect. We were well on track with behavior habits, but change came along. My husband and I separated, each one to find his own pathway and spiritual work on the planet.

Divorce is a word that became commonplace during the seventies, eighties and nineties. What happened to individuals has caused another great change. Responsibilities for our actions seem to be someone else's. Dishonesty and greed for the dollar has caused the roaches to come out of the woodwork. Responsibility and commitment were lost, and the family unit dislocated. Look around today—turn on television and see killings, con-men schemes, drugs and addictions, abuse to children and women, incest, shootings on the highways, innocent victims, injustice after injustice. An awakened society can promote good from an awareness, of what we have become.

People have gathered in the United States to claim the American myth—getting all you can get, while the getting is good. We are all people from many nationalities, forgetting that we are One, forgetting we are brothers and sisters, forgetting we form a united nation based on helping other nations. Many are wanting to get something for nothing. The change will come! But oh, are we really ready for what we may bring upon us? Do we realize we are responsible for the changes?

Mother Earth is hurting. The masses of people aren't working together. Honesty and integrity are forgotten words. However, there is a rise of spiritual growth—individuals searching, the explosion of awareness books on the market. Workshops facilitate role playing on any inner child hurts. Many are waking up, remembering from long ago some need, some thought, something to jog the memory—the original myth!

My waking up was a need for answers to understand a divorce. What is your waking up?

An inner part of me was identifying with the hurts of Mother Earth. I kept thinking, "If I could just put my arms around the planet, around someone who is in pain, I could make it all better." That may have been my own inner pain. I was guided into taking Reiki—my first opportunity of acknowledged awareness, and of being on a pathway. Reiki helped me to meditate, to hold close the sense of belonging, the inner guidance, the reawakening, to claim my spiritual rights. Reiki gave me strength for each day, no matter what was happening, getting me through the thoughts of suicide, through a divorce, through relationship endings, through losing everything. Now, people that know me see an inner strength. They tell me about the angel on my shoulder.

The many years of Reiki in my life led me through my angel death experience, my needing to be jogged big time. Books came that reawakened something in my cells to remember the original instructions—intuition heightened—confirmations came.

My concern for individuals and for our planet, I realized is not a new concept to me. My concern is about how I can help others make their connection, their wake up call. Reading about the Rainbow Legend, the Medicine Wheel, the Circles of Life, the connection to Divine Source, helped me realize my part in the Legend—more and more are awakening.

Much work is to be done. Our planet is hurting from the toxic wastes we have dumped onto and into her gasoline, oils, and fumes, and six billion tons of garbage yearly. If we think that our actions won't have a reaction we have our heads in the sand. The dolphins and whales have cried out by beaching themselves, the earthquakes have protested the drilling of holes in Earth's body, and weather patterns have changed.

Yes, we can do something!

Prayer

Really deep committed prayer can help heal a certain portion of the earth, i.e., rain forests, waters, drugs, addictions, famine, plague, health, government agencies, injustices, peoples and nationalities who work against the whole. Prayer helped change the direction of a hurricane.

United we stand together as one, if we choose to.

Responsibility and Intention

Become aware of your personal attitude in your driving habits, in your work habits and with coworkers, with your friends and community, with your nation and your lands. Remember the original instructions: the process of healing begins with us, and our efforts and accomplishments affect all future generations. The process begins with what is in our hearts.

Become a part of the Rainbow Legend
The original myth!
Become part of the Earth people generation.

A Stroke in Time

by C. E. 'Lefty' Hamblin

It was one of those Indian summer days that make life such a joy, a morning that literally begs to be noticed. I went into the company kitchen for coffee, and as I walked into my office, I found I could not grip the cup. My right hand had lost all strength and I felt pain in my shoulder. I thought I had a pinched nerve, and just tried to work it out through some movement. After an hour, my hand and arm felt weakened and had no sensation. Something was wrong, and I finally decided to go home.

My wife, a Reiki practitioner, started a Reiki treatment. We called my teacher Jeanne whom I had taken Reiki from and for whom I had great respect and trust. The two worked with me for four hours using their spiritual guidance and clairvoyant talents.

A dear friend and psychic minister called and said, "I think you need to go to the hospital to be checked out." Off we went to the hospital. We drove ourselves, since I was feeling so much better. I went through the battery of tests, and was diagnosed as having had a mild stroke. I was then referred back to another doctor, who examined me using an echocardiogram. This doctor told me to take an aspirin a day, and he gave me some exercises to perform, using my arm and shoulder.

Back at home we organized a Reiki Team to provide me with treatment twice a week for the next four weeks. Friends, Reiki students, and others gathered to offer their support and help. Others, unable to make it physically, prayed and visualized my recovery. Talk about energy coming in, talk about the strength of love, and talk about realizing how good friendship felt!

After a few days of the Reiki treatments, the exercises, and the aspirin, I went back to get reexamined. The doctor said he didn't know what it was I was doing, but whatever it was, I was healed and ready to go back to work. My whole range of motion had returned, my pain was gone, and the stroke had left no clue as to its presence. It was indeed a miracle. I noticed, felt, and experienced angels around me during my Reiki treatment. Their wings brushed against my body, and from that moment, not only was I healed, but I also knew that I was healed beyond a doubt. This experience opened my awareness in a way that is beyond mere knowing. This changed my life.

Angels at Work

by Katherine Thiele Jones

Angels are working full time to help mankind and their needs!

When there is a need and a deep desire for healing, then angels will help if asked. Also, we must consciously create the atmosphere for receiving such a loving response to our needs. My own specific need had to do with a heavy mucous condition in my throat. This had existed for years, and I thought I had to live with it and the added annoyance.

The answer came when a group of us met for weekly sessions of meditation and prayer. After a prayer to be willing to be open, we were directed to mentally put ourselves into a favorite room. I sat in a large armchair facing large windows, while the following scene unfolded. Outside the window, I could see trees and the bright sunshine flowing through the leaves. All was quiet. Presently, a beautiful angel appeared before me, smiling. The angel asked the exact nature of my need. I explained my throat condition and asked if it could be healed.

The angel turned into a huge beautiful butterfly. "Yes, this is not difficult. Twist a medium size bath towel tightly, dampen it with water, and fold it into a curve the size of your neck. Put the towel into the freezer on waxed paper. In the morning, wrap the towel around your neck and sit quietly until the cold is gone. Do this each morning until the condition is cured." The butterfly and the whole scene vanished.

I felt relaxed, thrilled, and blessed. I had the answer. I followed the instructions faithfully for eight days, until my throat became normal. Never again, have I been bothered with that condition. This healing experience and my gratitude are still with me from many years ago.

A Quantum Outlook
by Marius J. Broekhuizen

A centered existence is marked by the interconnectedness of mind and body. Evidence proving that the one can, and does, influence the other is growing. Enough nonmedical healings have taken place to allow us to consider abandoning the label of chance applied to them. There is a substantial case history of quantum healing, wherein conscious, purposeful, directed thought could be applied through the brain to cause physical healing.

However, we're not concerned with numbers. Significance lies not in numbers but in remembering that these healings were the opposite of chance; they were not accidental remissions. The quantum healing occurred only after a decision had been made to reverse disease and to heal.

The subjects accepted the presence of the invasive disease in their bodies, but absolutely refused to accept its inevitable devastation. They in effect said, "I know you're there but I refuse to submit to your indignity." That quantum step, moving up radically to a higher level of accepting the relation between one's mind and body, was the beginning of the cure in each case.

The ability to embrace such a belief—and it is a belief, not a laboratory-proven medical technique—understandably is not popular with the medical profession. Doctors in most medical fields are not committed to simple healing; they are committed to healing through medicine. Consider the shambles in the medical field if the belief in quantum healing were to be universally accepted as the basis for healing.

It's interesting to conjecture how many doctors in any field of expertise would stand aside as medical experts in the face of such a quantum healing. How many would be willing to submit themselves along with the patient to the conviction that the healing was the overpowering consideration, and not how it was brought about. I dare say very few at this point could resist the urge either subtly or overtly to nudge the patient back into the channel carved by traditional use of medicine.

That Dr. Deepak Chopra's book, *Quantum Healing, Exploring the Frontiers of Mind/Body Medicine*, is a national bestseller simply reflects national interest in this expanding field. Dr. Chopra is not a pie-in-the-sky theorist but a practicing endocrinologist, and thus able to describe authoritatively the latest experiments illustrating chemical reactions in the body produced by the brain, i.e., by a thought pattern. Nor is he by any means alone in this work. Nationally recognized and respected scientists, like the renowned Dr. Edelman, are working to determine where thought begins in the brain.

It is not a great step anymore from brain to body, as evidenced by what is being learned from high-tech electrophotography of the brain cells' actual functions and corresponding cell responses elsewhere in the body. Since choice is given to all, the choice to accept or reject the limitless benefits of quantum healing could mean the difference between life and death. What is there to lose?

Healing in a Beyond Space
by DuLois Lee

It seems as if there is an explosion of personal healing and transformation these days. Much of it is facilitated by the use of our minds, and our hands, and very importantly, our intuitions. As a structural integrator practitioner (Rolfer), I'm in a constant state of awe at just how quickly the body adapts, incorporates change, and heals itself; almost instantly it seems. With our intuition, and our heart as the navigator, we are able to communicate with the body's own intelligence and send healing energy directly into human tissue.

My own experience with the power of the mind happened about ten years ago. I lay in an awake state, still exhausted from a night of pain and interrupted sleep caused by my weak lower back. The pain had been fairly constant for five years, and I worried that I would become incapacitated, need surgery, or face some other, equally horrible future. Nothing brings you down in the dumps like constant pain.

This particular morning, I tried to get into a comfortable position. I was playing a little film in my mind. I saw myself running on the beach and turning cartwheels like a child, totally free of pain, and strong again. Then, to get a little further out of my body pain, I meditated on leaving this earthly plane and traveled out into the wonderful quiet of space. My house became further away, and then I saw the whole earth below me. Suddenly I was out in space with planets and stars floating around me.

I was moving outward into space and saw a very bright spot. When I got closer, it appeared to be an opening of light. I started into it. I felt I moved very fast, and I was suddenly in a place similar to a hospital. There on the table lay my spine. My bones were huge, and were a very phosphorus, bright color. Just over the right kidney region were two little volcano-shaped spots. Then a voice that I heard, yet which seemed to come from me, spoke, "just move your hand over them," which I did. The volcanoes closed up, and I soon awoke totally free of pain and feeling more refreshed and calm than I had felt in years. I just sat in my chair for a long time, and felt how good it was to just sit and not have my back hurting.

I still don't know what happened, but it was real. I had touched my own power. I had a renewed faith that I would get well. I started searching for the way, and Structural Integration was the answer for me. In this field, I am constantly amazed at the healing power we all have, as demonstrated in Reiki and other fields of healing, using energy, intent, and our hands.

The transformation that occurs from these health-restoring modalities was expressed by my esteemed Rolfing instructor, Emmett Hutchins of Boulder, Colorado, as, "the sensation of moving from weakness into strength and the exhilaration of owning a new part of oneself." That is exactly how I felt right after my dream vision, a sort of prophetic premonition of a cure for me. I had been allowed to feel this and know that I could become well again.

As I continue on the path, I see this power emanate from my clients as they discover the wonderful sensation and strength of finally being on their line of gravity, their Hara, as visualized by Reiki and other healing practitioners. It is this balance the body yearns and strives for, the unbroken flow of energy that lifts us up and holds us erect, to receive and utilize ourselves to our potential. We are empowered. Imagine the healing and growth that can be accomplished in these states of awareness.

We are uniquely ourselves—fascinating, wonderful, also irritating,
and very different—but very much the same—
tightly woven together in this vast web of humanity.
Earth People - Gateway to Inheriting the Universe

Someday, after we have mastered the winds, the waves, the tide and gravity,
we shall harness for God the energies of love.
Then for the second time, man will have discovered fire.
Teihard De Chardin

Chapter Twelve

Nature and the Sacred Space of Man

The Rainbow Legend

by Wind Dancer

Turtle Island (North America).

Light skinned peoples come from the East in boats with wings.

The people will have two types of feet. One like a dove. One like an eagle. Dove represents new freedoms, love and kindness towards all life. Eagle represents strength, technologies, warring attitudes, and greediness. The Eagle will dominate the new world and the light skinned ones will claw at the Red Nations.

The Red Nations will lose their lands and their spirits.

Later times, the Mother, Earth will become sick and will lose the virgin forests, clean waters, and fresh air, all necessary for man to have life. Greed, dishonesty, and technology will rule man's heart, all for the sake of wealth. Our short-sightedness will vote for technology, and greed will have ruled our lands.

How will the Mother cleanse herself of this sickness?
- Rumblings from deep within (unsettled angry energy - earthquakes).
- Lack of food and famines (man playing with viruses).
- Signs from the heavens (eclipses, asteroids, and planetary weather extremes).
- Weather changes (floods, drought, winds, and lightening).
- Many people will awaken spiritually to what is happening. Groups will form to work and educate people to wake up—to save Mother Earth and mankind. Many teachers within the framework of business will start becoming aware of their responsibility

The Reawakening. The Original Instructions. The Legend. The Myth.

Reincarnated souls, the elders, the thunder stick stories, the memories.
Together, the teachings of all of the peoples of all of the lands.
Learning to Honor the place upon which we dwell, Mother Earth.

The Symbol of the Rainbow:

Represents—All Peoples, All Races, All Religions working together.
Harmony, Healing and Wisdom will spread throughout the lands.

The Teachers are the *Rainbow Warriors*.
Peace, Harmony, and Abundance for All is the goal. The Golden Age.

My Goal—The Sacred Earth Center, this Book, and other spiritual writings.
Healing and Loving Nature is my way of helping our Planet.
Helping to create a universal bond of all Earth people towards
One Planet ♥ One People

The Challenge Continues

The Thunder had come, the lightning too,
The command was given to just a few
Out into the quadrants: earth, air, fire, and sea
God's calling out and not just to me!

The Thunder People heard the decree,
To pass on the knowledge to you and to me;
From all directions, out into the universe, a start
Reaching out with the lessons of the One-Heart.

Whether white, black, yellow or red,
"The brotherhood of man is required," he said.
Reach out to your Guides and your Angels so Bright
Still your mind with God's purpose, become the Light.

The Rainbow Legacy, The Thunder, The Challenge, The Plan
All of us needing to be the best that we can.
Are we meeting the Challenge, following The Great Plan?
Or are we caught off guard, with our heads in the sand?

The Spirit Clan communicated with the Great Life Force
Beings beyond the Thunder in the rain clouds of course.
The ones who ride Star Vehicles creating sonic booms,
Are they waiting for acknowledgment too soon?

O Thunder People, the holy ones of the tribe
You, who bring great truth, along with our Guides,
I acknowledge your power, your peace, and the Great White Source
I join you today with my heart and spirit, of course!

by Wind Dancer

Meditation by the Trees
by Lumis Two Hawks

Start: Relax in a comfortable position. Take a long, slow, deep breath. Exhale slowly through the mouth. Relax and repeat three times.

Envision yourself on a path in a dense, lush forest with green-leafed trees all around you.
The path is winding, deeper and deeper into the foliage.
You are aware of the scent of honeysuckle and jasmine. The birds are singing.
A gentle breeze rustles the leaves on the trees and the branches of the trees.
The sun filters down through the trees in beautiful patterns of light.
You are coming to a small clearing.
The ground is cool and soft. You sit down, feeling totally relaxed.
You look up to the sky and see a small rainbow of colors that appears to be swirling above your head.
Watch this circle of colors. Allow yourself to experience this for a few minutes.
Now you see the circle of rainbow colors becoming a funnel of energy descending towards you.
You feel wonderful as the funnel of light travels down through your body.
In the center of the circle, you are the center of your self.
Trust your knowing. Trust your intuition. The colors fill you, yet extend from you.
You feel at one with all the colors, the energy.
Trust this connection of energy within your heart and mind of knowing.
Allow yourself to totally "sense" this energy.
Take the time to receive each color from every sense. See it. Taste the flavor.
Touch it. Listen for the sound of the color. Catch the fragrance of the color.
Take time to remember the colors that you have chosen.
As you begin to sense the colors lifting up and away from you, release them, gently.
See the pattern and circles as they leave your body, becoming a tighter pattern of circles as they go.
Watch them blending—becoming the most beautiful colors you have ever seen.
(You could see one of the new colors that are forming in the ethers.)

As you send this energy up and out into the universe, you sense a greater love and connection than ever before, a connection of helping to heal yourself, the forests, the waters, the air, the planet.

You have a sense of being whole, at peace, healed, energized.
Allow the essence of the colors and the energies to stay with you.
Experience it.
Now start becoming aware of your surroundings,
The clearing in the midst of trees, where we sat, the birds singing, and the sweet smell of the air.
Take a deep long breath, now exhale.
You are completely in the now, grounded and balanced.

Opening Your Heart Meditation
by Wind Dancer

Start: Relax in a comfortable position. Take a long, slow, deep breath. Exhale slowly through the mouth. Relax and repeat three times.

In this centered, calm state of being, you are going to pull the golden light from your connection with Divine Source/Great Spirit and your angelic self down through the top of your head into the crown chakra and going to your Heart Center.

And now you are going to visualize bringing up the silver light energy from Mother Earth, the grounding level, up through your feet, legs and lower chakras, coming up into and meeting the golden light at the Heart Center.

Breathe in this mixture of golden and silver light
- a) into all of the cells, atoms, electrons and molecules of your being
- b) now surround and fill yourself with this light
- c) now fill the room and surrounding areas with this light

Now, place a door at the center of your heart chakra.

Now open the door and see, sitting before you, your higher self.

Step into your higher self and become one with this energy.

Now see before you a large chart of written information.

This chart represents all of the brilliance and talents that you were born with.

This chart also shows you your eccentricities looking back at you. See how these types of thought forms fit into patterns of attitudes, actions of aloofness, poor me, the interrogator or the manipulator; these patterns affect your journey in this lifetime, the lessons you will need to overcome and accomplish.

Discover within yourself all of the discontentments you may have allowed to exist because of your need to be approved of by our society, like guilt, perfection, control, anger, judgments, justice, anything else. Now see yourself detaching (see these cords being cut by Archangel Michael) from all of these discontentments, and see yourself moving towards a lightness and feeling of personal freedom.

Now see yourself expressing all of your freedoms, letting your brilliance show, knowing this release has allowed you to feel lighter in mind, body, and spirit. Now see the brilliance of Archangel Michael's blue light surrounding you filling you. The blue light is now moving from your body up to the crown chakra and out into the world, merging you and your new energy patterns into an electric blue light of change, becoming again one with the All.

Now slowly breathe yourself back into your body.

Know that you have conquered and claimed your personal freedom.

Write and journal the work you see for yourself in the future.

Remember the tools you have been given to work with—from the Greatness of the All, the One-Heart.

Angelic Connection Remembered
by Wind Dancer

Start: Relax in a comfortable position. Take a long, slow, deep breath. Exhale slowly through the mouth. Relax and repeat three times.

We are standing in a meadow with wild flowers and tall gentle grasses swaying in the breeze, the sun is streaming down, and we are following this clear and smooth pathway through these meadow lands, to a patch of woods, just a small distance away.

As we enter the mild coolness of the woods, we immediately feel the sense of quietness and peacefulness. We continue to walk along this pathway, and now we see the vibrant colored greens of the moss and ferns growing along the pathway, beautiful and lush and peaceful.

Soon we see a small pool of water before us, a gentle stream of water running over some rocks. Splashing and cascading down from a high waterfall, the waters fill the pond of water before us. This water is clear and crystal colored. We are now going to step into this shallow pool of water, and allow the water to cover our feet, legs, and knees. We immediately feel the trappings of everyday life, the material things that hold us back, starting to let go, and now flowing away with the stream.

This beautiful energized water is clearing away all thoughts of anger, tiredness, doubts and hurts. We are beginning to feel lighter and lighter, from the burdens being lifted and washed away. This energized water is removing the heaviness from our emotional/mental bodies, purifying us. The water has now cleansed and purified our being, as we sit in this shallow pool of warm water.

As we are sitting in this wonderful energized water, we begin to see the reflection of an angel. This vibrant light angel is handing us a beautiful white rose with pink feathered edges, and is placing this beautiful flower into our One-Heart Center; this vital force energy of the flower is now glowing within.

This vital life force energy is reminding us that we are perfect beings, and one with our Divine Source. We are reminded that we are the earthly part of an angel, and the heavenly part of the angel is with us at all times. We are forever connected to this Divine Source.

The heavenly angel will always be keeping us aware, and watching over us. The more we can stay in tune to the Divine Love connection and stay out of the fears, worries, and stresses of everyday life on this planet, then the more our heavenly angel can help us.

At this time, decide to take a vow of commitment and intention to remember. Remember that we are always watched over, remember this energy is always with us, and remember we are a part of our heavenly angel. Why do we take this vow to remember?

Because when we go back into our daily lives we get caught up in our daily routines.

Our angel is now placing a cloak of intense white, silver and gold energy around us; it looks like angel wings.

Whenever you feel lonely or stressed, remember your cloak of Divine Love, this shimmering silver and gold given to you into the forever.

Children of Fifth Solar Culture

by Wind Dancer

Start: Relax in a comfortable position. Take a long, slow, deep breath. Exhale slowly through the mouth. Relax and repeat three times. Ground yourself.

On the planet Earth we are of the fifth generation, the balance between Divine Source and the planet Earth. This is the marriage between God/mind and God/heart and soul.

The balance between Intuition/Heart/Nature and Sun/Moon/Earth.

As such, we represent a vibrating wheel of energy, a balance in this universe.

Our inner wheel (divine source) and we are one. This inner wheel of unity will help hold us in a vibration of awareness, for the times ahead.

Go slowly:

We are going to take a journey out into the universe, so let's mark the reference point of planet Earth, the country of the United States, the state we dwell in, and this room. Let each of us mount up on a winged bird, and allow ourselves to soar up and up and up, out into the universe, to other galaxies of stars and planets. Our winged friend and our self become one, one source of energy.

As we look around now, we can see the grand scheme of the universe. Allow the energy of the stars to bring us a message of our small part in this great scheme called life. Let us check out one or two of the galaxies, let us connect with the Pleiadian galaxy, allow them to give us a message for the coming days and their part in this universe. Now let us connect with the Sirius galaxy, and allow them to give us a message for the coming days, and their part in this universe.

Let us remind them that we are the Children of the Fifth Solar culture. We are here to help mend and bring forth the Rainbow Legend of the Earth people, working together towards unity and peace.

- a) we are the bridge between God and Mother Earth
- b) we are the only planet of free will; our planet holds the energy library of universal information
- c) we are the culture of spiritual human beings
- d) we are the generation merging into the Aquarian age
- e) we are to bring forth the Light, we are to awaken others, by living loving thoughts
- f) we are the Age of Remembering who we are, and what our purpose is

From here we can look around our universe where the veil allows us to see more clearly. Let us vow to remember upon returning home to Planet Earth, just what we are doing here. Remember what is left for us to finish. Let us realize our potential and our connection to Divine Source. Remember that any attunement or initiation can bring forth changes in attitude or a method of healing self and others.

It is our inheritance.

Now let us slowly return home, back to Earth upon our winged friend, back to our country, back into this room, and now back into this body, rejuvenated, relaxed, and with our purpose of life fulfilled.

Galactic Meditation
by Wind Dancer

1) Sit next to a partner for a joint healing/planetary meditation
2) Align and enclose yourself in a bubble of protected light
3) Ask your spiritual guides to direct your thoughts to stay with the program
4) Close your eyes, breath gently and deeply to quiet yourself

Now that you are centered and enclosed in a bubble of light and your spiritual guides are with you, we are going on a journey. Adjust yourself with your partner and align the joint energies with the color of the chakras: *Root/Red* being grounded or relaxed, responding in practical ways to our daily needs; moving upward to below the *Navel/Orange,* where we have feelings of safety, protection, sexuality; now moving upward to *Solar Plexus/Yellow,* the mental and emotional centers, needing to allow ourselves time to meditate and connect with our source; *Heart/Thymus/Green,* the immune and Divine One-Heart center, drawing the Father Sky and Mother Earth energy into this central core, this central sun within us; *Throat/Light Blue,* communicating with Nature and each other; *Third Eye/Indigo,* visions and awareness flowing, being directed with the coincidences of life; *Crown/Violet,* the bloom of Divine Source flowing through us, clearing and inspiring our Earth bodies into action.

Now we have this spectrum of rainbow healing colors, flowing throughout our body and our partners. Take a moment to send this rainbow of healing colors out into the universe, to our Mother Earth for the healing of the waters, the air, the forests needed for health, and for all the peoples throughout the lands who are not aware. Now that you have surrounded and filled Mother Earth with this healing, send this rainbow of healing colors throughout the universes, into the unknown.

Now let us send this rainbow of healing colors into the center of this circle for special requests. Say quietly to yourself any names of people from your prayer list, visualize their names in the circle, and their receiving this healing energy. Or, if arranged beforehand, you may call out the names into the circle.

With eyes closed, I want you to focus healing streams of energy towards your partner and their needs. Each one directs this loving Divine Source, the Chi, the Reiki, surrounding and filling their physical bodies, radiating atoms of light infused with the rainbow of colors. If your partner has a special need in their physical body, focus the laser jets of energy towards that area, beams and rays of rainbow colors to heal and align the body. Keep the jet streams of light flowing, lasering molecules, atoms, and electrons, working with each of the cells of the physical body. Allow your intuitive vision to see the area cleared, healed, and realigned in light, the golden radiance of Divine Love and Light.

And now take a couple of slow breaths. Each of us is going on this journey alone, but also together as One. The journey is to another dimension, for the healing of our soul. Allow yourself to settle down quietly, in a warm secure-feeling place. We can now start our journey and the story of life.

We have long carried within us precoded messages in our cellular memory banks, our sealed order, so to speak, from the time we descended into matter. The fulfillment of our divine mission is the reason we chose to come to Earth in the first place.

The story begins here

Planet Earth has given us a place to labor, prepare, study and serve, the call to awaken has been sounded throughout the lands, and throughout the celestial vastness. The call to awaken and to activate our memories is now. Choices are to be made; great times require both greatness of spirit and greatness of action. Mother Earth herself is nearing a time of graduation from the third dimensional patterning and needs our help.

Prior to our descent into matter on the Earth plane, we chose our destiny pattern and became aligned with either a first wave or second wave patterning.

The first wave beings choose to come to Earth to anchor the new. They are the ones who have experienced countless embodiments upon this planet; they are the founders and holders of ancient wisdom. They will not manifest on Earth, but on the other side of the Doorway, thus uniting the first and second waves. This is of great importance if we are to move through into a divine dispensation.

The second wave beings' purpose is to build on the new once it is firmly anchored. They have had less earthly experience. They are the visionaries, the architects, and the ones with new forms of healing, music and community awareness. They are bristling with energy to manifest their impatience to create.

Let us now ready ourselves for the journey.

Gently mount yourself on a white dove (your starbird) and take a ride into the vastness of the universe, where we shall soar into knowingness. Stay with the story and the journey.

Our first task is to transform ourselves, by merging the fourth and fifth dimension into the third dimension; this is Earth ascending and Heaven descending together. This sacred merger is our birthright and our heritage, the remembrance that we are angels incarnated, that we are starry beings of light who are no longer limited to, or bound by, the illusions of time, space, and matter.

We are now going into a new Doorway, a step beyond the known dimensional universe, into a new patterning of octaves. This journey into the unknown shall lead us closer to home.

Allow yourself time to feel the peacefulness and safety in this place, the longing.

The starborne here all understand we originate from somewhere beyond this planet. That part of our purpose and job in serving is the transmutation of matter, to help evolve this planet and portions of humanity into an entirely new evolutionary template, returning home to the consciousness of the One.

The Rainbow Warriors have come to be the bridge between these two spirals.

The old spiral is illusion and separation, feeling abandoned, looking for the material world to fulfill all the needs of life, feeling separated from the Source, searching for God and purpose of life.

The new spiral is the bridge, the anchoring of feminine energy to balance the material third dimensional world of planet Earth, the channel of information and knowingness, the transmutation of dark energy into light, and creating the way for all the peoples to become aware of the mass ascension.

Archangel Michael and his legions have been overseeing this spiral of duality, preparing the way for this vast quantum leap for humanity. We are on full alert. Be aware of a state of grace, the imprint of pulsations of light frequencies, transmissions from the beyond. If you place yourself into a state of receptivity, the invisible will be made visible.

The new spiral is to manifest. The key is created by all of us joining together as one. All fragments must be placed together for the door to open. Know your service, and work as one, rather than separately. One thousand years of peace will come, with a feeling of truly knowing we are one. We will no longer feel separated from the Source. Only one shall pass through the door, all as one. Most who journey from the starbird to Octave 7 will remain to build on the new. So gently now, see and feel yourself in this space and what it has to offer. Some may feel a sense of what is going on. Others may stay here and work for these moments. Some of you may ask for clarification at this point. If so, find a quiet place to rest here, and allow the thoughts to come through. We shall wait for you.

Now we shall go on. A few shall take the starbird leading to Octave 11 and to the Beyond, towards the Greater Central Sun System. Our dove is not a spaceship; it is an expression of our unified presence. Our white bird is so immensely vast, that it shall take twenty years once the Doorway is open to pass through the portals into the new spiral patterning. All as one is the heart of our dove. The One-Heart energy flows upwards and outward, like a fountain of light, becoming ever larger, as more unite together for this journey home.

We are for the moment staying here and resting on Octave 7.

Later tonight, as you rest, you may get more clarification about your destination, and if you are a first or second wave being. Or even now, an answer may come as we rest here, before returning.

To prepare ourselves for the return journey, again as a whole, we begin by cleaning out our lives, discarding outmoded habits and thought forms, which are rooted in illusion of separation and denial. Go through the closets of your mind, and then our real closets, and literally shed ourselves of anything that no longer resonates or serves us, with the truth of your being.

Simplify everything, so it vibrates in accordance with you, and leaves space for the introduction of the new. Allow yourself the coincidences, the awareness, to hear nature talking, the crop circles showing the spirals and the Doorway, the hum of vibrations heard through our lands. Stay in attunement; allow the visions and knowingness to guide and strengthen you. Lay your foundation. By organizing your life into greater efficiency, you nourish yourself; be silent and listen to the beyond transmissions. Take time to relax and play, to clear up any fears, any issues of power. Set aside any guilt, forgive yourself and others; thus we create, continuing our venture of awakening. Ask for your angelic or starry name. When you receive it, begin to use it. These names are triggers, which aid in our transformational process. These names are a tool available to us. This is our unique vibration; it strengthens us for the pathway home.

At this time, we have been given our final instructions. Now climb back onto your white dove for the journey back to Earth. As we are descending, let us find our country, this room, and slowly merge into our bodies. Start breathing slowly, become more and more alert that our journey has ended and we are back in our bodies. Now slowly open your eyes, emerge fully into your body, knowing you have been given purposeful life instructions, and awaken to your soul purpose.

Meditation Between Two Worlds

by Wind Dancer
These are thoughts to ponder!

The energy for these years will be one of taking a leap of faith, a time for each of us to face our greatest fears, acknowledge them, and to find alternative ways to overcome these fears. Trust is also a key word. We will be challenged by experiences over and over, repeated until we hold fast onto trust. For intuitiveness and inner truth, turn inward for the learning. The trust comes from within.

Spiritual assistance will be there for those humans that are open, and accepting from within their own inner truth center. Each person must seek harmony, individually, for it to be attained and maintained.

Those who have the ability to see the past and the future, creating stepping stones for getting from one place to another—these people will be in great demand. These visionaries will be sought by those afraid of trusting their own inner truth. Some will choose wisely the pathfinders and empowered ones, gaining their inner personal strength, independence, and spiritual freedom.

Others will unwisely choose those who talk the loudest, and who are willing to say what the masses want to hear. This choice will teach you about giving away your power, the lesson called discernment.

The vision of perfection will glow strong in the ethers and etheric structure around the globe as the planets and the comets are working with Earth.

There is a pyramid of new, higher vibrational energy flowing towards our planet; take time to listen to this new inner Harmony. This energy will stay with us for a long time. This is our Earth people's opportunity to take advantage of balancing our spiritual life, our health, our planetary attitude, and our neighborly attitude.

The moon represents opening the door to wisdom and truth. These energies assist with the manifestation of the triadic energies being focused upon Earth. We will no longer be trapped by separation, opposites, or taking sides. Limitations will be in the past. Each Earth person will choose consciously what energies to express and how it is no longer necessary for anyone to take one extreme or another. Balance and harmony have been needed for a long time. Our planet is our life, and the balance and harmony are needed not only for humans, the Earth people, but also for the very existence of the planet upon which we live. Genuine love heals all.

Genuine love is self-replenishing
The more you nurture the spiritual growth of others,
The more your own spiritual growth is nurtured.
Excerpts from *Meditations from The Road* by M. Scott Peck

If you want to learn to live peacefully,
You should place yourself in an environment
Where the principles of conscious living
Are actualized on a day-to-day basis.

by Wind Dancer

Spiral Dance Technique

Breathing, moving, rhythms, along with toning, music, or drumming, help move the kundalini into the first chakra, thereby producing energy or power at the base, ready for movement into the other chakras.

Kundalini is our primary means of sensing life and our physical reality. Secondary is our nervous system, which transmits the energy or experience in the kundalini to the brain via the spinal cord. Kundalini is our primary energy source for our spiritual vehicle. Each time a person has an initiation or breakthrough experience, the kundalini opens in a new way to the next frequency or harmonic of red.

As you do the Spiral Dance, you feel the energy moving upward from Mother Earth into your feet, up into your legs, into the root chakra, and then along the looseness of your hips. If you feel any tenseness, keep on moving and letting go, rocking back and forth. If you begin to feel lightheaded, the energy has accumulated at the top of your head; reach up and pull the energy away with your hands. Breathing produces movement. Breathe from the hips; this helps expand our trunk, and then our entire body. Practice until you feel this.

There are regular exercises and breathwork to help the kundalini rise and control the energy. Refer to *Wheels of Light,* by Rosalyn L. Bruyere, a book of advanced information about the chakra systems. Kundalini power was taught in the mystery schools. Also check out the books on "breathwork."

Two Channels

When you first sense or feel energy, when working on a client, this awareness lasts for a short time. Then this system ceases to record. That is why in Reiki you don't always feel what is happening during the whole time you are channeling energy. You only stop feeling it. That is because culture has taught us to think as one channel. When we become aware of the kundalini, our mind begins to work on two channels.

Example: We can feel what is going on and still think about something else. The first chakra enables us to think and feel on several channels with awareness; this is what the kundalini is all about, to awaken and stimulate our conscious awareness on several levels at once, to open the flow of energy on several channels.

One Eye Technique

This is an intuitive whole body technique. It is a technique that helps us be a whole-body third eye, rather than a limited three-eye (two physical, one physic).

Place hands on top of crown chakra (above head) with elbows pointing to the side. Lift your hands up slightly so you are just above the crown chakra. If you look into a mirror it will look like you have one eye above your shoulders (your head being the eyeball).

The idea is to practice thinking with your whole being as one eye, rather than with the psychic approach. The one eye leads you towards superconsciousness. Intuition is our sixth sense; it is a normal function that all people may tap into. It is our birthright, our inheritance. Our Divine Source would not have put us here without the knowledge of being in touch with our creator.

Sacred Ceremony

Sources: Earth Medicine *by Kenneth Meadows and* Dancing with the Wheel *by Sun Bear*
Call Upon: As Above—Father Sky (Blue) and So Below—Mother Earth (Green)

East	Archangel Raphael	West	Archangel Gabriel
South	Archangel Michael	North	Archangel Uriel

East	Element of Air	Animal—Eagle	Illumination/Awareness
South	Element of Fire	Animal—Mouse	Transmuting/Purification
West	Element of Water	Animal—Bear	Strength/Inner Knowing
North	Element of Earth	Animal—Buffalo	Wisdom/Sacred Knowledge

Relationships—Four Directions/Seasons/Man's Spiritual Responsibility to Self and to Nature:

East	Yellow Man	(Spirit)	Spring	Being born	Determining
South	Red Man	(Emotion)	Summer	Youth	Giving/Emotions/Feelings/Love
West	Black Man	(Body)	Fall	Adulthood	Steadfastness/Strength
North	White Man	(Mind)	Winter	Maturity	Sustenance/Receiving/Knowing

Place crystals in medicine wheel center for energy and cleansing in Lakota language —
Chant each of the following three times to make your connection with the spirits to empower your crystals:

Wa Kan Kin (waconkin)	Inpi (innippee)	Ya Ma Kan (yemawcon)
Great Spirit, Great Mystery	To Cleanse Impurities	It Is Sacred, It Is Done

Native American Story: White Buffalo Woman gave the people the peace pipe ceremony and a rich spiritual tradition. The white buffalo calf signals a time of hope, rebirth and unity; a time of purity, of mind, body, spirit, and unification; of all nations of the four directions. The birth of the white buffalo signals a time of moving past our differences, past our own infancy. We are challenged to grow and mature as a species, through our mutual awakening into a new sense of our interconnectedness with all of creation. In this ceremony we pray for the fulfillment of these ancient prophecies and offer up this prayer.

We ask White Buffalo Woman, who gave birth to the peace pipe ceremony for all the people, to enter our heart and purify our mind. Heal our being, mind, body and soul. We ask that we may each live and grow in harmony with all of creation, earthlings and beyond into the universe. Many of us have been wounded and hurt during our cycles here, in this dimension of Earth. We ask that each one of us accept the past for what it is; an experience along the pathway. Help us to move towards the future, with healing, love, and peace in our heart, our center of oneness.

Help us join together now and remember our oneness.
Teach us how to be enriched by our diversity and our unity.
Show us how to live together in our community.

Help us to speak the truth, to have honor and honesty, integrity, compassion, giving and receiving with an open hand and an open heart. Guide our sharing of gifts and abundance, in a good and honorable way. May we each leave this world a better place for our children and their children till the sun no longer sets and the moon no longer rises.

Sacred Earth Healing Ritual

This ceremony is based on concepts from Earth Spirit's Medicine Wheel.

We will call in: Four Directions, the Four Archangels, the Four Elements, the Power Animals.

We will send out: Healing to the waters of the planet, to the trees, to the animals, the wind, earth, sun, moon, stars and all the peoples of this planet and the universe.

We will take part in: The rhythms and breathing of Mother Earth and her spirals of dance.

We will learn: About sage, our blessings, our connection to Mother Earth and to all of mankind, our purpose on this planet—through prayer and meditation.

This ceremony helps promote all Earth People toward…One Planet ♥ One People!

The Lakota Ten Levels of Consciousness

Sources: **Lakota Belief and Ritual** *by James R. Walker and Reiki handout*

These symbols reawaken your memory. They are a massage of the soul, soul memory retrieval, going beyond the fears or limits of man. They are remembrance of no beginning and no end, the foreverness. The words/definitions or translations work with these symbols, acting as catalysts for going outward and inward at the same time. They are the foreverness of who and what we are in the universe.

The Ten Levels in Lakota Language

1) Wa Kan Kin   (waconkin)   Great Spirit or The Great Mystery

2) Kan La   (conla)   Almost Sacred

3) Wa Ni Ya   (wakneeyah)   Spirit of Man or Woman

4) Wo Pe   (woe pay)   Legendary Beautiful Woman Who gave First Counsel and Pipe; She who Builds or Destroys

5) Ni Ya   (knee a)   That which Causes the Soul from the Beginning, the Birth

6) Ta Ku Wa Kan   (takoowahcon)   Pertaining to Great Spirit; One of Aspects of Great Mystery

7) Akicita Wi Kan   (acahseeta wecon)   Messenger of the Sun

8) Inipi   (innippee)   To Make the Spirit Strong; To Cleanse the Impurities of Body/Mind/Soul

9) Ni Ton   (kneetawn)   Gives Spirit Power, Intuitive Power, Healing Power; Connected to Great Mystery

10) Wo Ma Kan   (womawcon)   Doing for the Good of the Land; Sacred Energy Given out to All

To activate symbol -
Ya Ma Kan   (yemawcon)   It Is Changed, It Is Sacred, It Is Done

Ten Levels of Consciousness Technique and Notes

1) Concentric lines for each circle not spiral, vibrate to your own center/being when doing.
2) Keep your mind with the program of what you are doing, or you aren't connected to the process.
3) Placement crown chakra. Starting at outside of head area and moving inward to center of crown.
   Use three middle fingers to form line, start at one o'clock position, stand behind client.
   Concentric circles. Do not overlap.
   Remove hand after each circle and reposition for next circle.
   Draw in a clockwise direction.
   Speak each of the chants with the drawing of each circle, vibrational expression.
   Creates a vortex of funneled energy into body.
   Outside circle is the largest, inside the smallest.
4) Silver Level divine source; changing all you perceive, worldly things falling away.
5) Essence: you don't need to give direction to symbol, stay in the essence of flow, a self-contained foundation, ever flowing, ever continuing.
6) Light turning up the Light, symbol works beyond the level of the disease.
7) In doing this ancient symbol, I have found that when a group or individual is really with the program, each one has an experience of connectedness. You can see the difference when they are just going through the motions.

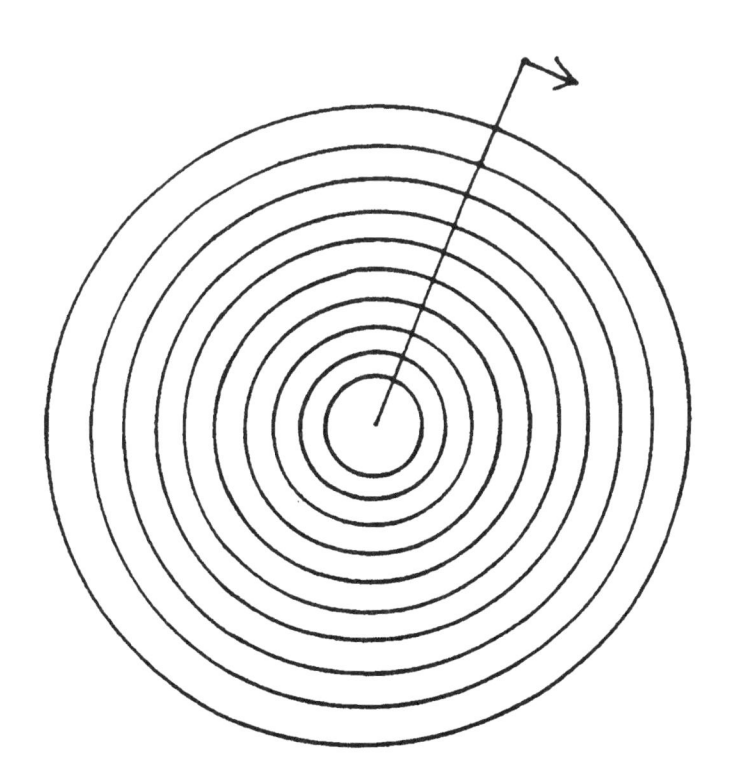

Golden Light Alignment

The Golden Light Alignment came in a revelation, what I call a mystical experience. It was the second of three experiences during a six month period of time, right after I was given direction to put together a "healing book," including the natural method of Reiki.

Three of us had gathered together to do some healing work with the eastern coastline. Later we understood this was preliminary work, right before a hurricane was to arrive in our area.

The three of us were not prepared for the wonderful golden light energy that filled the room, nor was I prepared to channel, especially when I found myself sitting on my shoulder wondering what was happening. I was able to watch, but was just as interested as the others in the information that was coming out of my mouth. We were awestruck, confused at first; but then confirmation came when we realized an antique coin I was holding had changed from silver to gold.

A council of ascended ones gave direction and these symbols were given to "open the pathway" for many peoples in the future days. The vibrational energies on our planet are changing, and affecting us all. With these changes, the Brotherhood of Light, Angelic Ones and Rainbow Warriors are working with many people, opening the doorway for our planet Earth on her voyage of evolution, and ours.

I share these symbols with you with the blessing of the ones who brought this information to planet Earth; please use discernment and conscious intention.

Directions:

This alignment is done with both the client and the facilitator standing.

1) Start on back of body and above the head; work your way down the body to the feet, representing Mother Earth. Then reverse.
2) Move to front of client and, starting at base, work your way up the body, finishing with angelic wings over the head—base, root, sacral, solar plexus, heart, throat, third eye, crown, and above head moving into upper chakras.

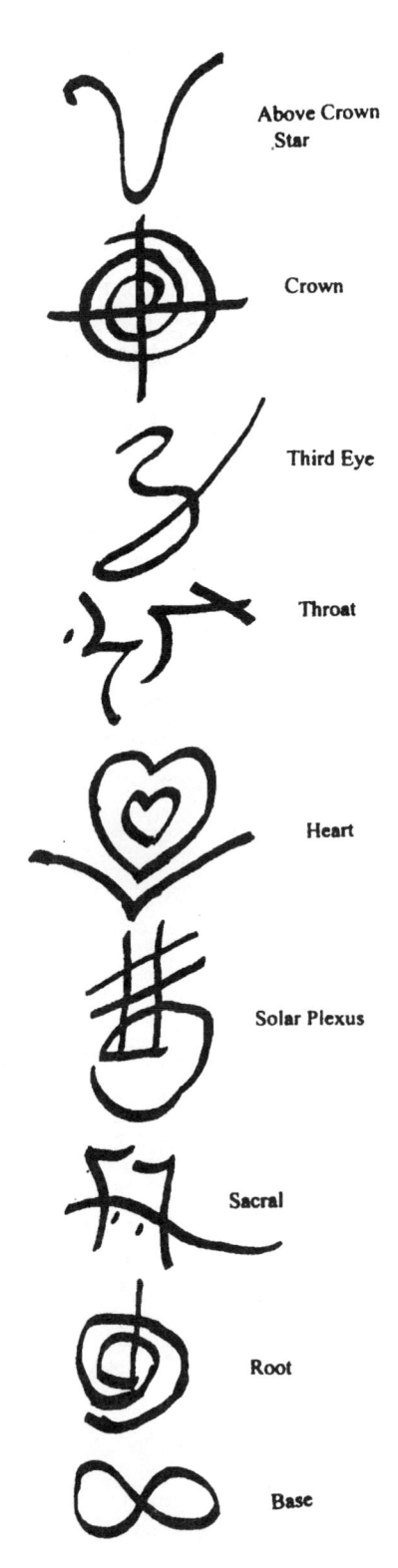

Creating Our Own Sacred Space

Creating sacred space is a dedication to creating harmony for self and anyone who enters this space!

Remember that everything has consciousness. This vast flowing energy field fills the empty spaces around us, is everything in the universe. The Ancient Ones knew this and treated "the all" with respect. The rivers were thanked for the fish they would yield, the plants and trees were thanked for the shade and for the fruit, nuts and wood that were provided. The animals were thanked before the hunt and after the hunt, for providing food and clothing.

Land

Several years ago, I built a house on twenty-five acres, way out in the woods. The first thing I did was to walk the land. I talked to the trees and asked permission to build. I told the trees and the land what kind of a house I wanted to build, a home that was environmentally designed. I explained how many trees would need to be removed. I told the land about planting an orchard, pretty flowers, a garden; and that I was into recycling. All went well. In fact, I discovered later the land had deer ticks and chiggers, but I had never been bothered. When it was time to sell, I sold the property to people that ended up bulldozing the trees and the orchard. When I went to visit the land again, the trees were gone. I felt an immediate headache and sickness, and I could feel the pain of the land.

Home

Our homes, whether solid or empty space, are filled with infinite vibrating energy fields. Our homes consist of the physical vibrations of structure and furniture, plus the emotional vibrations of spiritual and etheric energies, that constantly move and swirl. The types of materials used to build the home also have their own unique vibrations, even the way the materials were handled. Colors, fabrics, pictures, lights, air quality, smells, size of rooms, and pets all contribute to the vibrations of the home. The way you feel about your home and the types of visitors coming into your home also have an affect. If your home has been owned before, previous owners' personalities and activities resonate. If a home is erected over old grave sites, an underground stream, or the location of a torn-down building, they also affect the vibrations, as does the person who built the home.

Your home has an aura just like you do. The physical form of the building and the objects within the home influence the aura of your home. Also, the spiritual energy fields from the trees, earth, and landscape convey the angelic and devic kingdoms present. Primal Earth energy, called ley lines, also affects your home's spiritual aura. The most important thing that influences the spiritual energy is the love that is given and received within the walls of your home. Your home is an extension of your thoughts and feelings; you are not separate from the home anymore than you are separate from the air you breathe. Your home reflects and mirrors your consciousness. Just as the body is symbolic of our inner states, your home reflects your inner state. Your home is nourished by how you hold it in your heart. The home has a living spirit that is sustained through the reverence and love you hold for it. Otherwise the home spirit resides in an inanimate and lifeless atmosphere.

Rooms

The home and the individual rooms need a balance of the yin and yang. This way a room will not feel restrictive, cold and dark or too yin, where one could become ill. A room that is very open, with lots of windows, painted stark white, and where the sun shines all day, would be too yang. The main entrance to your home is the major entry point for energy to flow into the dwelling. It is important that the approach to the main entrance is not obstructed. Any door that opens into a wall, rather than opening into free space, will impede the energy flow. High ceilings or low ceilings, house plants, windows, furniture, mirrors, etc. all have energy vibrations that affect the house. Check out yours!

Creating Sacred Space in your Environment

The Art of Placement is called Feng Shui.

The ancient art of Feng Shui balances the energies inside rooms, positively affecting aspects of life including family, health, wealth and happiness. The concept is called Bagua, an eight-sided diagram that is derived from the Chinese book of divination. Each side represents a different aspect of life. The entire diagram is overlaid on a floor plan for a house or individual room to determine which area needs enhancing. You would always align the Bagua with the wall containing the front door or main entrance to a room or house. Projections can cause either an enhancement or depletion of energy. Feng Shui is an eclectic mix of design sense, esoteric wisdom and physics or sacred geometry; when used properly, it can offer people new methods in dealing with daily stresses.

I am sure you have visited places where, upon entering, you immediately felt this person was a decorator, or had a special knack for design or unusual things, places where you always felt peacefulness and serenity, places where it was always a joy to be. You could even have been places where you were uncomfortable, felt nervous and jittery, were afraid to sit down or even accept something to drink. The art of placement is to help these situations, to even out and balance the energies.

Attitude

Peace is a feeling of tranquillity and warmth that can be enhanced through love, self-knowledge, and your home. Harmony is the feeling of togetherness created by people, thoughts, impressions, and the atmosphere of your home. Together the two allow for feelings of freedom and serenity, a place of retreat and refuge, a reminiscence of warmth felt from the secure embrace of a loved one.

Entrance

Upon acceptance of an invitation to enter someone's sacred space (their abode), the first thing that is appealing would be the yard, walkway, porch or entryway, an inviting front door, chimes, flowers, welcome mat and rug. All of this would have an immediate effect upon your personal energy field of a positive or negative nature. Just think of your reaction if you walked up to an abode where trash was littered around the yard, and paint was peeling on the house; you could feel unwelcome or even unsafe, if you did not know the occupants.

Upon entering the home, the first impression is what lasts in your memory. The warmth or coolness, which is really the energy of the house, speaks to you. This energy is generated from windows, mirrors, plants, colors, placement of furniture, pictures, and the general all-round attitude of the people living within the walls.

Placement

What do these aspects represent? Windows and mirrors promote openness and a feeling of being welcome. Artificial lighting should be soft and pale to create a passionate mood or warmth. Bright lighting evokes knowledge and excitement. Books, portraits, toys, collections, and particular designs pertinent to this family bring the history of the family forth. There is definitely a difference in the feeling within a home that is lived in, and one that has all the furnishings of great wealth or prosperity but is not lived in. Children within the home need to have a feeling of where things belong, what space they are allowed to feel freedom of movement in, and what areas are off limits—everyone needs to learn boundaries, this helps teach responsibility. The placement of furniture should be practical, functional, and yet encourage conversation. You may actually have several small areas of furniture placed for social interaction. Natural fibers, such as cotton, linens, and muslin, seem to offer great comfort to the surrounding areas, whether used for window treatments, throw pillows, or a sofa throw.

As laid out in I Ching, there are eight basic ways in which these energies interact. So we have eight different positions in any location corresponding to the eight configurations of Yin and Yang. By adjusting any one area in the physical space we can effect a change in the corresponding area of our life.

Examples

A healthy plant enhances the relationship area. Putting the color yellow in an educational area of the home brings forth knowledge and mental alertness. If the wealth area of the home is a closet or bathroom, place a mirror on the outside of the door and crystals in the room, thereby reflecting back the energy (chi) to create wealth.

If your home is at the top of a T intersection, you will feel the unbalanced energy from cars approaching on a regular basis. This keeps stress at your location on a constant basis, and could lead to health problems. Trees or a hedge will cut down on the negative effects of such a site.

Electromagnetic Energies

More modern Feng Shui experts may use a Gauss meter to measure any electromagnetic pollution that could be generated by nearby power lines, faulty building wiring, or appliances. Although the scientific community continues to debate the subject, there has been an enormous amount of both anecdotal and empirical evidence that associates health problems with high electromagnetic fields (see chapter 6). The link between healing our sacred space and healing ourselves could help bring us one step closer to creating a peaceful and healthy planet.

Book Resources

Sacred Space by Denise Linn
The Art of Placement by Sarah Rossbach
The Complete Illustrated Guide to Feng Shui by Lillian Too

> *Each of us carries our sacred space within us.*
> *Our challenge is to live from this peaceful center*
> *throughout our life journey.*
>
> Twylah Nitsch

Feng Shui Diagrams

The following are diagrams used in Feng Shui (which use an eight-sided Bagua). Compare to your own home diagram. The balance of Yin (all that is still, heavy, receptive and cool) and Yang (all that is active, light, hot and outgoing in the environment) is what we achieve with our own sacred space.

```
                    FAME
   WEALTH          Fire, red        MARRIAGE
   Green, red, purple, blue  SOUTH  Red, pink, white

   FAMILY         The BA-GUA        CHILDREN
   Wood, green   Earth, yellow     Creativity,
   EAST          CENTER             metal, silver,
                                    white, WEST

   Cultivation, black,  Foundation, water,  Travel, white, grey, black
   blue, green          black                BENEFACTORS
   KNOWLEDGE            NORTH
                        CAREER
```

Diagram of a house floor plan showing WEALTH, FAME, MARRIAGE along the top (with FAME and MARRIAGE labeled as "missing areas"), FAMILY and CHILDREN in the middle, KNOWLEDGE, CAREER, BENEFACTORS along the bottom.

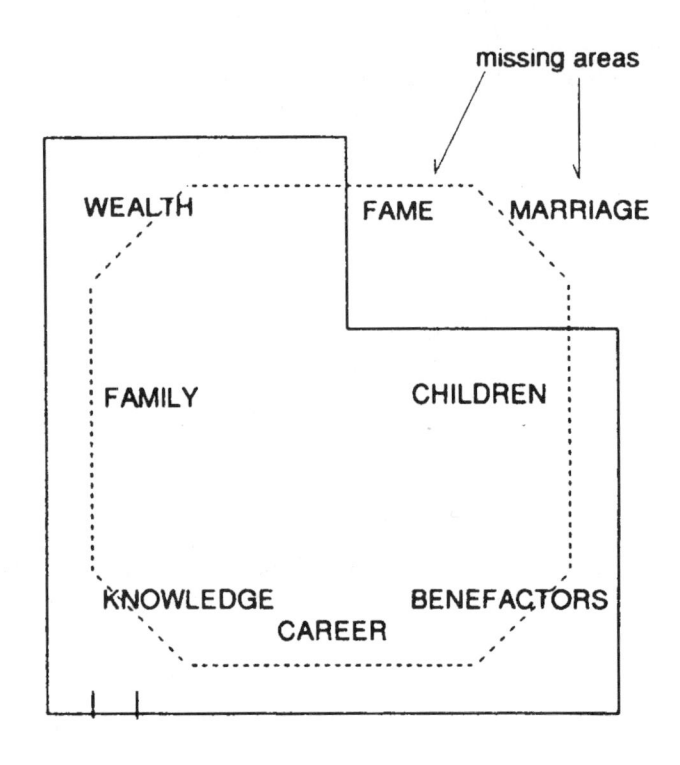

Appendix A—Dental Chart

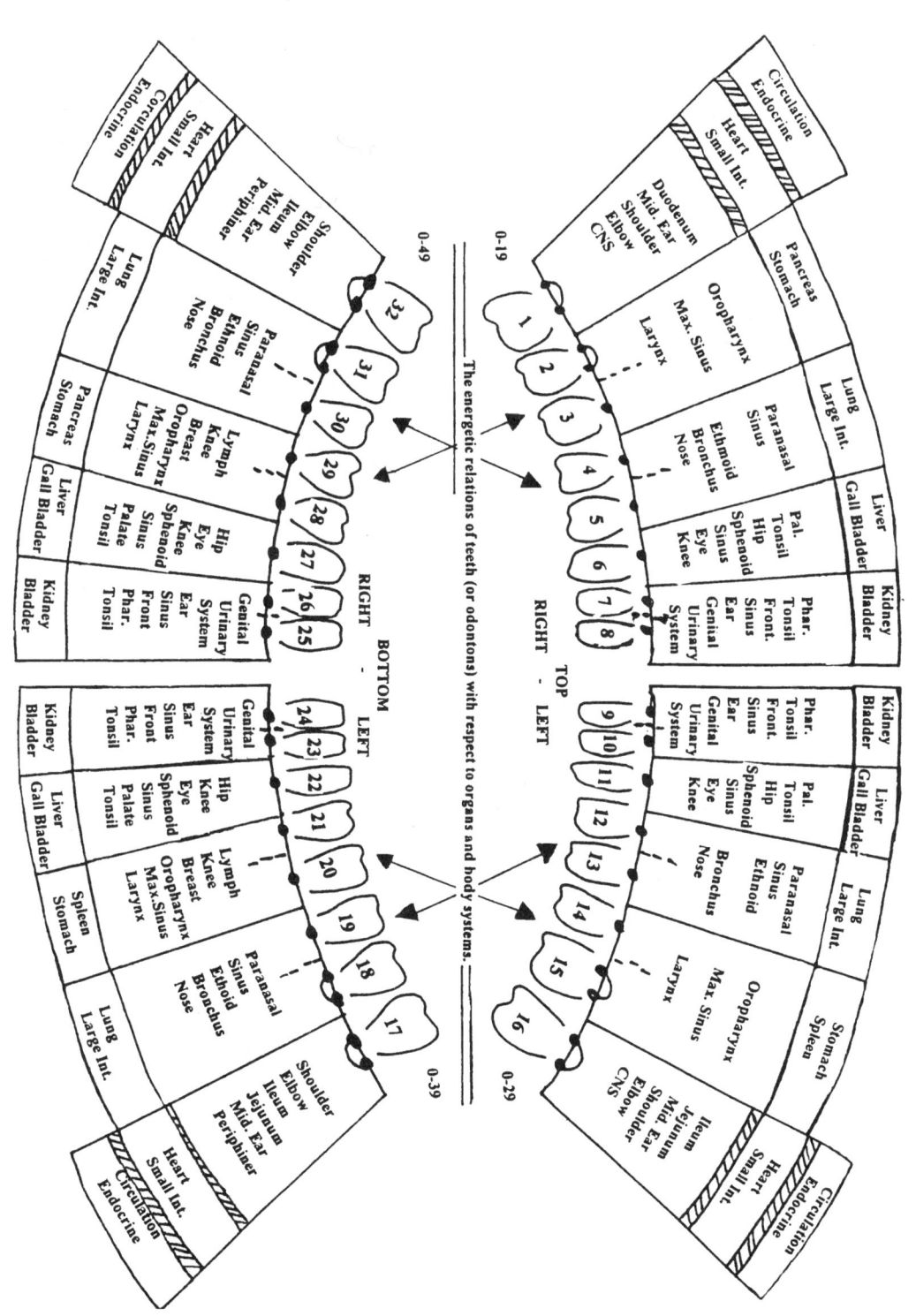

Appendix B—Chart of Effects of Spinal Misalignments

"The nervous system controls and coordinates all organs and structures of the human body" (Gray's Anatomy, 29th ed., page 4). Misalignments of spinal vertebrae and discs may cause irritation to the nervous system, which could affect the structures, organs, and functions listed under "areas." The effects listed are conditions or symptoms that may be associated with malfunctions of the areas noted.

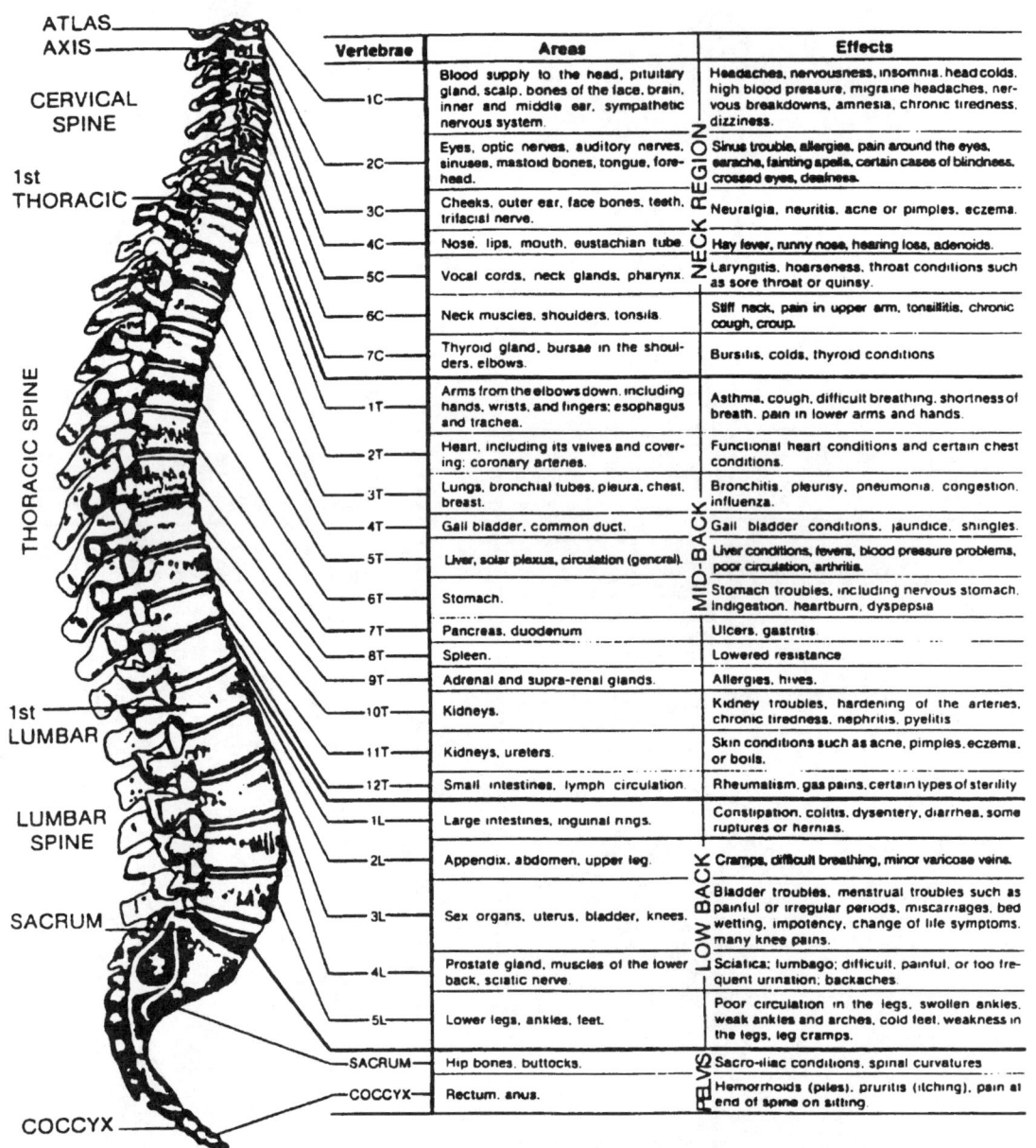

Vertebrae	Areas	Effects
1C	Blood supply to the head, pituitary gland, scalp, bones of the face, brain, inner and middle ear, sympathetic nervous system.	Headaches, nervousness, insomnia, head colds, high blood pressure, migraine headaches, nervous breakdowns, amnesia, chronic tiredness, dizziness.
2C	Eyes, optic nerves, auditory nerves, sinuses, mastoid bones, tongue, forehead.	Sinus trouble, allergies, pain around the eyes, earache, fainting spells, certain cases of blindness, crossed eyes, deafness.
3C	Cheeks, outer ear, face bones, teeth, trifacial nerve.	Neuralgia, neuritis, acne or pimples, eczema.
4C	Nose, lips, mouth, eustachian tube.	Hay fever, runny nose, hearing loss, adenoids.
5C	Vocal cords, neck glands, pharynx.	Laryngitis, hoarseness, throat conditions such as sore throat or quinsy.
6C	Neck muscles, shoulders, tonsils.	Stiff neck, pain in upper arm, tonsillitis, chronic cough, croup.
7C	Thyroid gland, bursae in the shoulders, elbows.	Bursitis, colds, thyroid conditions.
1T	Arms from the elbows down, including hands, wrists, and fingers; esophagus and trachea.	Asthma, cough, difficult breathing, shortness of breath, pain in lower arms and hands.
2T	Heart, including its valves and covering; coronary arteries.	Functional heart conditions and certain chest conditions.
3T	Lungs, bronchial tubes, pleura, chest, breast.	Bronchitis, pleurisy, pneumonia, congestion, influenza.
4T	Gall bladder, common duct.	Gall bladder conditions, jaundice, shingles.
5T	Liver, solar plexus, circulation (general).	Liver conditions, fevers, blood pressure problems, poor circulation, arthritis.
6T	Stomach.	Stomach troubles, including nervous stomach, indigestion, heartburn, dyspepsia.
7T	Pancreas, duodenum.	Ulcers, gastritis.
8T	Spleen.	Lowered resistance.
9T	Adrenal and supra-renal glands.	Allergies, hives.
10T	Kidneys.	Kidney troubles, hardening of the arteries, chronic tiredness, nephritis, pyelitis.
11T	Kidneys, ureters.	Skin conditions such as acne, pimples, eczema, or boils.
12T	Small intestines, lymph circulation.	Rheumatism, gas pains, certain types of sterility.
1L	Large intestines, inguinal rings.	Constipation, colitis, dysentery, diarrhea, some ruptures or hernias.
2L	Appendix, abdomen, upper leg.	Cramps, difficult breathing, minor varicose veins.
3L	Sex organs, uterus, bladder, knees.	Bladder troubles, menstrual troubles such as painful or irregular periods, miscarriages, bed wetting, impotency, change of life symptoms, many knee pains.
4L	Prostate gland, muscles of the lower back, sciatic nerve.	Sciatica; lumbago; difficult, painful, or too frequent urination; backaches.
5L	Lower legs, ankles, feet.	Poor circulation in the legs, swollen ankles, weak ankles and arches, cold feet, weakness in the legs, leg cramps.
SACRUM	Hip bones, buttocks.	Sacro-iliac conditions, spinal curvatures.
COCCYX	Rectum, anus.	Hemorrhoids (piles), pruritis (itching), pain at end of spine on sitting.

For further explanation of the conditions shown above, and information about those not shown, ask your Doctor of Chiropractic.

Appendix C—Location of Major Body Organs—Front View

- Parahyroid
- Thyroid
- Thymus
- Lungs
- Heart
- Liver
- Stomach
- Gallbladder
- Descending colon (large intestine)
- Ascending colon (large intestine)
- Small Intestine
- Cecum
- Appendix
- Urinary bladder

Appendix D—Location of Major of Body Organs—Back View

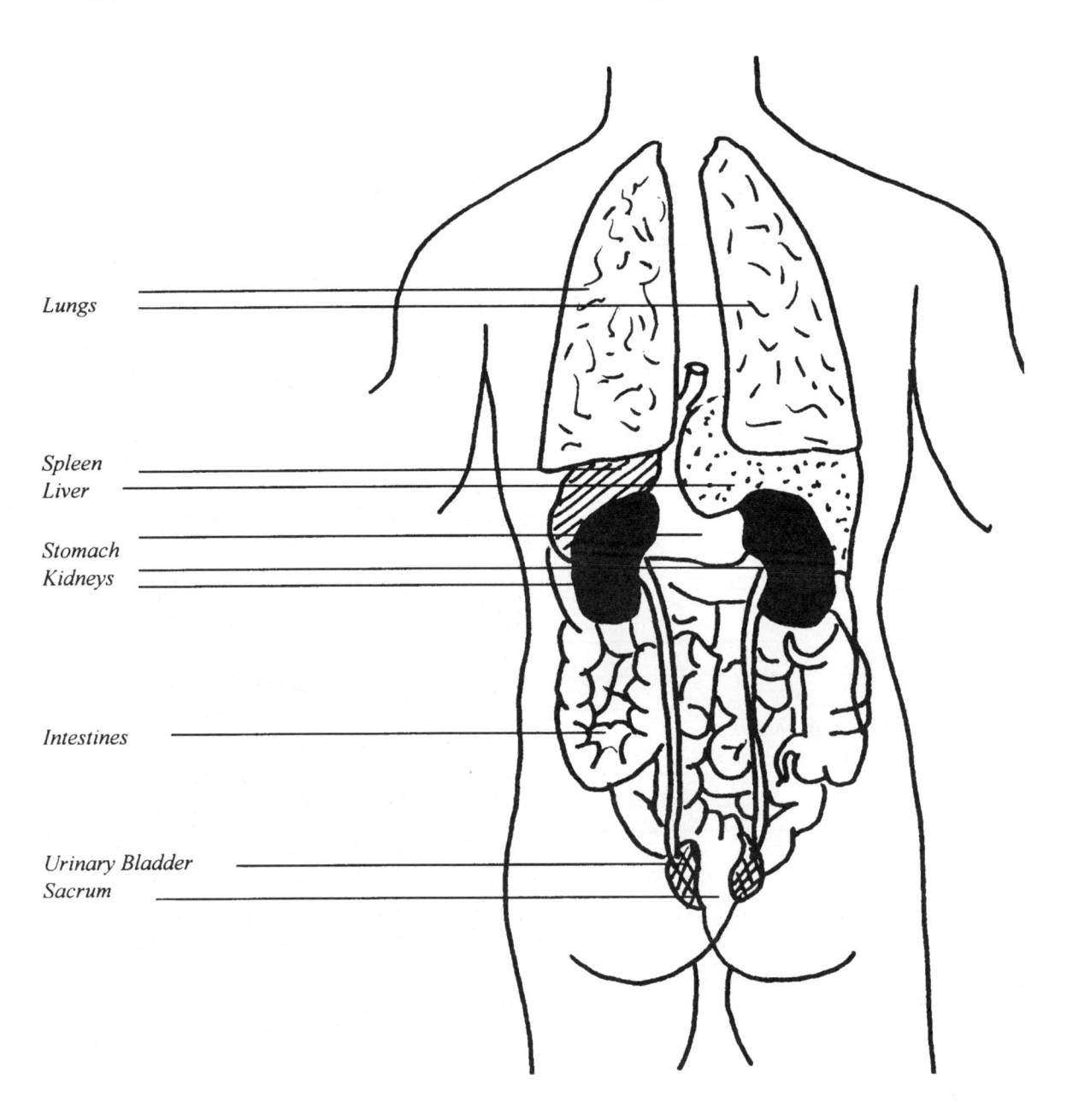

Lungs

Spleen
Liver

Stomach
Kidneys

Intestines

Urinary Bladder
Sacrum

Appendix E—The Lymph System

A circulating system of clear fluid that helps clean the blood and protect against illness. It relies on bodily muscle movement to circulate its vital fluid. The darker areas are lymph nodes and glands.

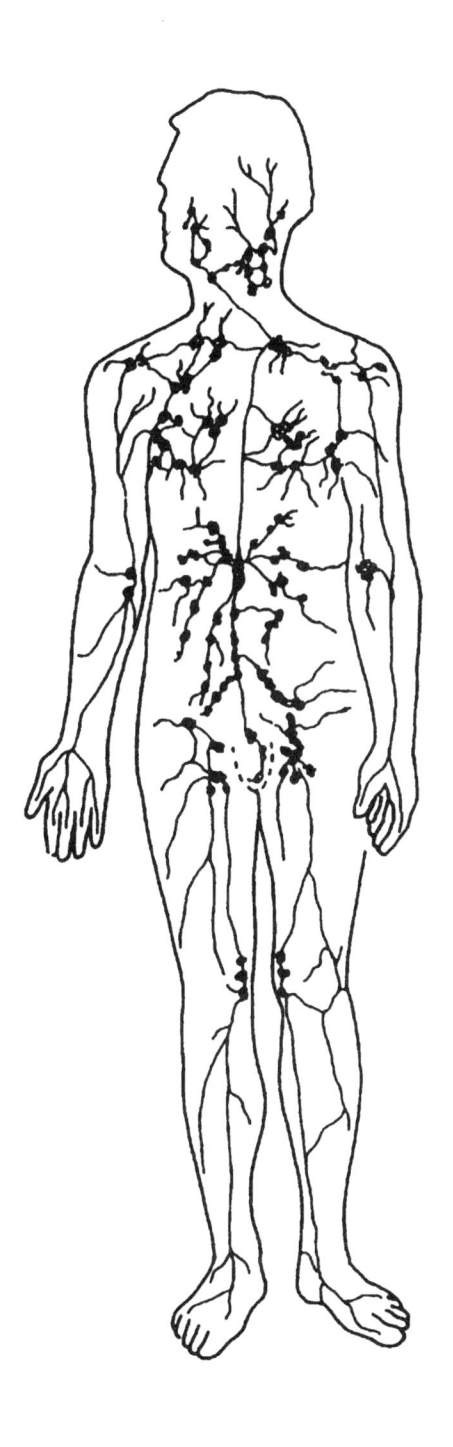

Appendix 7—The Endocrine System

Note: The cells of Leydig are in sexual glands and the adrenal glands.

1) Heart
2) Thymus gland
3) Parathyroid gland
4) Thyroid gland
5) Pituitary gland
6) Pineal gland
7) Adrenal gland
8) Pancreas
9) Ovaries (female)
10) Testes (male)
11) Brain and spinal cord
12) Trachea and bronchus
13) Lungs
14) Stomach
15) Kidneys
16) Uterus and Fallopian tubes (female)
17) Scrotum (male)

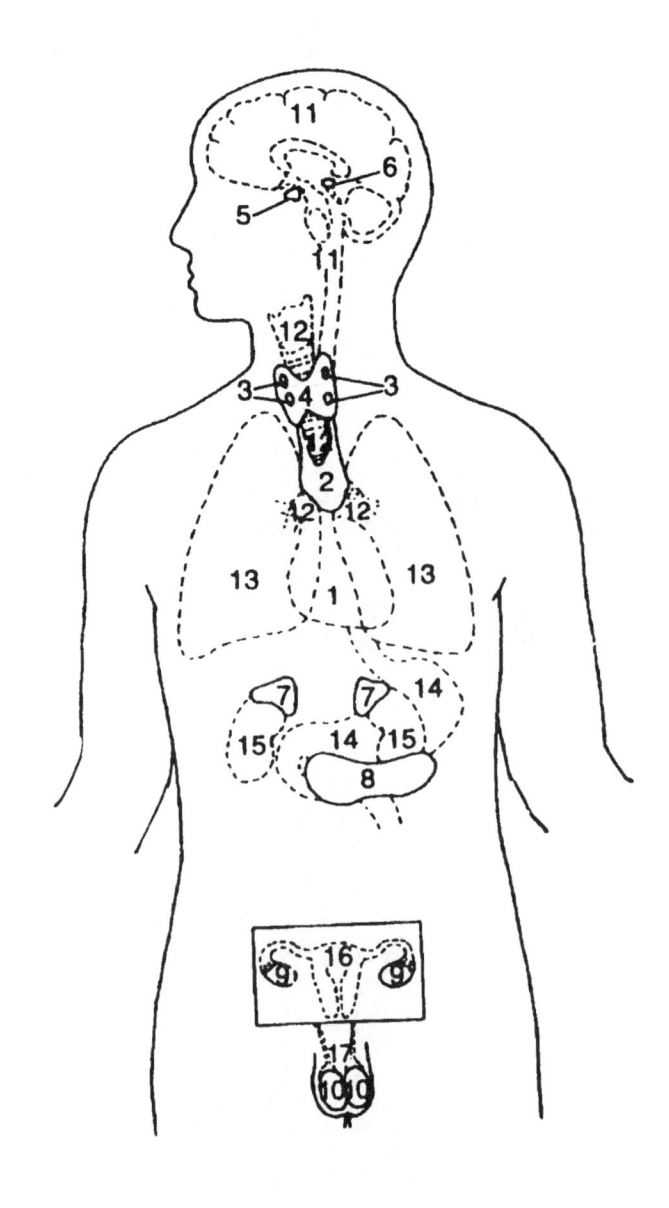

Appendix G—Reflexology—Hands

Reflexology is an ancient therapy used for healing physical ills. Compression on various hand/foot parts, using fingers or a pencil eraser tip, releases a flow of electrical energy to blocked nerve endings, which show up in the hand/foot when the responding parts of the body are congested. This compression normalizes the cells of the diseased area, and hastens the ability of the cells to heal themselves. Because of gravity, your body's metabolic wastes can settle in your feet, like dirt settles to the bottom in a glass of water. The breaking up of these metabolic wastes in hand/foot areas opens the energy flow to the corresponding organs. Reflexology should be included in a person's general health plan to enhance their overall health and state of being. Receiving massage therapy, chiropractic adjustments, and a change in diet are all great additions in the role of good health or recovery from surgery.

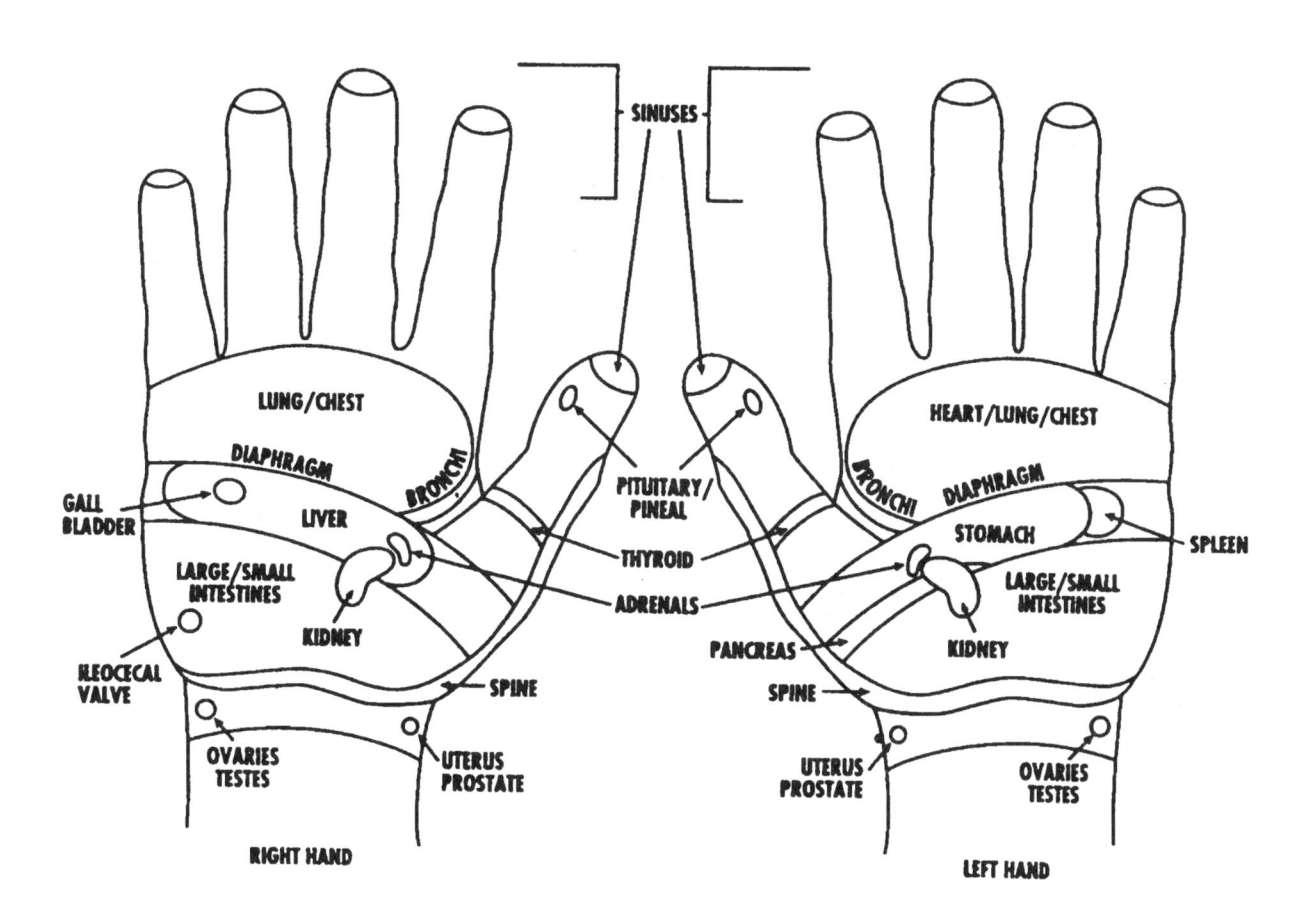

Appendix H—Reflexology—Feet

I find that soaking the hands or feet in warm water, with lavender oil, before massaging and using the compression points, helps to release the tension in the whole body.

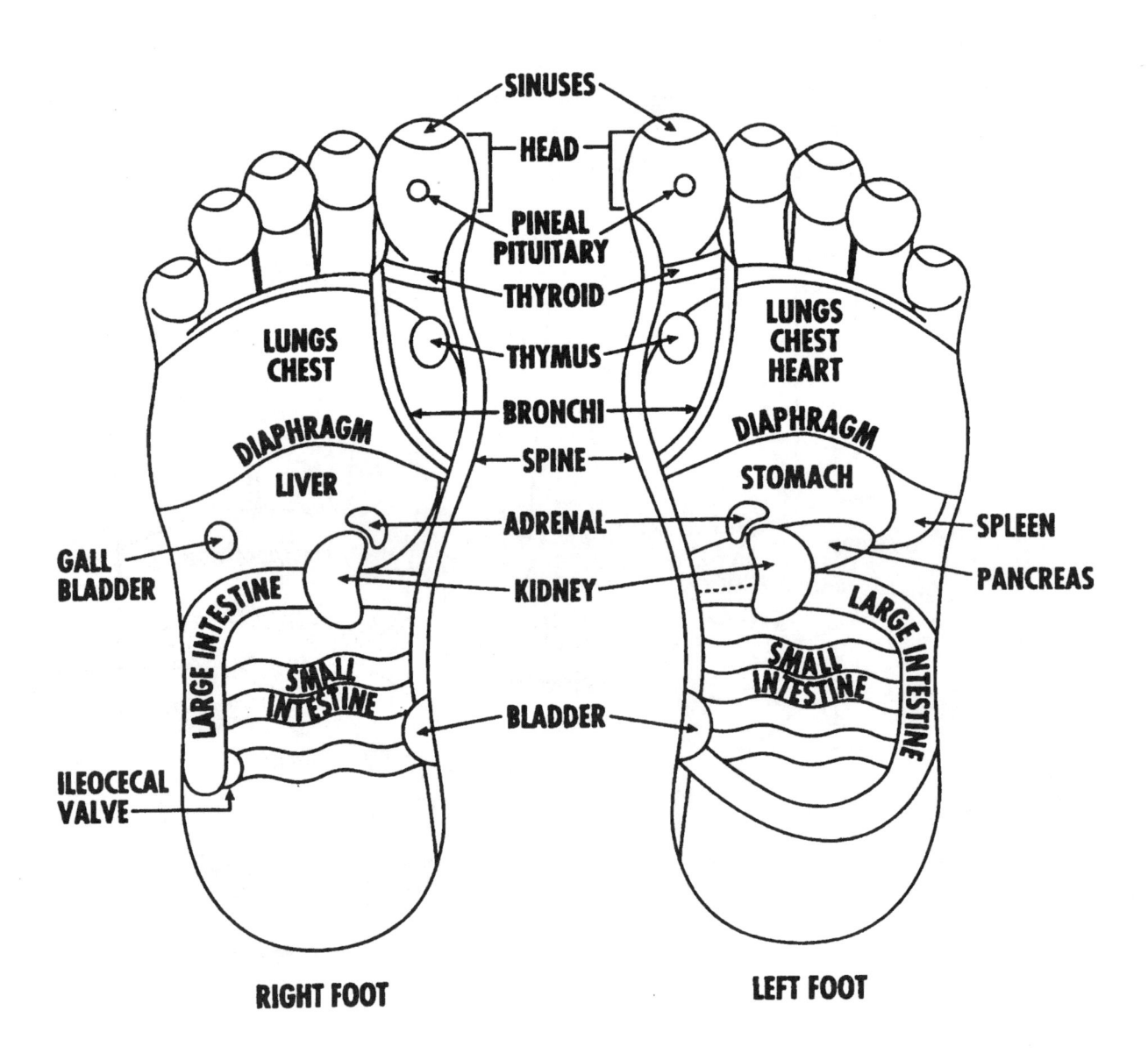

RIGHT FOOT — SINUSES, HEAD, PINEAL, PITUITARY, THYROID, THYMUS, BRONCHI, SPINE, ADRENAL, KIDNEY, BLADDER, LUNGS CHEST, DIAPHRAGM, LIVER, GALL BLADDER, LARGE INTESTINE, SMALL INTESTINE, ILEOCECAL VALVE

LEFT FOOT — LUNGS CHEST HEART, DIAPHRAGM, STOMACH, SPLEEN, PANCREAS, LARGE INTESTINE, SMALL INTESTINE

Glossary

Absorption—A process by which nutrients are absorbed through the intestinal tract into the bloodstream to be used by the body. If the nutrients are not absorbed, the body becomes deficient in building and healing substances.

Adrenal Glands—Produce many hormones, part of the endocrine system, located above the kidney.

Akashic Record of Earth—(esoteric) An ethereal energy force field surrounding Earth containing detailed pictures of every person and event on Earth and, arranged in order according to Earth's history; can be perceived by some of the better psychics.

Akashic Records—That which out of all things is formed; tiny ethereal records that store attitudes, emotions, and concepts from the mental mind as the physical body experiences the five senses, thoughts during each earthly incarnation. Utilize the law "for every action there is a reaction."

Alchemist—Alchemy is the study of how to transmute energy and learn to transmute the self from one vibrational frequency to another. An alchemist is an etheric world intelligence serving as a guide in each person's inner band, whose main function is to keep a chemical balance in the body. Capable of attaching to the pineal gland to help with one's psychic/intuitive development.

Alveoli—Tiny sacks, shaped like grapes, which actually deposit the air we breathe into the blood vessels.

Ama—Ayurvedic word for the buildup of toxins.

Antioxidant—A substance that slows oxidation (see oxidation). Examples include vitamins C and E, the minerals selenium and germanium, superoxide dismutase (SOD), coenzyme Q10 catalase, and some amino acids.

Aromatic—Plants with volatile oils.

Astral—Refers to the energy/matter frequency band just beyond the etheric. The astral body is strongly affected by emotion. It is the plane in which we dream, the body of the fourth chakra.

Attunements—To still the conscious mind and allow the subconscious mind and the superconsciousness to connect with the higher planes of reality. This expands and extends our fields of energy.

Aura—The electromagnetic field surrounding life forms; the soul's light force as it manifests through the body; the extended energy around the human body which alters in radiance and color depending upon the state of physical, mental, emotional and spiritual health.

Ayurveda—Science of life. Wisdom of the ancients. Eastern Indian medical system.

Catarrh—Inflammation of the mucous membrane.

Celestial Plane—The realm of light, visualization, and archetype. The body of the sixth chakra.

Chakra—(Sanskrit) Wheel of Light. One of the energy centers within the body, the spinning of which generates an electromagnetic or auric field around the body. Associated with various states of evolution, consciousness, physical organs, glands, colors, and stones.

Channeling—A term used to describe the healing technique in which one person acts as a channel to transfer various frequencies of energy to another person. The purpose is rebalancing chakras, thereby facilitating stress

Cholesterol—A crystalline substance, consisting of various fats, that is naturally produced by all vertebrate animals and humans. Cholesterol is widely distributed and manufactured in the body and facilitates the transport and absorption of fatty acids.

Clairvoyance—The ability to perceive matters or images beyond the range of normal perception, including subtle body energies, chakras, and auric fields.

Cocarcinogen—An environmental agent that acts with another to cause cancer.

Crystals—Nature's three-dimensional geometric forms whose outward appearance mirrors the internalized perfect ordering of atoms. Crystals are capable of reflecting pure light and color that can be channeled in numerous ways.

Detoxification—The process of reducing the body's toxic buildup of various poisonous substances.

DNA—Genetic blueprint for the entire organism, contained in every cell. The substance in the cell nucleus that genetically codes amino acids and their peptide chain pattern. Determines the type of life form into which a cell will develop.

Dosha—Blueprint of Ayurveda medicine, body type (Vata, Pitta, Kapha, or combination).

Earth Chakras—Huge, concentrated fields of energy and intelligence hovering close to the earth, absorbing the spirit in the air and transmuting it into material energy, to be utilized by the earth, e.g., Glastonbury in England. Functions in a fashion similar to the chakras of the human body.

Earth Medicine—Life science based on Native American Indian medicine teachings, whose origin in even more ancient wisdom was lost, and now can be regained. These teachings are the essence of knowledge impregnated through all the tribes' medicine. A person's medicine meant their power or expression of their own life energy system, a system of self-discovery.

Earth People—Humans living on planet Earth. The opportunity of becoming aware of the life force energy surrounding all living organisms upon this planet, and the evolutionary cycles within this planet's energy and all surrounding planets and universes. This is a planet of free will. This free will, or how we play the game of life, is what directs our spiritual attainment. Materialism, greed, dishonor, fear, and anger are lessons we each must overcome—the working together in harmony for the good of all mankind is what makes us an Earth people. Our future lies in the brotherhood of man, and our environmental awareness.

Earth Walk—Way you live out your dreams, aspirations, hopes, and also fears. It is the way you live your life and express your personality.

Electrolyte—A chemical substance with an available electron in its structure that enables it to transmit electrical impulses when dissolved in fluids.

Electromagnetic Field—The space around a charged object where an electric field exists in a perpendicular direction to a magnetic field.

Energy—(Ancient Egyptian) Primeval spirit of the universe; fundamental life force, an innate law from the beginning of creation that makes all particles comprehend. Vibrates at different speeds. (Eastern Indian) A limited manifestation of the Almighty, the changeless aspect of the One. Energy is magnetism, and found everywhere—moving throughout all the universes, in all directions.

Enzymes—Specific protein catalysts that increase chemical reaction time in the body without being consumed.

Essential Fatty Acids—Substances that the body cannot manufacture, which therefore must be supplied in the diet.

Essential Nutrients—Any of the forty-five different nutrients needed by the body for building and repairing.

Eternal Rhythm—(esoteric) The internal pulsating rhythm of the earth as a continuation of the rhythms of the universe. Everything in the earth, the particular tempo of a human's heartbeats, beats to the same rhythm, making everything all one system.

Ether—(esoteric) A very fine indefinable matter or substance believed to support the earth and atoms of the air, the energy necessary for all life and things found in the atmosphere since creation, vital life force energy.

Etheric—Energy field of the body, works under the law of intelligence.

Etheric Plane—The realm of pure sound and pure thought, devoid of light, the spiritual template for the physical world. The body of the fifth chakra.

Family Karma—(Sanskrit) A series of happenings, a collective result of the family's past actions made from members individually and from attitudes of all members, which gives the actions energy to react as a whole.

Fifth Dimension—(esoteric) A faster rate of vibration than Earth's that makes a transparent plane running through the Earth plane and throughout the atmosphere. Artists and composers receive inspirational thought and work from this plane.

Free Choice—To think thoughts of one's own preference. Earth is a planet of free choice. A human is the only organism that does everything of his own accord and has complete charge of his or her own body, affairs and choices. Choices made over many incarnations make our world today. A different choice today can change our energy fields. A free choice is utilizing the law of karma, and so one must live by their decisions. Free choice is a sacred universal law and one should not be deprived of it.

Free Radical—A free radical is an atom or group of atoms that has at least one unpaired electron. Because another element can easily pick up this free electron and cause a chemical reaction, these free radicals can effect dramatic and destructive changes in the body. Free radicals are activated in heated and rancid oils and by radiation in the atmosphere, among other things.

Free Radical Scavenger—A substance that removes or destroys free radicals.

Fungus—One-celled organism, part of the plant kingdom. Its members contain a number of species, including Candida albicans (yeast), which are capable of causing severe disease in immune compromised hosts.

Galactic Confederation—(esoteric) Believed to be a brotherhood of intelligences that restored order to Earth's solar system between the Lemurian and Atlantean periods, leaving large antenna systems, e.g., pyramids, to monitor the planet. These could be seen from other planets, and Earth could then be monitored from the air;

Galaxy—(esoteric) A constant transformation of energy divided into four parts: active, receptive, function, and result; a large system of stars held together by mutual gravitation revolving around a Central Sun, which is part of a supergalaxy.

Great Awakening—Time when the alchemist accomplishes the transmutation of his/her internal organs.

Great Central Sun—The omnipotent eternal source of light existing in the center of the infinite universe out of which radiates the entire panoramic creation: the power that creates the infinite universe.

Great Soul—Involving and evolving "total" motivated by the potential within to perfect and purify itself through its many universes.

Great White Brotherhood—A group of soul minds in the etheric world who lived long incarnations on planet Earth and other planets. They became advanced, with stern self-discipline, extraordinary capabilities, and ability to control the natural forces, etheric and mundane. They understood alchemy and could transmute their bodies. They were able to prolong their lives for centuries. Truth seekers. Jesus was both an adept and master in the Great White Brotherhood.

Guardians—Highly evolved soul-minds who are now incarnated in the Earth vibration and who are entrusted with knowledge of secret vaults scattered around the earth; these vaults hold sacred knowledge of the universes which will be released when the time is right.

Herbal Therapy—Uses various herbal combinations for healing as well as cleansing purposes. Herbs are used in the form of tablets, capsules, tinctures, extracts, and herbal baths with poultices. Herbs are a valuable adjunct to many therapies.

Higher Consciousness—Attuned and aligned with the source of power and truth within the self; the neutral aspect of awareness that identifies with spiritual light and is fulfilled by creatively manifesting that light through thoughts, feelings, words and actions.

Hormones—Essential substances produced by the endocrine glands that regulate many bodily functions.

Hydrogenated Foods—Contain fats that have been chemically processed into another form, and when consumed change back into original form, causing free radicals to form in the body's system.

Hydrotherapy—A form of water therapy.

Immune System—A combination of cells and proteins that assists in the host's ability to fight (resist) foreign substances such as viruses and harmful bacteria. The liver, spleen, thymus, bone marrow, and lymphatic system are interrelated in the immune system's normal function.

Infused oil—The process of steeping herbs or flowers for one or more months, then straining to obtain an oil-extracted concentrate.

Intestinal Flora—The "friendly" bacteria present in the intestines that are essential for the digestion and metabolism of certain nutrients.

Ketheric Plane—Realm of pure energy and spirit. Emergence with Deity. Body of the seventh chakra.

Kirlian Photography—A method of capturing on a photographic plate an image which records energy patterns or emanations from living organisms, i.e. people, animals and plants, and captures changes in accordance with physiological or emotional changes.

Kundalini—Spiral of concentrated intelligent cosmic invisible energy, vital to life. Beginning at base of the spine (first chakra), fed by all the chakras along the spine and by the cosmic energy entering through the feet from Mother Earth. Kundalini is directed by the speed of the soul-mind, according to the needs and thinking of the individual. Kundalini is feminine polarity in nature, sometimes called serpent, cosmic fire, chi, bioplasma, and Holy Spirit.

Kundalini Prana—An energy emanating from the sun and moon to the earth, where it is transformed into negative Mother Earth polarity. It then travels up the feet of mankind to the base of the spine, feeding power to the kundalini.

Laser—A device which produces coherent lights, directed to stimulate particular acupoints for relief of illness. These are now available for the public.

Laying On of Hands—A general term for a type of direct, hands-on healing sometimes referred to as psychic healing or magnetic healing, e.g., Reiki.

Left Brain—Refers to the left cerebral hemisphere, which operates in analytical, logical, and linear modes of thought.

Ley Lines—Path of power extending around the world and marked on the earth's surface by the great megalithic sites, like the pyramids and Stonehenge, which were built thousands of years ago. Megalithic sites have mysterious properties ascribed to the locations where they intersect, implying that these ley lines have special powers, and were used for their power in ancient ritual. This is the major energy network of Earth's gridlines.

Lymph—A clear fluid that flows through lymph vessels, and is collected from the tissues throughout the body. Its function is to nourish tissue cells and return waste matter to the bloodstream. The lymph system eventually connects with and adds to venous (vein) circulation.

Lymph Glands—Located in the lymph vessels of the body, these glands trap foreign material and produce lymphocytes. These glands act as filters in the lymph system, and contain and form lymphocytes and permit lymphatic cells to destroy certain foreign agents (see list of illustrations for location of chart).

Matrix—(Sanskrit) The mother goddesses of early Hinduism, means that which gives form to a thing, so it is used as a term to name the Aura.

Medicine Wheel—(Native American) A wheel that depicts the total universe. A sacred way that all Creation balances. A tool to gain wisdom, guidance and growth from external clues. The wheel teaches gentle dealing and respect for nature, its creatures and people. Wheel teaches one to sing the song of the world, to become whole people and one with the universe. Wheel tells the responsibilities of all, to return good to Earth Mother, in order to keep Earth balanced, and prevent her from becoming sick (from earthquakes, war, floods, hurricanes, anger, and greed).

Oversoul—Those who exist in the etheric plane, and are aligned and attuned to the source of spiritual light. Those serving as nonphysical spiritual guides, in the evolutionary process, of individuals and the planet. Advanced beings that originally inhabited the earth, and seeded the root races. They formed the Brotherhood of Light.

Oxidation—Chemical reaction that occurs when oxygen is added, resulting in a chemical transformation.

Parasite—Organism that lives off another organism.

Peristalsis—Rhythmic involuntary contractions of the muscle fibers of the intestinal canal, whereby the contents are mixed with the digestive juices and forced along the canal.

PH—acid/alkaline measurement: 0–7 acid, 7 neutral, 7–14 alkaline.

Prana—Also known as chi or ki. Name given to the vital life force or energy in the body.

Psychic Block—A wall made in one's auric atmosphere that prevents a psychic from tuning into that person by (1) good cloak of insulation made with affirmations, positive thoughts and prayer, (2) cloak of skepticism, (3) closing off in normal life of personal attitudes and thoughts to any outside intrusion.

Quantum Physics—(esoteric) The branch of physics that studies the energetic characteristics of matter at the subatomic level.

Right Brain—The right cerebral hemisphere, associated with spatial, intuitive, artistic, symbolic, and nonlinear thought.

Sacred Shield—The shield is a mirror image into self-discovery. Painted and decorated with feathers, fur, bones, stones, etc. Each shield represents the past and present aspects of the individual, not only who he was, but what he sought to be. Skills, achievements, goals, aspirations, strengths, weakness, and fears are shown in the design of his own circle of life.

Sanskrit—Ancient Indo-European, Indic language. The most important religious and literary language of India, a mystery language of the Brahman.

Scanning—A healing technique in which the healer moves his or her hand over the edges of the client's aura field in an attempt to obtain necessary information about the energy flow.

Second Sight—Capacity to see auras, chakras, energy, as well as remote past or future objects, or events.

Silver Cord—Extends from the Sushumna in the human spine to the human being seed (monad). Cord serves as a person's connecting link to the universe; making the two all one unit. Cord connects the soul-mind to the physical body during an astral projection, seen coming out of the top of head. A vital energy source, necessary to sustain the physical body, which exists to perfect the human being seed.

Soul—The spark of infinite spirit existing within each individual; that which holds the key to ultimate truth and power, the unique personalized aspect of the cosmic force.

Spirit—The omnipresent intelligent life force comprising and creating all manifest and nonmanifest states of reality; the cosmic force which is eternally existent, changeless, true, the common denominator throughout the entire creation, the spark of life, the light, the truth and the source of all that is.

Star Children—Those beings incarnated on the earth that originate from other planets and/or galaxies, those light-workers who have come to teach the higher laws and principles of the universe.

Star People—Soul-minds, who were born of earthly parents, but who have had past incarnations on other planets which were more evolved than Earth. They are here as planetary helpers for the coming age. They show these similarities: unusual blood type, low body temperature, urgency to accomplish goals, feel displaced here, were unplanned children, are good artists and musicians, and hear buzzing when doing psychic work. They work with healing, and usually perform their best work when sleeping.

Subconscious—That part of the personality which dwells below the surface of waking consciousness and controls automatic human functions. It subliminally records all information taken in by the senses and is conditioned, programmed by rewards, punishments, and messages that subtly build up our internal picture of self-worthiness.

Sun Astrology—Founded on the principle "As Above, So Below." Our Earth Walk is influenced by another ancient concept, "As Within, So Without." Whatever thinking is within is what we portray to the outside world. Planetary astrology probably originated with the Chaldeans, since its starting place is your time of birth, with twelve divisions that correspond to the sun sign months.

Superconsciousness—That part of the higher soul structure that is usually unconscious but accessible to the personality. The superconsciousness contains higher wisdom, whereas the subconscious relates with the personality of a six-year-old child.

Tantra—The weaving of energy expansion. Initiate must unlearn time and space. Highly developed magical-mystical religion.

Tincture—Herbal extract using alcohol or glycerin.

Toxicity—A poisonous reaction in the body that impairs bodily functions and/or damages cells. Caused from ingesting any substance with a toxicity higher than one's level of tolerance. Can be caused by exposure to chemicals from household cleaning supplies, gasoline fumes, paint products, or other environmentally unsafe products.

Toxins—Poisons to the body, that impair bodily functions.

Transmutation—To change the basic structure of physical matter, from its current vibrational frequency to a higher frequency. To dematerialize an object by rearranging the atomic structure, until it is ethereal in nature. To rematerialize these atoms into the mundane plane in a higher frequency, so it does not appear to be the same object. An alchemist can travel in the etheric world while in this ethereal state. Distance and time span are not barriers. Capable of then changing back into a body, according to the chronological time; can function intelligently under the laws of each frequency.

Vedas—Scriptures that form the basis of the Hindu religion, composed by Seers and Rishis of an indeterminable antiquity; philosophy teaches mind over matter, advanced psychology, and that there are invisible threads that will help transform the earth into a sublime harmonious family, contributes to the wisdom of the mysteries. Aryan race, earliest ancestors of India are responsible for writing the Vedas, the sacred books; believed to be the first subrace inhabiting India and Egypt.

Vibration—Constantly moving particles and interlacing tiny weblike connections; extending from dense earth to celestial planes. An innate characteristic of the atom usually referred to as spirit or energy.

Violet Flame—(alchemy) Violet vibrations in the etheric world which are believed will eventually transmute unwanted conditions and balance all by the Light. Saint Germaine emanates this violet ray; call upon him for help.

Vision Quest—An essential part of a young Native American's initiation into adulthood. The youth is sent on a vigil involving fasting and praying in order to gain some sign of the presence and nature of his guardian spirit. Often the sign is a dream in which his guardian spirit appears to him—usually in animal form—instructs him, and takes him on a visionary journey.

Vitamins—Approximately fifteen essential nutrients that the body cannot manufacture and that need to be supplied for life and health.

Wheel—When an American Indian shaman constructed a circle that contained any representation of physical things, forces, or energies, he was actually putting together a symbolic model of how the universal mind operates, the human mind, for instance. The Earth Wheel is based upon the natural cycles of the year and the four seasons as the earth orbits the sun, which in turn govern the environment in which we find ourselves living—this physical dimension of existence. There are no straight lines in nature. The sun, moon and earth are round. The rising and setting of the sun is in a circular motion, the moon traces a circular pattern in the sky. Birds, trees, animals all exist in a living circle. Only the white man thought mechanistically in straight lines.

    The wheel, the circle, is a container. It represents the Great Everything—the All, the universe, the totality of space. It also represents the individual and everything around the individual, so this is our own personal space or personal universe. Take a circle and put a dot in the middle. This is an ancient symbol that represents the cosmic center, the heart of infinity.

Yeast—Yeast is a single-cell organism that may cause infection in the mouth, vagina, gastrointestinal tract, and any or all body parts. Common yeast infections include candidiasis and thrush. This continuous infection in the body gradually breaks down the body's immune system.

Yang—(China) Polarity is active, male, sunlight, strength, fire, and heaven.

Yin—(China) Polarity is receptive, female, darkness, weakness, water, and moon.

Index

A

Acupuncture... 7, 13, 21, 31, 122, 170
Air quality.............. 96, 241
Algae, plant food 41, 44, 47-48, 53, 67
.... 77, 88, 116, 127
Alternative therapies 14, 15, 23
  aromatherapy 6-7, 13, 34, 66, 69
  .... 71, 73, 80, 84, 92, 100 161-162
  acupressure 7, 21
  acupuncture .. 7, 13, 21, 31, 122, 170
  biofeedback 7, 21
  breathwork 24, 28, 161, 236
  chiropractic 8, 15-16, 19-21, 23
  .... 170, 251
  colon therapy 8
  color 8
  contact healing 7-8
  core energetics 9, 28, 150, 163
  dreams 9
  hair analysis 9
  herbal medicine 6, 10, 41-42
  hypnotherapy 10
  iridology 8, 10-11
  kinesiology 11
  massage 6-7, 11, 13-16, 21-24
  .... 27-28, 30, 34-35, 39-70, 73
  .... 76, 78-79, 81-82, 84, 86
  .... 120, 130, 162, 170, 255
  meditation ... 11-14, 21, 83, 131, 135
  .... 161, 220, 229, 232, 234
  nutrition..... 6, 10-12, 16, 21, 34, 45
  .... 56, 61, 66, 76
  past lives 32-33, 159
  polarity 12, 19, 21, 24, 26, 28
  rebirthing 13, 28, 161, 170
  reflexology 11, 13, 21, 24, 70
  251-252
  Reiki............ 13, 16-25, 28-34
  .... 158, 162, 170, 172
  .... 175-225, 238, 256
  Rolfing 13, 15, 21-24, 29, 34
  sleep learning................ 14
  toning 14
  touch............ 8, 14-15, 19, 34
Angel....... 27, 163, 171, 185, 224
.... 230-231, 269
  meditations 232-234
Anger.................... 172-173
Amino acids 40, 42, 44, 46
Antioxidants............ 42-43, 253

B

Auric field, see also 8, 130, 158
  blockages................ 167
  chakras 130-133, 148-149, 257
  clearing 69
  core level 153
  hara line................... 152
Ayurveda..... 7, 21, 34, 81-84, 86-89
  .... 92, 120-122, 253-254
Kapha......... 21, 82-84, 86-89, 254
Pitta 21, 82-84, 86-89, 254
Vata 21, 82-84, 86-89, 254

B

Baths 75, 137, 162, 256
Betrayal 151
Blessings.................... 162
Body oils 70
Boundaries 136
Breathing ... 21, 28, 81, 125, 235-236

C

Calcium........ 35, 39-40, 43-44, 50
.... 61, 64, 90, 95, 111, 124, 126
Cancer ... 11, 39, 41, 43-44, 49-50, 52
.... 58-59, 62, 87-88, 95, 100
.... 103, 108-115, 123, 173
.... 200-201, 220, 253
Candida....... 32, 107-108, 111, 117
.... 120, 255
chakra(s), ... 121, 130-133, 167, 253
  aromatics 69-70
  auric field 121-122, 130-133, 149
  balancing of 148
  color 8
  disease 167
  fifth (throat)...... 140-143, 150, 159
  first (root) 133-135, 150, 159
  fourth (heart) . 139-140, 147, 150, 159
  second (sacral).... 135-137, 150, 159
  seventh (crown) ... 145-147, 150, 160
  sixth (brow)...... 143-145, 150, 159
  third (solar plexus). 137-139, 150, 159
  tones, healing................ 14
Channeling 187, 253
Character structures 150-151
Chelation 47, 116, 126-127
Chemicals 80, 112, 117-118
  air 97
  foods 45, 260
  household 99-103, 258
  water................... 94-96
Chiropractic chart 246
Closure technique 209

C

Coffee, organic 51, 67
Colonics 8, 11, 122
Cookware 51, 100
Cords 131, 148, 149-150, 232
Core star 154-155, 175-176
Creative energy.............. 154
Crystals....... 26, 158-160, 163, 254
  fifth chakra.............. 143, 159
  first chakra 135, 159
  fourth chakra 141, 159
  second chakra............ 137, 159
  seventh chakra 147, 160
  sixth chakra 145, 159
  third chakra 139, 159

D

Dance, spiral 170, 235
Diseases .. 83, 124, 128, 148, 167-170
  animals and emotions.......... 214
  emotional sources . 172-173, 194, 213
Denial......... 8, 136, 151, 165-166
  .... 172-173, 185
Dental 20, 115
  amalgams 100, 107, 112-115, 117
  chart..................... 21, 245
Divine love 3, 175, 231, 233
Deodorants 74-76, 100, 108, 109
Detoxification 124, 254

E

Earth........... 221-223, 227, 237
EMRs 98
energy............. 129, 230, 256
people................... 2-3, 254
recycling............... 102-104
Ego 136, 173
Elements 82-83
  air 3, 7, 13-14, 81-82, 160-161
  earth 3, 7, 13-14, 81, 83, 160-161
  fire 3, 7, 13-14, 81-83, 160-161
  water 3, 7, 13-14, 81-83, 160-161
Elimination .. 77, 83-84, 122-123, 127
Endocrine system... 119, 132, 134, 138
.... 144, 146, 167, 200, 250, 253, 256
Universal energy fields ....
  auric field.. 8, 120, 128-129, 130, 158
  chakras..... 121, 130-133, 163, 253
  healing 3, 5, 8, 15, 20, 22, 25, 27
  .... 81-82, 128, 157-158, 175-180
  .... 2198, 220
  negative 69
Energy blocks 167
Environmental pollution ... 96-97, 102

Enzymes.........42-45, 60- 61, 110
................118, 121, 254
Essential oils.....6, 10-11, 38-39, 66
........74-74, 76--80, 84, 121-122
Exercise.......15, 21, 24, 42, 61, 84
................112, 119, 124-125
dance............28, 144, 146-147
one eye....................236

F

Facial lotions..................74
Fear.....12, 16, 17, 19, 24, 130, 133
........136, 143, 149, 151, 160-161
........165, 168-169, 172-173, 175
................213, 234, 238
clearing....................168
denial......................165
facing..................151, 171
Feelings...5, 12-13, 18, 24, 121, 131
........133, 140, 151, 160-161
....................172-173
Fees......................179
Feng Shui............100, 242-244
Flukes................108-110
Foot chart, reflexology.........252
Fragrances..70, 84, 94, 100, 102, 146
Free will.....142, 182, 212, 231, 254

G

Galactic.............219, 232, 255
Garlic......36-38, 41-42, 46, 49, 54
............64, 66, 77, 86, 90, 99
....................102, 112, 127
Grounding....132, 134-135, 148, 158
............161, 197, 217, 230
Guardian angels..............149
Guidance........175, 192, 200, 224
angelic.....135, 137, 139, 141, 143
....................145, 147
spiritual guides..........184-185

H

Hair and scalp...9, 37, 38, 40, 60, 69
................75-77, 80, 93, 98
Hand chart, reflexology.........251
Hand positions............204-208
Hara............152-153, 211-212
Healer
physician........5-6, 9-10, 16, 23
....................129, 171
dentist..15, 20, 95, 107, 110, 112-118
chiropractic.....8, 15-16, 19-21, 23
....................170, 251
naturopathic...5, 10, 21, 23, 41, 195

nurse.............13, 15-18, 34
physicians assistant..........16-17
Rolfing.......13, 15, 21-24, 29, 34
Healing................
blockages........160, 167-168, 170
fears....24, 130, 149, 151, 165, 168
................172-173, 231, 234
meditations..11-14, 21, 83, 131, 135
........161, 220, 229, 232, 234
resistance to.................160
spiritual guidance.........200, 224
Health foods....................
acid forming........57, 63-64, 120
alkaline forming........63-64, 120
basic herbs..........41-42, 48, 71
basic spices..................50
combining..........46, 61-62, 66
Heart......37, 39, 41, 44, 46, 48
.....50, 52, 58-60, 62, 87, 110-112
........114-116, 122-120, 147-149
............173, 200-201, 205, 254
One-Heart.....5, 216, 230-232, 234
thymus..................147-148
Herbs......10, 21, 36-38, 41-42, 46
............49-50, 66-61, 71-73, 75
................78-80, 84, 86, 111
................121, 127, 256
basic kitchen..................50
reference chart.............36-38
teas....................51, 64

I

Illness, see emotional............
Imbalances.............7, 83, 124
Inner child..........30, 214, 222
Intention.......13-14, 18, 25-26, 29
............140, 152, 158, 184-185,
............199, 210, 212-215, 222

J

Judgments...................230

K

Kapha.........21, 82-84, 86-89, 254
Karma........10, 32, 33, 146, 168
....................194, 211, 255
Kidney.......35, 37, 40, 47, 58, 69
........77, 93, 101, 111-112, 114
........118, 121-122, 124, 126, 250
Kundalini......8, 133, 159, 211-213
................235-236, 256

L

Life force.....6, 10, 13, 20, 119, 129

....132-133, 147, 160, 167, 170-171
....175-178, 184, 191, 198, 203, 221
................254, 255, 257
Liver.....35, 37, 39, 40-412, 44, 46
........51, 57, 60, 64-65, 76-77, 83
........87-88, 91, 93, 101, 108-109
........114, 121-122, 124-125, 127
................200, 202, 256
Love........25, 139-141, 147-148
........150-151, 159-160, 168-169
........173, 175, 196, 241-242
Lung.........30, 37, 48, 52, 83, 101
........113, 115, 121-122, 124-126
........136, 140-142, 200, 250
................173, 254
Lymph.......11, 24, 31, 37, 70, 74
........102, 116-117, 124-126
................249, 256, 257

M

Masks....................5, 133
self..................165-168
Massage........6-7, 11, 13-16, 21-24
........27-28, 30, 34-35, 39-70, 73
........76, 78-79, 81-82, 84, 86
........120, 130, 162, 170, 255
Meat....45, 47, 51, 56, 61, 77, 90-91
........100, 107, 109, 111, 116118
Mediterranean diet........62, 63, 66
Menus, quick.............53-55
Mercury.....37, 94, 97, 99, 101, 108
................110, 112-118, 126
Meditations.............229-235
Meridian...7, 11-12, 26, 75,122, 145
Minerals......6, 9, 11, 12, 30, 42-45
........47-49, 66, 72, 86, 89-91, 96,
........110, 114, 119, 123, 126, 253

N

Natural.......................
pest control.............101-102
food supplements..............46
Natural products................78
air filters................97, 100
baths..38, 69-70, 73-75, 78, 162, 256
cosmetics................75, 80
essential oils.....6, 10-11, 38-39, 66
........70-74, 76--80, 84, 121-122
facial lotions..................74
hair................69-70, 76-77
herbs.......10, 41-42, 50, 71-72, 78
................111, 121, 127
oil......39-40, 44-45, 58-59, 70-76

soaps 71-73, 75

O

Oils . . . .
  body 70-74, 46
  essential 6, 10-11, 38-39, 66
  . . . . 70-74, 76--80, 84, 121-122
  cooking 58-59
Organic foods . . . 48-49, 51-52, 56, 67

P

Pancreas 37, 44, 114, 122, 250
Parasites 8, 37, 104, 108-112, 125, 214
  herbs for 37, 42, 99, 109
  what to do 109-112
Pesticides 96, 99, 102-103
  . . . . 108, 121, 125
Pitta 21, 82-84, 86-89, 254
Planes, energy . . . .
  astral 120, 130, 253
  cosmic 131, 256
  physical 130-131
  spiritual 131
Poems . . . .
  Lumis 190
  Wind Dancer 157, 189, 190
  . . . . 228, 234
Polarity chart 156
Purification technique 160-161

R

Rainbow warrior . . 222, 228, 233, 240
Reflexology 11, 13, 21
  feet 252
  hands 251
Regression 24, 170
Reiki 13, 21, 175-176, 183
  application 189
  beaming 196
  chronology 180-181
  closure 209-210
  guidance 184-185, 211
  hand positions 203-208
  hugs 185
  initiation 1210, 211, 218
  no-fault 184
  preparation 193
  masters 181
  origin 177-180
  scanning 195
  symbols 175, 199, 210, 212-217
  treatments three point 197
Rolfing 12, 15, 21-23, 29, 34

S

Sacred . . . .
  ceremonies 211, 236-237
  space 99, 211-212, 220, 241-244
Sea salt 75, 91, 98, 110, 162
Seeds, organic 67
Smudging 158, 163
Spiral dance 235
Spiritual guides 184-185
Spiritual purpose 28, 152
Smoking, ... 10, 42
  cigarettes 108
Structural Integration . . . 13, 15, 22-23
  . . . . 29, 170, 226
Sweeteners . . . .
  additives 59
  natural 60
Symbols 210
Ten levels 239-239
  emotional 214, 218
  master 216-217

T

Tan tien 152
Thymus 109, 112, 133, 140-141
  . . . . 147-148, 205, 250, 256

U

Unhealthy digestive tract 123

V

Vata 21, 82-84, 86-89, 254
Vegetables 39-40, 43, 45, 48-52
  . . . . 56-57, 61-66, 84, 123
  cooking 51
Vinegar 48, 49, 60, 64, 66, 73
  . . . . 76, 97, 99, 102, 137
Vitamins 40-44, 47-49, 76-77
Natural Vitamin chart 39-40
Ayurvedic Vitamin and
Mineral Chart 86-89

W

Water 45, 71, 94, 99. 102, 107
  . . . . 123, 126, 137
  bottled 96
  chemicals 95
  filters 94, 110
  fluoridation 97-95
  pollution 96
Wormwood 37, 71, 109, 111

Resources—Organizations

Consumer Product Safety Commission
East West Towers, 4330 East West Hwy.
Bethesda, MD 20814
1-800-638-2772

Environmental Protection Agency
401 M Street SW, Washington, DC 20460
(202) 260-2090
  Bureau Air and Radiation
  Water 1-800-426-4791 (hotline)
  Solid Waste and Emergency
  Prevention Pesticides and Toxic Substances
  Asbestos 1-800-368-5888

Department of Health and Human Services
200 Independence Avenue SW
Washington, DC 20201
(202) 619-0257
  Food and Drug
  Public Health Services
  Center for Disease Control
  Indian Health Services
  Substance Abuse
  Center for Food Safety and Applied Nutrition
  National Library of Medicine
  National Institute of Dental Research

Department of the Interior
1849 C Street, NW, Washington, DC 20240
(202) 208-3100
  Water
  Science
  Land and Minerals
  Bureau of Indian Affairs
  National Parks

US Government Printing Office
North Capitol and H Street, NW
Washington, DC 20401
(202) 512-0000
Superintendent of Documents Publications
(202) 512-1800

Department of the Treasury
Bureau of Alcohol, Tobacco and Firearms

Department of Commerce
(202) 482-2985
National Oceanic and Atmospheric Administration

Department of Public Affairs
(202) 208-3171

Department of Agriculture
14th Street and Independence Avenue, SW
Washington, DC 20250
(202) 720-2791
  National Resources and Environment
  75% Forest Reserve
  Wetlands

Rainforest Action Network
(415) 398-4404
http://www.igc.apc.org/ran
 (defender of the rainforest)

Environmental News Network
http://www.enn.com
 (latest events affecting the planet)

Natural Resources Defense Council
(212) 727-2700, http://www.nrdc.org/nrdc/
 (using law to defend the environment)

National Institutes of Health
Office of Alternative Medicine
(301) 402-2466, (888) 644-6226

National Institute of Environmental Health
Sciences (NIH)
Triangle Park, NC 22709
(919) 541-3211

National Cooperative Business Association
Washington, D.C.
(202) 638-6222;

Greenpeace
(202) 462-1177, http://greenpeace.org
 (preserve and protect the planet)

Friends of the Earth (202) 783-7400
Friends of the River (916) 442-3155

Peace Corps
1990 K Street, NW, Washington, DC 20526
(202) 606-3886

Earth Island Institute
http://www.earthisland.org

Book Resources (Library)

Alternative Medicine: The Definitive Guide
by Burton Goldberg group

The Encyclopedia of Natural Medicine
by Pizzorno and Murray, ND

Encyclopedia of Common Natural Ingredients Used in Food, Drugs and Cosmetics
by Leung and Foster, American Botanical Council

Merck Manual: Reference Book for Physicians

Schools

Bastyr University (425) 823-1300
14500 Juanita Drive, NE, Bothell, WA 98011
Accredited education and research center for alternative and natural medicine.

Southwest College of Naturopathic Medicine
Health Sciences (602) 829-9286
6535 East Osborn Road, Suite 703, Tempe, AZ 85251
Naturopathy, nutrition, botanical and homeopathic medicines, manipulation and physiotherapy, acupuncture and counseling.

Rocky Mountain Center for Botanical Studies
(303) 442-6861
PO Box 19254, Boulder, CO 80308-2254
North American bioregional plant medicines.

National College of Naturopathic Medicine
(503) 255-4860, 11231 SE Market Street, Portland, OR 97216
Degree in Naturopathic medicine.

National Organizations
American Menopause Foundation, Inc.
(212) 714-2398, Madison Square Station
P.O. Box 2013, New York, NY 10010

American Holistic Medical Association
(Send $5.00 for national referral directory)
4101 Lake Boone Trail, Suite 201,
Raleigh, NC 27610

American Association of Naturopathic Physicians
(Send $5.00 for list of licensed naturopaths)
2366 Eastlake Avenue East, Suite 322, Seattle, WA 98102
(206) 298-0126

Ayurveda Product Resources

Earth's Essential Oils and Aroma-therapeutics
1695 10th St., #111B, Sarasota, FL 34236
(941) 316-0920, Fax orders: (941) 316-0860
oils, treatments, training workshops
Book: Ayurveda and Aromatherapy

Natures Care Products Company
#6 Charles Place, Guilderland, NY 12084
(518) 464-6002

Ayurvedic Institute and Learning
11311 Menual NE, Suite A,
Albuquerque, NM 87112, (505) 291-9698

Infinite Possibilities 1-800-858-1808
#60 Union Ave., Sudbury, MA 01776
books, herbs, seminars

Ayush Herbs, Inc.
Belwood Office Park #4, 2115 112th NE
Bellevue, WA 98004, 1-800-925-1371

Environmental and Ecology

Alpine Industries 1-800-989-2299
310-T Elmer Cox Road, Greeneville, TN 37743
 (air purifier eliminates toxins, mold, etc

Clarus Systems Group
1120 Calle Cordillera, San Clemente, CA 92673
1-800-4Clarus, Fax: (714) 498-3952
products converting harmful electromagnetic rays
to pure subtle energies for home/office

Holy Earth Foundation (Earthstewards Network)
PO Box 10697 Bainbridge Island, WA 98110
(206) 842-7986

Int'l Institute for BauBiologie and Ecology, Inc.
Box 387, Clearwater, FL 33757
(727) 461-4371
http://www.bau-biologieusa.com
e-mail: baubiologie@earthlink.net
art/science of holistic interactions between life and
our environment, natural building designs

The Millennium Whole Earth Catalog
1-800-628-7493
PO Box 38, Sausalito, CA 94966-9932
http://www.well.net/nwec/wer.html
access to tools and ideas for the 21st Century

An Earthling Mission—To All Earth People

*We are all being called for the greatest mission we have ever known
The entire power of Heaven, the Galaxies beyond Galaxies
And the Suns beyond Suns have focused throughout infinity on this Great Star
Called Planet Earth, for the way of rebirthing and healing will be shown.*

*Beware of the darkness, less it creep into your life
Whether it is a person, an attitude, or a book that brings strife.
Part of the mission is to keep a watchful eye and learn the lessons
Of discernment, divine love, and egos that may mislead.*

*Remember that "intention" in all that you do will bring forth its just rewards
Whether you send forth greed and anger or integrity and love
It'll come back to you like sowing what you reap with a shove.
It's our values and our honor that we should be working towards.*

*How long will it take for all of us to wake up to this mission?
When somehow, we forgot to allow the sixth sense called intuition.
Our attitudes affect the rebirthing of our planets crystal energy grid lines
It's all part of the healing and ascension of Earth and mankind.*

*As the Elders of the Rainbow Legends have said,
We have only Mother Earth, upon which we live.
One body to inhabit, so let your inner knowing wake up to the Realms of Above,
Set your sights on the goal of One Planet ♥ One People instead!*

by Wind Dancer

Angelic Guidance through a Time and Space Warp!

My story and why this book:
Time: spring. Place: New York State.

It was late one night and my plans to stay overnight had suddenly been changed.

Here I was put in the boonies with no place to stay and extremely tired. It had been a long trip to New York and an intensive three days, and I was just starting my long journey home to Virginia. Needless to say, when you are emotionally upset, you should try to center yourself before getting into an automobile. I didn't.

I was traveling along this very hilly two-lane, winding road and saw lights up ahead where a vehicle was off to the side of the road. Since it had only been five minutes since I had been upset, my mind wasn't thinking of danger ahead.

Very soon my eyes saw the full panoramic view: on my left a house and a car sitting in the road, on the right a dead deer, a deep ditch and a mountainside coming down to meet the ditch. I knew immediately the way was blocked, there was no way through.

I heard a deep groan come from within and heard myself say, "Oh my God!" I hit my brakes and immediately lost control of my truck. I was aware of trying to maneuver the truck to keep from rolling over, struggling with the wheel and feeling the vehicle rocking back and forth.

My next awareness was driving straight down the road. Tears already had welled up and run down to my chin. I saw no lights, nothing behind me. I felt only quiet and peacefulness. There were stars out and I heard myself saying, "What happened? I'm going straight. How could I possibly be going straight?"

Sensing an intense urgency to look at the seat next to me, although I knew no one was riding with me, I felt impelled to look anyway. I saw a beautiful angelic light being. I heard myself softly whisper, "Thank you, oh thank you."

Logic was trying to figure out what happened. What was it—a time lapse, or a space warp? It was definitely a miracle! I had been moved through the obstruction on the highway. Many times, in the last few months, I have rethought the experience. I had been taken through this obstruction. What glorious opportunities there will be for our future. We are just beginning to tap the well.

My next cognizance was, "Well, you must have something left for me to do on this planet," knowing that grace had been given to me. Again, only much louder and claiming the action, I said, "Tell me what it is you want me to do. I will do it!"

A picture flashed before my eyes, and I knew I was to put together a book of information, including Reiki, a book that would be helpful on many levels, including information for a journey toward our personal pathway. Just as I had been helped this night and over many years, I am fulfilling my commitment. I am grateful for this opportunity.

Goal—helping our community to become One Planet ♥ One People!

A wild card—a blessing. What a way to be reawakened!

About the Author

S. Jeanne Gunn

Background
Sacred Shield Art
Angelic Channeling
Reiki Master and Teacher
Therapeutic Bodywork Massage

S. Jeanne Gunn is an artist from the Virginia area. She works with Earth Mother and the healing energies of the Universe. Part of her purpose in life is to help humanity dance the sacred dance, helping to awaken the conscious mind. To honor each other's chosen path, and to recognize our Oneness, rather than our differences. She is a certified healer, therapist in bodywork, Reiki teacher, and a published poet. She has three children, three grandchildren, and a white lab puppy nicknamed "Mutt-boy."

Jeanne Gunn's Website can be visited at http://members.tripod.com/~jwinddancer.

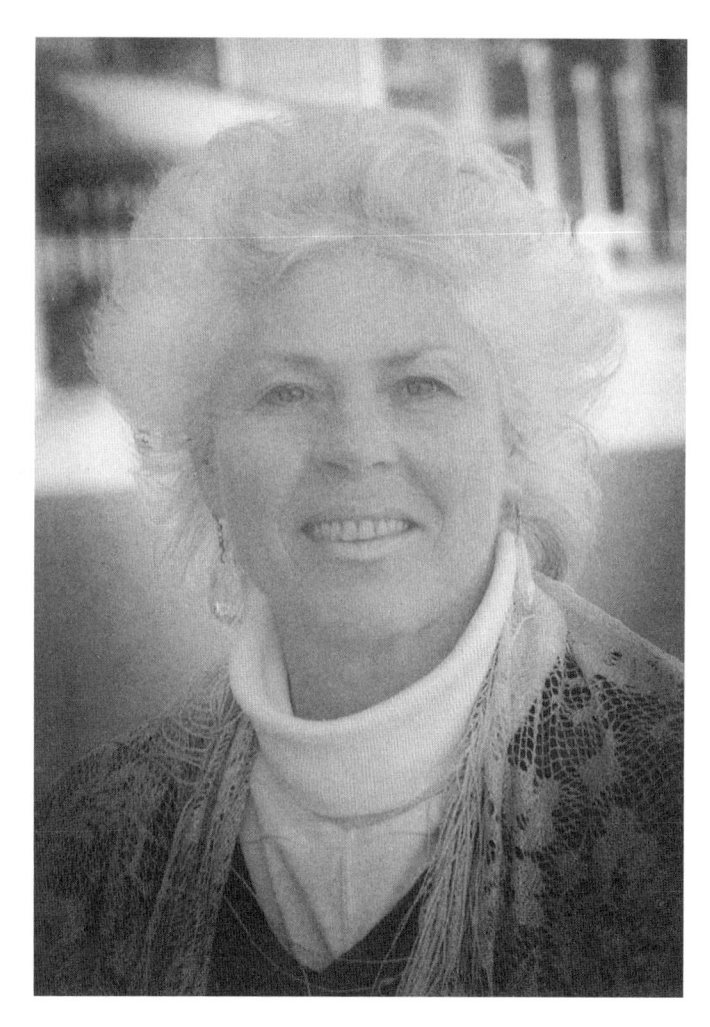

To order additional copies of

Natural Healing

Book: $19.95   Shipping/Handling: $3.50

Contact: ***BookPartners, Inc.***
P.O. Box 922, Wilsonville, OR 97070
Fax: 503-682-8684
Phone: 503-682-9821
Phone: 1-800-895-7323